Jalaja Bonheim

A FIRESIDE BOOK

Published by Simon & Schuster

APHRODITE'S DAUGHTERS

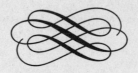

Women's Sexual Stories

and the Journey of the Soul

FIRESIDE
Rockefeller Center
1230 Avenue of the Americas
New York, NY 10020

Library of Congress Cataloging-in-Publication Data

Bonheim, Jalaja.
Aphrodite's daughters : women's sexual stories and the journey of the soul / Jalaja Bonheim.
p. cm.
"A Fireside book."
Includes bibliographical references.
1. Women—Sexual behavior.   2. Intimacy (Psychology).   3. Women—Communication.
I. Title.
HQ29.B664   1997
306.7'082—dc21   96-53615
ISBN 0-684-83080-9

"I have felt the swaying of the elephant's shoulders . . ." from Mirabai, "Why Mira Can't Go Back to her Old House." In Robert Bly, *News of the Universe*. San Francisco: Sierra Club Books, 1980. Reprinted by permission.

Marion Woodman's story of ritual for Krishna's birthday from Marion Woodman, *The Pregnant Virgin: A Process of Psychological Transformation*. Toronto: Inner City Books, 1985. Reprinted by permission.

Poetry by Lalla from *Lalla: Naked Song*. Translated by Coleman Barks. Athens, Ga.: Maypop Books, 1992. Reprinted by permission.

Verse by Hildegard of Bingen from *St. Hildegard of Bingen: Symphonia; A critical Edition of the Symphonia armonie celestium revelationum*. Edited and translated by Barbara Newman. Ithaca, N.Y.: Cornell University Press, 1989. Reprinted by permission.

Poem by Thich Nhat Hanh from Thich Nhat Hanh, *Being Peace*. Berkeley, Ca.: Parallax Press, 1987. Reprinted by permission.

"salt" and "she is dreaming" from Lucille Clifton, *Good Woman: Poems and a Memoir, 1969–1980*. Rochester, N.Y.: BOA Editions, Ltd., 1987. Reprinted by permission.

Poems by Sumangalamata ("At last free . . .") and Mirabai ("O friends, I am mad") from Jane Hirshfield, ed., *Women in Praise of the Sacred*. New York: HarperCollins, 1994. Reprinted by permission.

"For I am the first and the last . . ." from James M. Robinson, ed., *The Nag Hammadi Library in English*. 3d ed. New York: HarperCollins, 1990. Reprinted by permission.

"Deep in love . . . ," "Even though she was awake . . . ," "Holy sixth day . . . ," and "Praise to Vishnu . . . ," from W. S. Merwin and Jeffrey Mousaieff Masson, trans., *The Peacocks Egg: Love Poems from Ancient India*. 1977. Reprinted by permission.

The author wishes to thank Diane Wolkstein and Samuel Noah Kramer for their book *Inanna: Queen of Heaven and Earth; Her Stories and Hymns from Sumer* (New York: Harper & Row, 1983).

ACKNOWLEDGMENTS

My deepest gratitude goes to all the women who recognized the healing potential of this project and dared to share their stories with such courage and honesty. Your stories are the lifeblood of this book, its passion, strength, and vitality. I offer *Aphrodite's Daughters* into your hands as a piece of your own flesh, a spark of your own soul, and a mirror in which to contemplate your own miraculous nature.

Writing this book has been much like giving birth—exciting and tedious, terrifying and exhilarating. I was fortunate to have the help and encouragement of a number of good midwives. Special thanks to Sherry Anderson, Betsy Blakeslee, Virginia Logan, Rose Najia, and Rosanne Annoni for their invaluable support and feedback. Gratitude to Natasha Kern for her enthusiasm, faith, and commitment, and to Cindy Gitter for her dedicated editorial support.

Thanks, now and forever, to Skip, beloved soul mate. Your love never ceases to humble, awe, and delight me. Without you, this book would not be.

I have drawn poetry from many sources. Any use of copyrighted material for which I have not obtained permission was inadvertent. Please contact me through my publisher to rectify.

To my father, who gave me his love of books,
and my mother, who gave me her love of people.

CONTENTS

INTRODUCTION

We are all engaged in the task of peeling off the false selves, the programmed selves, the selves created by our families, our culture, our religions. It is an enormous task because the history of women has been as incompletely told as the history of blacks.

Anaïs Nin

When women get together, they tell stories. This is how it has always been. Telling stories is our way of saying who we are, where we have come from, what we know, and where we might be headed.

We have many different kinds of stories. Some we share without a moment's hesitation, like plums from a tree laden with more fruit than we can possibly use. Others are like prize roses that we save for special friends. And then there are the stories we never tell, the ones we pack away in boxes and shove into the very back corner of our psychic basement.

Most women find that their sexual stories fall somewhere between the second category and the third. "Well," you may say, "isn't that as it should be? Isn't sex a very private matter? Don't we have enough sexual titillation in our society? What good can it do to probe the most intimate nooks and crannies of our life?"

My interest in women's sexual journeys is based on my belief that sex is an inherently sacred and soulful force, and that if we look carefully, with an open mind, we will find that our sexual stories yield rich spiritual nourishment. Women have always found sacredness in the midst of the ordinary, harvesting spiritual wisdom from the fields and forests of their everyday embodied experience.

Yet, especially in sexual matters, our knowledge has remained largely unspoken, as if we were creatures of the sea who float and turn silently in the depths, graceful but mute. The stories you will find in the following pages reveal what rich treasure lies concealed beneath the blanket of silence. They bear witness to the beauty of the feminine spirit, and to the magnificent flowering of maturity, insight, and soulfulness that sexual experience can elicit in our lives.

We have often been told that our sexual nature has no relevance to our spirituality. I do not believe this is true. Yes, the Great Mystery transcends gender, as it transcends all dualities. Nonetheless, our spiritual paths unfold along very different lines, depending on whether we enter the world in a male or a female body. Our soul (by which I mean the portion of our greater Self that is engaged in a process of blossoming through time and space) does not simply sit in a body like water in a jar. Rather, it merges with the body, so that each permeates the other as the golden color of a sunflower permeates its petals. You cannot separate a sunflower from its color. In the same way, our soul acquires a particular coloring and fragrance by virtue of inhabiting a feminine or a masculine body. The soul of a woman vibrates with a different frequency than that of a man, emits a different quality of light, and sings a different song. Men and women may be headed for the same ultimate destination, but we travel different paths.

I started gathering women's sexual stories in 1994. But in a deeper sense, the foundation for this book was laid during three extended trips I took to India in 1981, 1984, and 1987. There I was first introduced to a playful, erotic god*; a voluptuous, sensual goddess; and an ancient tradition of sexual priestesses. India taught me about the many faces and forms of god and goddess and gave me a spiritual education my Western upbringing had failed to provide. Most important, it totally transformed my sense of who I am as a woman and sexual being.

All my life, Indian culture had fascinated me, but I had never experienced classical Indian temple dance until one rainy evening in

---

*Throughout this book, the words *god, goddess,* and *spirit* have not been capitalized. This decision reflects the author's understanding that god and the world, matter and spirit, are so inseparably entwined that no one can say where one ends and the other begins.

1981, when I went to see the performance of a young Indian dancer. The minute she stepped onto the stage, I felt transported to another world. She wore a rich purple and emerald-green silk costume sumptuously embroidered with gold brocade; on her ankles were rows of delicate bells, and in her jet-black hair were delicate white jasmine blossoms. In a soft voice, she us that she was about to perform very ancient dances that had been passed down through an oral tradition. Nobody knew their exact age, but gestures and postures on thousand-year-old temple walls suggested that a millennium ago, Indian temple dance was already a well-established tradition.

Through the silent auditorium, the deep, earthy pulse of the drums began to sound while the dancer stood motionless, looking herself like a temple statue. Then, slowly, as if coming to life in response to the call of the drum, she began to dance, leaving me breathless with amazement. Never in all my life had I seen such grace, strength, and sensuousness. With her stamping feet, she seemed to be calling forth the spirit of the earth, while her arms and hands moved like snakes to the plaintive melodies of the flute.

I returned home later that night determined to learn this dance, and with every day that passed, my infatuation grew stronger. I began to dream of going to India, and the dream soon became an obsession. Like a dog whose nose has picked up an intoxicating scent, my soul was quivering with excitement and straining at the leash. All the while, my more rational side protested. "This is ridiculous," it said. "You can't be serious. What about your job? You are not a dancer, you're an academic. This is crazy." But the other voice would not let me be. "Go," it said, speaking with an authority that left no room for argument. I knew I had to follow this trail, wherever it might lead. And so, just a few months later, I was on my way to India.

From the moment of my arrival, I felt as if I had returned to a long-lost home. All my senses felt hungry for the chaos of smells, colors, and teeming life that now surrounded me. Delighted as a child in a zoo, I wandered through the tangled jungle of gods and goddesses, demons and deities, saints and sacred animals who inhabited every street corner, serenely showering their blessings on the madness of modern India. Within a few weeks of my arrival, an

Indian family adopted me, and simultaneously I found my dance teacher. The sharp sound of her stick beating out the rhythms of the dance soon became dear to me, and I would listen for it as I walked up the narrow alleyway to her tiny apartment.

And every day, I danced. At first, I felt foolish and awkward next to almond-eyed four-year-olds and fluid-limbed young women who seemed to have stepped straight from the sculpted walls of an Indian temple. But soon, my body began to absorb the movements, almost as if remembering what it once had known. "Many past lives," my teacher would remark in a matter-of-fact way.

As a student of Indian dance, I was taken to thousand-year-old temples on whose sculpted walls voluptuous dancers mingled with lovemaking couples. Gazing at these breathtakingly erotic sculptures, I realized that though modern Indian women seemed to be just as repressed as Western women—or more so—their ancestors were obviously not. On the temple walls, they artfully arrange their necklaces to show off their full breasts. They turn their luscious backsides to the viewer, tossing radiant smiles back over their shoulders. They stand with a lover, arms thrown around his neck as they kiss him fervently. They gaze at you with peaceful eyes as they squat, letting their menstrual blood flow into the earth.

One day, I asked one of my spiritual teachers about the fascination with sex and erotic play that is so evident in the sacred art of India but contrasts so strikingly with the more austere attitudes of Christian religion. In response, he told me an ancient Indian creation myth.

In the beginning was the One, and It was infinite in all directions, neither male or female. But It was alone, and loneliness is not good for the soul. Alone, the divine being yearned to love and be loved, to know and be known, to touch and be touched. And so It split Itself in two. One half was male and the other female. The male half we call Shiva—pure, formless, unmoving spirit. The female half we call Shakti, our mother, who is matter and energy and form. Shiva and Shakti have always been one and will always be one, but to our eyes, they appear as two.

The minute those two caught sight of each other, they fell

in love and had no greater desire than to reunite. Always, we desire the opposite of what we have. This is how things are, even with the gods. The one wanted to become two, and the two wanted to return to their former oneness. Shiva desired Shakti, and she desired him. And so, they made love, and the goddess gave birth. She gave birth to sun, moon, and stars, to animals and plants, and also to people like you and me. And because we are the children of these lovers, we too yearn for sacred union. "Tat twam asi," say the scriptures—"you are That." You are that divine light playing with itself, always creating, always molding, always seeking shape and form and expression. Therefore, you see, we must honor desire. Without desire there is no creation. This is why we tell stories about desire and love.

But India is a land of extremes. While ancient India gave me the vision of an erotic universe lost in ecstatic love play, modern India is suffocating in a swamp of sexual repression that shrouds sexual truths in silence, obstructs sex education, and glorifies female virginity and chastity. Anyone who cares to peek behind the façade of rigid moralism will uncover shame, hypocrisy, and horrendous sexual abuse. Many Western people have heard of the barbaric bride-burnings that are still common in India, but few know about India's shocking epidemic of sexual slavery. Of India's 10 million prostitutes, Bombay alone shelters more than 100,000. Ninety percent of them are indentured slaves, and more than half of them are infected with HIV. Many prominent politicians are in league with the organized crime factions that run the highly lucrative flesh trade, so the Indian government virtually ignores the situation. Indian AIDS experts predict that within the next decade, "AIDS will pull the country into a black hole of despair unlike anything seen in this century."[1]

Given this state of affairs, one can see how contemporary Indians might tend to shamefacedly deny the amazing erotic freedom their ancestors possessed. Whenever I asked about the sexual customs of the temple dancers, my friends would respond evasively and with obvious embarrassment. Several times I was told that over the last centuries, the temples had fallen into disarray, and that poverty and corruption had forced the dancers into prostitution. But originally, they hastened to assure me, the dancers had been chaste and celibate, much like Christian nuns.

I listened and said nothing, but I knew this could not be true. One look at the fluid, languid sensuality of the dancers on the temple walls was enough to convince me that these women had not lived celibate lives. Naked except for the jeweled belts that circled their hips and the necklaces that snaked around their ample breasts, these were obviously women who rejoiced in their sexuality and had no sense of shame about doing so. On the contrary, they were accustomed to being revered and even worshipped as vessels of sexual power. Their bodies radiated a lush eroticism along with an exquisite sense of elegance and sophistication.

As time passed, I yearned for more information about these sensuous performers of Indian temple dance. Who were they? How did they live? What were their beliefs, rituals, and practices? Naively, I assumed that contemporary Indian dancers would be eager to tell me about the lives and customs of their foremothers. I soon realized how wrong I was. The deliciously erotic tradition that had spawned Indian dance had fallen into such disgrace that few people were willing to discuss it, least of all the dancers themselves. My primary dance teacher, for example, was terrified of doing anything that might stain her reputation as a "virtuous" woman. Evidently she, too, thought of the former temple priestesses as prostitutes and felt the need to distance herself from their scandalous ways. I also observed how many of her most talented students would suddenly stop dancing once they got married. "My husband said no," they would tell me. This puzzled me for a long time. What husband, I wondered, would not want his wife to practice such a graceful, enchanting art? But gradually, I understood how many Indians still associate temple dance with prostitution.[2]

What little information I eventually gathered raised more questions than it answered. Most historical records about the sexual customs of the temple dancers date back no more than two or three centuries and reflect a tradition redefined by centuries of patriarchal rule, the caste system, and many other repressive factors. Nonetheless, what I did learn intrigued and touched me deeply. I discovered that the temple dancers were priestesses whose sexual energy was held sacred, and that traditions similar to theirs had once existed in Japan, in Egypt, in Europe, and throughout the Middle East. I also learned that these cultures valued sexual intercourse as both a spiritual practice and a potent method of restoring balance to the psyche, harmonizing the disturbed soul, and healing the sick. To know that such sexual priestesses had once existed meant a lot to me. It assured me that my own sexual energy, too, might be sacred, and that I, too, might be something beyond what my culture encouraged me to be.

Emphasizing the sacred function of the ancient sexual priestesses, feminist writers have called them sacred prostitutes. While the term has been used with the best intentions, I find it inappropriate and sadly misleading. It perpetuates a false image of the sexual priestess as a woman who catered to men's desires, and whose livelihood depended on doing so. Though some of them received rich gifts from lovers and worshippers, they did not depend on such gifts for their survival. Like the shamans and healers of many other cultures, they were go-betweens, messengers between heaven and earth—not prostitutes but priestesses. Let us therefore call them by their true names.

In India, these sexual priestesses were called devadasis, which can be translated as "servants of the divine" or "servants of the Light." They were raised within the temple compound, where they received an excellent education, a rare gift in those times. From early childhood, they were trained in all the arts: dance, rhythm, and music, as well as ritual and meditation, reading and writing, philosophy, religion and mythology. They were ritually worshipped as embodiments of the goddess who, according to Hindu mythology, birthed the world and its many creatures, and some of them became renowned mystics and spiritual teachers. At puberty, a devadasi would marry god in an elaborate marriage ceremony, much as a Catholic nun marries Christ. Henceforth, marriage to a human partner would be forbidden to her. Instead, she related to god as her most intimate friend, her teacher, lover, and mate, and saw herself as his beloved, his spokeswoman, his servant, and his queen.

Unlike their Western counterparts, the devadasis never adopted the Christian ideal of celibacy. In their eyes, every man was an incarnation of their divine husband. During their marriage ceremony, they might pick up a handful of sand or mustard seed and pray that their lovers be as numerous as the grains in their hands. He who ritually made love to a devadasi became the god; together, the couple enacted the sacred marriage of god and goddess.

When the devadasis danced in the temple, their dance itself was considered a form of lovemaking, a sensuous celebration of their union with the Beloved. In essence, their dance *was* the dance of love. At the same time, it was also a form of storytelling. To this day, Indian dancers are extraordinary storytellers who bring the ancient myths to life, and who taught me about the importance of storytelling for the life of a community. In this tradition, it is understood that the story of any individual man or woman is also the story of god or goddess. The heroine who goes on a quest for adventure, for hidden treasure, and for the love that endures, is none other than the goddess herself, and the hero who gets lost in the deep forest, who struggles with monsters and demons, and must summon all his courage and skill to find the way out is none other than the god. The sacred marriage between man and woman is therefore the marriage of the divine lovers who live within us, whispering their secret memories of the source beyond space and time.

Given the radical challenge the devadasis posed to patriarchal values, it is no wonder their traditions were eventually suppressed, especially as the sexually repressive values of the English took hold. The English, accustomed to thinking of god as a male, celibate, asexual being, perceived the devadasis as mere whores and convinced the Indian elite to think along similar lines. The sexual temple rituals so enraged the British that they outlawed the devadasis' customs; the practice of temple dance was made illegal and remained so until India gained its independence in 1947.

Nonetheless, the tradition is not yet entirely extinct. In India, a few temple dancers are still alive today, though their traditions are destined to die with them.[3] Tragically, they have been so humiliated that they are now quite reluctant to talk about their ways. Their fate reflects the collective descent of sexual priestesses worldwide, who, once worshipped as embodiments of the goddess, were later reviled and shamed as prostitutes.

Still, the presence of living devadasis in India allowed me to come into direct contact with a lineage of priestesses whose view of sexuality and spirituality differed radically from the Western norm. During my first visit to India, in 1982, I was introduced to a woman who had once been a very beautiful and renowned devadasi at the Mysore temple. My dance teacher and I visited her at her family home, a traditional Indian house consisting of a single, cavernous room segmented by carved wooden pillars. The devadasi was then in her eighties and had lost her eyesight, but the bearing of a dancer was evident in the pride and dignity of her posture.

Upon hearing that I was a young Western woman who had come to India to study temple dance, she became very excited. Though we had no common language, she communicated her welcome clearly and announced that she wanted to dance for me. Too frail to stand, she sang in the quivering voice of the aged. Her song was a love song to Krishna, the divine flute player, whom she begged to appear. As she sang, her hands and arms danced, illustrating the peacock feather over Krishna's head, the beauty of his face and smile. Her wrinkled face and blind eyes shone as if illuminated from within. I will always be grateful to her for teaching me, in that moment, that the dance of the priestess, unlike the dance of a stage performer, does not depend on physical fitness and youth. Her dance was the dance of the soul, and no physical frailty could obscure its radiance.

Before we left, the devadasi called me to her. I knelt in front of her. Immediately she fell into a light trance, her eyelids fluttering, as she began to mutter Sanskrit mantras. Then she took some of the red powder used in Indian temples and households for blessing and pressed it firmly into my forehead, all the while talking to me loudly and with great insistence. Uncomprehending, I looked to my dance teacher. "She says," my teacher responded, "you are blessed. She says you were one of us in many lifetimes and you have returned. She says to learn well and to serve god." At the time of this meeting, I did not understand the significance of the event. Later I realized that in this encounter I had reconnected with a lineage of priestesses to whom I was karmically linked, and I had received a direct initiation and transmission from one of them.

Learning the dance was merely the first of several initiatory gateways through which I was to pass. Shortly after returning from the first of several study trips to India, I had a dream. It was a short, simple dream, yet I would puzzle over it for many years. In the dream, a priestess appeared, whom I knew to be a devadasi. She was old, very old, and quite tiny, though she stood straight and proud. Her hair was white, her face furrowed with deep lines. Even so, I could see what a stunningly beautiful woman she had been in younger years. Looking me straight in the eye, she said, in a tone of great authority, "We want you to carry on the tradition." I was bewildered. "That is impossible," I stammered; "this is the twentieth century." The priestess shrugged. "I know nothing about your times," she replied, "but we want you to carry on the tradition." I woke up, instantly wide awake. The dream had the feeling of a real event, as real as the familiar walls of my room in the faint light of the moon. I turned on the light, wrote the dream down, and tried to go back to sleep. But I was too shaken. Like many of the dreams I was having, it seemed to point to a past world without showing me how to build a bridge to my present reality.

The challenge of bridging the vast gap between ancient India and modern America continued to haunt me for many years. India had given me priceless gifts, but was it possible to share these gifts with my community, and how could that happen? Following a pathless path, outside all formal traditions, I was being forced to live on the edge, in a state of radical unknowing. I was attempting to do the work of a priestess without knowing exactly what that meant. I had no job description, no list of my duties, no clear identity or role.

Today, I would describe a priestess as a woman who lives in two worlds at once, who perceives life on earth against the backdrop of a vast, timeless reality. Whether or not she is mated to a human partner, she is a woman in love, wedded to being, to life, to love itself. Having offered herself, body and soul, in service of spirit, she mediates between matter and spirit, between the human and divine realms. She may or may not be sexually active, but she will always honor sexual energy as a link to the source of life itself, and to the unseen dimensions from where her soul has come. Some of the women whose stories you will read in this book do not define themselves as priestesses; others do. But they all share the belief that their spirituality, their creativity, and their sexuality arise from the same source, and they all have experienced sexual love as a form of worship and meditation.

For several years after my return from India, I taught and performed Indian dance, but eventually I stopped, because I felt I was imitating a way that was not my own. Instead, I began using movement and dance in an unstructured, meditative way, allowing the movement to flow from within, rather than be dictated from without. My first book, *The Serpent and the Wave,* grew out of the work of this period. For a while, I felt satisfied. It seemed I had found a way to take what I had learned in India and translate it into a form appropriate to a Western audience.

Once in a while I would think about the old devadasi in my dream, still puzzled. In a limited way, I *was* carrying on the tradition by teaching women to enter into their bodies and to respect the deep wisdom within. "But," I would think to myself, "the devadasis did much more than dance." Then I would shrug. What did those ancient women expect from me? This was, after all the twentieth century, and the task they had assigned me was an impossible one.

But gradually, my work began to transform once again. Instead of leading groups for men and women, I chose to meet with women only. At least for the time being, it seemed that my task was to evoke women's long-buried knowledge of the sacred feminine. Movement meditation was no longer the primary focus. Instead, we would sit together in a circle. Inviting the presence of spirit, we would listen to whatever wanted to emerge from within ourselves, without imposing much structure on the process. Sometimes we would dance, drum, or chant; at other times, we would perform rituals together or meditate in silence. To me, a circle of women will always be a magical place, a place where miracles can happen, where truths long held in silence can be spoken and women can experience the joy and the beauty of the sacred feminine in a way words can never convey.

In these circles, women would often tell their stories. They would talk about their joy and their pain, their fears and their dreams. Some stories had us rolling with laughter; others left us feeling very quiet and thoughtful. One evening, as I was listening to a woman talking about the birth of her son, I suddenly realized: "This is what the devadasis did."

Our stories of birth and divorce and lovemaking and betrayal are, after all, no different from the sacred stories I heard in India.

Like the devadasis, we too tell stories of jealousy, anger, betrayal, and loss, as well as of tenderness and joy. The only difference is that we have forgotten how to honor the sacred and precious nature of our stories, how to treat them as rubies and emeralds that have fallen out of the crown of a goddess. Whether we dance is not the issue. What matters is that we gather in sacred space, speak our truth, and listen to our bodies. We may no longer have temples, but we still have our circles, sanctuary spaces carved not of stone but of our intention. Like the ancient priestesses, we know how to invoke spirit through ritual, sound, prayer, meditation, and movement, and we know how to tell our stories.

Finally, I felt I was doing what the old priestess had asked me to do. In my own way, I was continuing the tradition as well as I knew how. There was only one problem. The devadasis had not just been priestesses, but *sexual* priestesses. I, on the other hand, was acutely aware of how little I knew about women's sexual lives and about the impact of sexual experience on their spiritual journey. It seemed that I *should* know a lot about this subject. I had led hundreds of women's groups and retreats, during which women had shared themselves with great honesty and depth. As a counselor, I was privy to women's most intimate thoughts and emotions. And yes, I had heard women talk about relationship problems or about the difficulties of menopause. Still, it intrigued me how little we really talked about sex. On the few occasions when a woman did raise sexual issues, one could almost see women's ears perking up. The room would become very silent, charged with the intensity of our listening and our desire not to miss a word. I remember one woman talking about how she was having difficulties coming to orgasm and I remember thinking, "How brave of her to voice this, and how rare!"

If sex was rarely talked about in my workshops, it was *never* discussed at all by the Buddhist and Hindu teachers I listened to, or mentioned only as a troublesome and somewhat embarrassing problem. Rummaging through bookstores, I found plenty of titillation and plenty of advice on how to attract a mate, how to have great orgasms, and how to experience all-around sexual ecstasy. But the impact of ordinary sexual experience on a woman's life was rarely mentioned. It seemed that to warrant any attention, sex had to be either abusive, kinky, or supremely ecstatic.

In the meantime, my dreams continued to send me often cryptic and mysterious reminders of my task. One night I woke up with a jolt, disoriented. It took me a second to remember who and where I was. Then, vaulting across a dark expanse of time and space, I dropped back into the present. I groped in the dark for pen and paper and jotted down the dream of being in a different body, a different time, and a different place.

I am four years old, dark-skinned and barefoot, with anklets that tinkle as I walk. Like a puppy dog, I am circling a group of women, skipping and hopping around them as they walk across the compound. Until we come to the god's temple. Then, suddenly, I feel shy and apprehensive. I press against one of the women, trying to draw strength and reassurance from her body. As we step into the temple, all the bright outdoor noises fall off into a deep well of silence, broken only by the sound of water trickling down the walls. We are in a very dark cave inside a mountain, with rough, dark, unhewn walls. This temple is unlike the others I know. There are no sculptures, no images of gods and goddesses, nothing, just water dripping down the walls of the cave. The only object I see is a large black rock, perhaps three feet tall, that stands towards the back. I stare at that rock, entranced, and somehow it frightens me. It seems alive, stubborn, primitive, infinitely tenacious. It sits there like an alien creature, glistening wet, pulsing with primordial power.

Now, the women have surrounded me. One of them picks me up and points at the rock. "That is your husband," she says. "When you are bigger you will marry him." I say nothing but I feel scared and confused and strangely excited. Her words—"husband," "marriage"—mean nothing to me. Yet in some way, beyond words and concepts, I understand. The rock and I, we have recognized each other. Its dark power has pierced and penetrated me.

In our day and age, the long-dormant priestess is awakening, knocking loudly on the doors of our psyche, demanding entrance, and often bringing tumultuous change and upheaval to our lives.

Afraid, we may turn away and try to ignore her call. But she will not take no for an answer. "You have work to do," she insists. "Don't run away." As she called me to India and spoke to me through my dreams, so she is calling my sisters everywhere, reminding us of what we once knew. Today, many women are reporting dreams that reveal their ties to ancient spiritual traditions and priestess lineages and reflect their longing to reclaim a knowledge that our contemporary world has forgotten. One woman told me of a dream that made her understand, in no uncertain terms, that the old feminine roles no longer sufficed, and that the time had come to leave the safety of an old life behind:

> I was in a beauty shop, with rollers on my hair, looking at a scrapbook with pictures of myself. "Oh, what a nice person," I said. And then, all of a sudden, I felt outraged, just absolutely enraged. *"Nice person!"* I yelled. "That's it? That's all?" I woke up, and right away, I bought a plane ticket to Europe, called my landlord and gave notice, and quit my job. It was time for change. For a long time, I had not acted on the vision I held. Now, the time had come to follow it.

In the fall of 1994, I decided to stop leading workshops for a while and to devote my time to interviewing women on the spiritual path about their sexuality. Finally, I had to face that some vital and essential part of my own experience was crying out to be articulated. In vain I had searched for mirrors, hoping to find glimpses of the awareness I was struggling to articulate. Most books seemed to be interested in "fixing" something—in healing sexual wounds, improving sexual communication, or refining sexual technique. These were worthy goals, but I was looking for something else. Eventually, it became clear that the mirroring I hungered for would come not from experts but through the voices of women willing to share their personal experience in all its bewildering complexity.

What I wanted to know could not be studied in a scientific way, by doing traditional research or compiling statistics. Nor did I attempt to define precisely what I meant by "women on the spiritual path." The women I interviewed included Buddhists, Christians, Jews, and women affiliated with no particular religious tradition at all. They were single and married, heterosexual, bisexual, and lesbian. Roughly three quarters of them were white, middle-class women, and the others were of African or Latin origins. This book is based primarily upon thirty in-depth interviews. In addition, hundreds of clients and workshop participants have shared their stories with me and have taught me the ways of the sacred feminine.

My desire was not so much to hear about isolated sexual experiences as to get a sense of the entire journey each woman had traveled. It seemed important that she should have plenty of time to tell and ponder her story. In most cases, we spent two full days together. We would light candles, meditate, go for walks, and share meals. Sometimes, the nights would bring revealing dreams that led us deeper into sacred territory. The disadvantage of spending so much time with each woman was that it limited the number of women I was able to interview. Nonetheless, it seemed the right approach, given that my primary intention was not to represent a cross section of the American population but rather to initiate a change in the way we relate to our sexual stories, and to inspire both men and women to enter into respectful and honest dialogue about their sexuality, their spirituality, and the journey of the soul.

In each woman I looked for authenticity, a commitment to her path, thoughtfulness, and—last but not least—the willingness to speak honestly and openly about her sexuality. "What have you experienced?" I would ask. "What is your story? What does it mean to you? How do spirituality and sexuality relate for you? How has your experience changed you? How has being female affected your spiritual journey? What does it mean to be a woman?"

The answers I received were so powerful and varied that I was stunned. Every woman without exception acknowledged what an important aspect of her spiritual path sex has been. "Sex is like a signpost in the desert," said one woman. "Every event of any significance in my life is keyed in sexually." Today, I know that sex is a great spiritual teacher, one of the greatest we have. Sexual experience teaches us about emotions, communication, creativity, good and evil, boundaries and their dissolution, love and hate, joy and suffering, birth and death.

Tantra, the Indian art of ecstasy, has long taught that sexual and spiritual energy are related. Many women I talked with confirmed that the Tantric premise is correct: sex *can* lead to states of ecstasy and to communion with the divine. This book, too, is about the Tantric way, not as many have come to understand Tantra in the West—as a set of techniques designed to enhance sexual pleasure—but in the sense that I have been inspired by the Tantric vision of the universe as the ecstatic play of cosmic sexuality. At the same time, I am uncomfortable with the implication that people who have "ordinary" sex are somehow less spiritual than people who have ecstatic sex. Ecstatic sex is wonderful, and I am grateful that we now have access to teachings that point the way for people who want to experiment with their sexual energy in this way. However, my goal, as I embarked on this project, was not to advertise sexuality as a means of achieving ecstasy. Rather, the question I wanted to explore was how our everyday sexual experience affects our spiritual unfolding.

What, I wondered as I set out to interview women, would they say about their not-so-ecstatic, run-of-the-mill sexual encounters? What about out-and-out bad sex? Worse still, what about sexual abuse or rape? What about abortion? Can all aspects of sexual experience be gateways to wholeness? After having spent hundreds of hours listening to women's sexual stories, I have come to believe that, yes, even the darkest experiences are important passages of the soul's journey and can serve as teachers, if we are willing to relate to them as such. Throughout this book, we will be hearing from women who did just that. For some, ecstasy, love, or joy was a gateway. For others, the gateway was loss, rage, jealousy, or the experience of violation.

Many of the women I approached were not only willing to tell their stories but delighted to have the rare opportunity to reflect on their entire sexual journeys, from their origins to the present moment. Even in these times of so-called sexual liberation, most of us hold our sexual stories in silence, alone. "I had no idea what a powerful experience this would be," one woman told me several days after our meeting. "I thought I would simply tell you my story and go back home. But I feel transformed."

Still, the telling itself was not always easy. There were moments of discomfort, of shame, moments when we would find ourselves rocking together in pain. Over and over, I watched women struggle with the challenge of breaking the ancient silence that has shrouded our sexuality. Many would start their story by passing judgment on themselves and devaluing their experience. "My story is boring," they would say, "it's not interesting. I don't really know anything about sex." One woman began her story with the words, "My life is not a good exemplary sexual model." Then we looked at each other and laughed. Does our story not deserve to be told unless it is an exemplary sexual model? And what does that mean, anyway?

Often, women contracted in fear as they acknowledged that in order to speak their sexual truth, they had to break old rules and unspoken prohibitions that had governed them for a long, long time. Though uncomfortable, this breaking of taboos turned out to be important work, soul work. Once they had pierced the barrier of silence, they often marveled at the flow of insight and healing that followed. The process of telling their personal stories and of mulling over their meaning helped them distill the precious essence of feminine spirit and wisdom.

As women began to talk, I would see them struggling to emerge out of an ancient wordlessness. I would watch them molding their language as a sculptor molds her clay, often shifting from hard prose to a more poetic language, a language of images, metaphors and symbols. "My sexual story is one thing," said Eva, an eighty-year-old wisewoman. "But there are levels of feeling tone, of imagination and metaphor, of subtle content that I feel vibrating there. I am not able to articulate them yet, but I feel myself almost trembling in relation to this whole dimension. It has to do with the Ultimate, with the coming together and connecting of all things far beyond the stricture of the body."

To contain the soul stories of so many women in my mind and heart has been a great honor, as well as an immense challenge, for women's stories are as powerful, inspiring, and terrifying as the goddess herself. And in fact, these *are* the stories of the goddess. As women, we know her because we are she. Each woman, no matter how powerless she might feel, is a cell within her vast form, an embodiment of her essence, and each woman's story is a chapter in the biography of the sacred feminine. By sharing our stories, we remember who we are, in the sense of rejoining a limb to the body from which it has been severed. We all share the same wounds and challenges and are struggling with the same demons. All too often, our isolation has made us lose sight of the fact that all our stories are segments of a greater story. But our individual wounds are collective wounds, our individual stories fragments of the larger collective story—the story of the sacred feminine, her descent, and her reemergence into our world.

Certain stories cannot be told lightly, but must be received and contained with total attentiveness and care. Fortunately, my work has taught me to hold sacred spaces for others, spaces in which men and women can safely drop into their depths, where they can give birth to new ways of perception and of being, and where the psyche's most vulnerable, raw parts can be witnessed with compassion. I entered into the interviews that provided the bulk of material for this book with little more than the intention to listen with all my heart and to hold sacred space for each woman. Together, we envisioned ourselves sitting in a *temenos,* a sanctuary space created of our intention to be truthful, respectful, compassionate, and open to the sacred presence.

Traditionally, a temple priestess always begins her dance by invoking the sacred presence. Then she proceeds to tell the stories of how god and goddess appear within our world. Our journey will follow the same pattern. We will begin with an invocation of the universal goddess; from there, we will proceed to tell the stories of her daughters and priestesses. In the eyes of temple priestesses, such stories are sacred offerings, and telling them is a sacred act. What makes a story sacred? Does it have to be about saintly beings or about the triumph of good over evil? No. What makes a story sacred is the healing intention behind the telling, the intention of fostering understanding and compassion. As the temple dancers offered their stories, so every woman whose voice you will hear in the following pages consciously told her story in the spirit of an offering made to all women, past and future, to men, and to the collective process of healing.

As you read, I invite you to imagine yourself stepping into the quiet, luminous interior of a sanctuary where the light glides down from high above in golden shafts. In the deep, compassionate stillness of sacred space, open your ears and your heart.

INVOCATION OF THE TWOFOLD GODDESS

Astarte, Ishtar, Inanna, Isis, Lakshmi, Shakti, Devi, Parvati, Yemaja and Yemanja, Erzulie, and Huitica—these are just a few of the names by which people across the world and throughout the ages have invoked the enchanting, infinitely seductive goddess of love. But here in the West, we know her best as radiant Aphrodite.

Who is Aphrodite? Standing on a seashell, symbol of the vulva, she arises from the ocean, fully formed, exquisitely graceful, her face aglow with enchanting beauty. In her presence, colors become deeper and more radiant, as if suffused with an otherworldly light. Dullness and boredom scatter as she approaches in a golden cloud, trailing flowers and pearls and wafting heavenly perfume. With her, she brings charm, magic, and grace, enlivening the sober fabric of daily life with frivolous strands of shimmering gold. In her presence, rippling, causeless joy and laughter bubble up from our hearts like champagne. When Aphrodite blesses our lovemaking, all sense of fragmentation vanishes and we feel healed, holy, and whole. Like a rocket shooting out beyond the earth's gravitational field, earthly pleasure then crosses over into heavenly joy, and sexual union blossoms into sacred communion.

The ancient Greeks did not worship Aphrodite merely for her flirtatious beauty and her power to infuse us with sexual desire. Rather, they recognized sexual energy as a sacred mystery and a guide to inner knowledge. Sex was, in their eyes, a universal, primordial form of sacred power. To them, Aphrodite embodied that mysterious pull that draws all creatures toward the threshold between the worlds, the Great Gateway, where spirit enters into material form, where inspiration is received and the spark of life is transmitted.

With her seductive powers and her irresistible magnetism, the goddess entices us to open to that divine spark, to become its instruments and channels, to let it stream through us, and to channel a current so strong it pushes against our edges and makes us grow larger. Beckoning with the promise of sweet pleasure, Aphrodite arouses our desire and calls us to that union whereby lovers become parents.

But though Aphrodite is the goddess of love, lovers are not her only worshippers. She is the source of our longing not only for sexual union but above all for sacred union. By her blessing, artists become creators, and through her touch, souls become intoxicated with the sweet wine of mystical love. She is present in the rush of a new friendship or in the transformative encounter with another person, an animal, or a landscape. Our sigh of pleasure at the scent of a rose, our surge of enthusiasm over a fresh insight, the way our heart leaps with excitement at the sight of wild geese flying across the pale blue evening sky—all these are tributes to the golden goddess.

And like all goddesses, Aphrodite mirrors an aspect of our own femininity. We are her children, but we are also She, embodiments of all her powers. Every woman is one of her daughters, no matter how awkwardly she might fit the stereotypical images. Aphrodite's beauty, joy, playfulness, magnetism, and capacity to give and receive deep, voluptuous pleasure are essential qualities of the feminine spirit. She is the fresh, shimmering presence we enjoy in young children and the sparkling aliveness we feel when body and spirit move in unison. She is the golden light hidden within our bodies, the secret radiance of our flesh. Shining from within the core of our being, she seeks to make every cell of the body her own and to fill it *with her luminous presence. This is why the Greeks called her the golden goddess, the shining one, streaming with light.*

But as there is no light without shadow, no spring without winter, so the golden goddess cannot be without her dark side, her twin sister, the black one. The Great Gateway between the worlds is, after all, not only the cosmic birth canal, but also the gaping maw that will swallow us all in due time. When new life streams from the goddess, we perceive her as golden and fair, but when she devours our loved ones, we call her dark and terrible. Yet the goddess is one, mother of both life and death. Even Aphrodite, epitome of life at its fairest, was also worshipped as Melaina, "the black one," or Skotia, "the dark one," as Tymborychos, "the Gravedigger," and as Epitymbidia, "she upon the graves."[4] Hindu images portray this black goddess wearing belts of severed arms and necklaces of skulls. Naked, intoxicated with blood, she dances in a frenzy upon the corpses of her children. Buddhist images show her crushing the world between her jaws. Middle Eastern myths describe her as the black queen of death. She is black like the reaches of outer space, invisible, unfathomable, and indefinable, unknown and unknowable. She is black as ebony; black as night, death, and the unconscious; black as the sun on a photographic negative. Her blackness has infinite shades—the black of velvet, the glittering, sparkling black of a river seen dimly at night, even a luminous shining black.

Her blackness reminds us of the many dark-skinned people whose spirituality was scorned and trampled by the white worshippers of the sky god, and the sight of her is a healing balm to all those who feel they have overdosed on images of white male gods. She, who in Asia is worshipped as the fierce destroyer of evil, appears in the West in the gentler, sorrowful form of the Black Madonna, who shares the suffering of her children. She is the goddess of the disempowered, the disenfranchised, the victims, the have-nots, those whom life has tossed into the underworld. She is the Destroyer who rips away the very objects and people we most love, but she is also the Great Liberator who slashes through the illusions and the falsehoods that bind us.

What endures after everything is stripped away? What is that formless, nameless essence that remains untouched through life and death? Only those who have died into the embrace of the dark

Mother know. Twin sister of the golden goddess, she is an equally great teacher and initiator. Inflicter of wounds, she is also the trainer of healers, and those who survive her harsh initiations become healers of others. This dark Aphrodite is the great mistress of nonduality, for in the depths of her dark body, all differences are erased. Until she initiates us, our outlook upon life remains dualistic: we run toward the light and fear the dark. The dark goddess teaches us how to say yes to existence in its totality; how to embrace our suffering, our rage, and our despair; how to value the dark valleys on our path as much as the light-filled peaks. And since the sexual journey brings us both light and darkness, pleasure and pain, life and death, we call upon the goddess in both her golden and her dark aspects to guide us along this journey.

How can we meet this dark mother? To find her, we need not shoot up into the starry firmament. We need only dig down into the moist earth, and into the hidden recesses of our own bodies. She is our own innermost essence, the mystery of incarnation manifest within every living cell. And though our mind may recoil at the thought of her, our bodies are hungry for her healing medicine. Her blackness is a cool, clear pool in which we can immerse our frenzied, feverish nervous system and allow it to rest. Lapping through our overworked brains, her black waters silence the mind, so that the body can let go into the sweet heaviness of its own weight, the heart can soften, and the soul can find its rightful place within the body. This black Aphrodite is as important a guide to the erotic mysteries as the golden one, for every ecstatic sexual encounter is also an encounter with death. It is she who erases tension in our body, who cuts through inhibitions with her crazy laughter, who teaches us to let go of control and to let our small, separate selves dissolve in her vastness. It is she who sets the lover's soul free to soar. Therefore black is one of the colors of ecstatic love, the color of freedom and of infinite expansion.

To this golden-black goddess, mistress of life and death, we offer our stories. May she bless us to know that we and she are one.

I

MOTHER, LOVER, PRIESTESS

Sexuality is the way we are intimate with our own feeling states; the way we are moved by the diamonds of rain on a spider web; our paintings and letters; our laughter and stews; our persuasions and politics. Sexuality is our moment-by-moment, changing relish for who we are. Sexuality is our willingness to let ourselves really show in the world.

Carolyne Edwards

Roseanne is a heavy, motherly woman in her late fifties, with a kind face and a deep passion for family and children. Her home in Portland, Oregon, is a symphony in pink and white, an orgy of creamy white lace-trimmed linens and plump billowing pillows, sparkling crystal vases filled with shamelessly huge roses from her garden, delicate china, comfortable furniture, family photographs, knick-knacks, and delicate perfume bottles—just the kind of luxuries Aphrodite is said to love dearly. Yet initially, I failed to recognize Roseanne as one of Aphrodite's priestesses. Looking back, I see, with some embarrassment, that her abundant motherliness clouded my vision and prevented me from recognizing her as the deeply sexual woman she is. Entrapped in the cultural prejudice that would deny mothers (and large women) their sexuality, I saw only the plump, kind housewife and the passionate mother.

One morning, while I was staying at Roseanne's house for a few days, I told her I was planning to write a book based on women's sexual stories. "I will tell you my story," Roseanne announced cheerfully. I was surprised and a little taken aback. Roseanne had attended one of my workshops, and we were just beginning to become friends. Still, I knew little about her, and what I knew led me

WEIGHT

I have a lot of issues about weight, but they are gradually falling away. Some of my most beautiful sexual moments with my husband have been when I was at my fattest stage. He really likes it. He is really passionate and lets me be wild with him, and in those moments I couldn't care less. I'm round. Women in general are round. So, I am learning to accept roundness more. I'm accepting being voluptuous, and I'm discovering my inner fullness.

PAMINA

Raising two very beautiful teenagers, who were sixteen and seventeen when I was around thirty-five, was hard. Compared to them, I felt so old, so fat, so ugly, so wrinkled. I'll never feel that old again. My meditation master kept saying, "Hannah, soon you'll be dead. Life is short. Why are you worried about what you look like! You are soon dead, soon dead!"

HANNAH

to believe that she had fairly little sexual experience. Each interview meant a great deal of work, so I tended to be very selective. What, I wondered, might Roseanne tell me that would warrant my interviewing her? But I was curious, and I liked Roseanne and enjoyed her company. "Okay," I said, a little doubtfully.

What I learned from my interview with Roseanne, and from many subsequent interviews, was that women who seemed very traditional and conventional would often surprise me by expressing insights and attitudes that ran contrary to everything they had ever been taught. My first surprise was to discover that Roseanne has received one of Aphrodite's greatest gifts—the gift of knowing her own beauty. To my great delight, I found that though she is one of the heavier women I interviewed, she is nonetheless truly pleased with her body, a rare phenomenon in a fat-phobic society.

When we are in touch with the radiance of our being, we experience ourselves as beautiful, not because our body conforms to con-

I like feeling deprived and gaunt. I have such discomfort with my belly. My lover put his hand on it and said, "This belly has borne children." But a part of me still believes he would rather be with someone flat. I have a lot of trouble with the womanly parts of my body. DIANE

I am in my fifties, and I weigh three hundred pounds. My lover, Patrick, is younger than I, and drop-dead gorgeous as well. We feel that we are living our love on behalf of the planet, on behalf of all its people, and on behalf of the possibility of sacred union. We are part of the healing of the whole. Once we went out to dinner with another couple, and I could see the guy was feeling really judgmental. All he saw was a fat older woman enamored of a handsome young man. "Who is she to you?" he asked Patrick in a challenging tone. And without a moment's hesitation, Patrick said, "She is my life's breath." Then the guy looked at me and said, "And who is he to you?" "He's my spiritual communion," I answered. It was a moment of spontaneously speaking our deepest truth. FRANCESCA

ventional standards, but because an inner beauty shines through us. We are rooted in our true nature and receive the same nourishment that gives plants and animals their luster—a word related to "light." Then we shine from the inside out, and our bodies begin to glow like plump fruits, delicious and sweet. Clearly, Roseanne is such a fruit. She has never allowed the media idols—the skinny child-women with their flat bellies; their firm, girlish breasts; and their emphatically unmotherly bodies—to affect her. "I am very comfortable with my body weight," she told me happily. "I like myself better heavy than thin. When I was thin, I had no breasts. I was so thrilled when I got pregnant and my breasts grew. I think it's really fun to be heavy and have these breasts. I really enjoy them. I touch them and I like the squishy feeling." When a friend asked Roseanne whether she didn't feel embarrassed to be naked around her lover, she laughed and told her, "Not in the least. I love my body the way it is, and so does my lover."

Roseanne's voluptuous body and radiant face reminded me of the stories about Aphrodite's magic girdle. Any woman to whom Aphrodite loans her girdle instantly becomes irresistibly attractive. It doesn't matter who she is or what she looks like. She may be young or old, fat or lean. If she is wearing Aphrodite's girdle, men will swarm around her like moths around the flame. The Greeks knew that sexual allure does not derive from conventional good looks, but has something to do with a quality of light that shines through us. Our stretch marks, our no longer young breasts, our wrinkles, and our scars in no way bar us from embodying the golden goddess. We have all seen beautiful women who have no sensual radiance. We have also seen other, less attractive women who are definitely wearing Aphrodite's girdle. They cast a spell, an enchantment, and men swarm around them like bees around the honey pot. Such women are truly beautiful and will be seen as such by those who have eyes to see, regardless of their physical appearance.

Though my initial assumption that Roseanne would not have much to say about sexuality proved wrong, her story is indeed a simple one. In her entire life, she has made love with only two men, both long-term partners. The first was her former husband of twenty years, an emotionally unavailable man who regularly rejected and belittled her. The second is her current lover, Jack, with whom she has been living for twelve years, and whom she describes as her soul mate. Yet in its very simplicity, Roseanne's story describes perfectly the transition we are all trying to make. Her two relationships have taken her from repression to liberation, from inequality to equality, and from sexual frustration to sexual fulfillment. She has done what women are collectively attempting to do, which is to leave the patriarchy behind and empower themselves to live in ways that honor the feminine spirit and the equality of men and women. Once an unhappy, frustrated wife, Roseanne is today a confident, radiant, joyful lover who knows her own value and takes obvious delight in her femininity.

Roseanne's description of her childhood and marriage seems almost like a caricature of a woman imprisoned in patriarchal constructs. Her mother was a hardworking, devout Mormon, as well as a frustrated, angry woman who believed that the only way to teach children their lessons was by hitting them. In her father's arms, Roseanne would find refuge from her mother's blows. But there was no place to hide from his derisive, sexist comments, which planted the seeds of shame in her young mind. Simultaneously, her Mormon upbringing instilled in her a deep fear of sexual pleasure:

> My grandmother still wore the garments Mormons are supposed to wear, which went from her neck to her ankles, and which were never to leave her. I still remember how she used to bathe, holding her garments in one hand while she washed herself with the other, and how she would get out of the bathtub and put them back on. I don't think they are supposed to take them off even to make love. My mother wears them underneath her bra and her panties, too. Now, my mother is eighty years old, and every time she goes to the temple, they still ask her, "Are you pure?" meaning, "Have you had sex?" I didn't have sex until I was twenty-six years old and married. I turned off my sexuality through all those years. I never even petted. It was too shameful and hard.

Obviously, nothing in Roseanne's upbringing had prepared her to value her body or her sexuality. And so she was conditioned to put up with a dire lack of sexual fulfillment in her marriage.

> I got married at twenty-six after dating for two years. We necked and petted a lot, but he would not have intercourse. I found it extremely frustrating. I was ready and wanted it, but he thought I was trying to trap him by getting pregnant. That should have been a warning, but I wasn't smart enough to pick up on it. I married him so that we could have sex, but we had a terrible sex life.

Even so, some rebellious streak would never let Roseanne totally capitulate to her husband's patriarchal dictates:

> My husband thought there was a way women were supposed to be, and if I wasn't that way, there was something wrong

with me. There was an expectation that I should help him have an orgasm, but that he would not do the same for me. Our wedding night was horrid. That night, I didn't want to have sex, and my husband was just furious. It set a chord of anguish in our marriage. We had sex anyway. The fact I didn't want to was irrelevant; this was my wedding night, and I had to do it. I could have refused, but I didn't.

One time my husband told me that I owed him sex because I had married him. I took my ring off and said, "Okay, then we are not married anymore." That ring sat on the nightstand for five years before I put it back on. He never changed his view, and I couldn't live with it. To me, it was so dehumanizing. The right to say no is so basic. If I were to name one thing that causes pain to women, it is this total discounting of who we are as human beings.

Later, I started working at Planned Parenthood and giving talks on the right to say no. After every talk, all these women in their forties and fifties would come to me. First, they would ask me how they could teach their kids to say no to sex. But then the conversation inevitably turned to how to say no to their husbands without ruining the relationship. It's a big problem, and it's sourced in women's belief that their own feelings and their own sexuality aren't important.

"If I told my husband I liked something he did in bed," Roseanne said as a frown creased her forehead, "he would tell me I was trying to control him, and he would never do it again." We both scowled in disgust, and for a minute, we sat in silence. Then, wondering at the immense chasm between Roseanne's past and her present, I asked, "How did you learn to honor yourself the way you do? Who taught you to approach sex as a sacred energy?" Roseanne considered my questions for a minute. Thoughtfully, she answered, "I am not sure, but something inside of me has always known."

Roseanne's response is not unusual. Something within us knows, no matter what we were told, that our sexuality is neither sinful nor dirty but, on the contrary, miraculous and sacred, and that our core nature is worthy of honor. Still, once this innate knowledge has been so thoroughly repressed, it usually takes a special key to unlock it. That key might be physical illness, which is often the body's way of shaking us awake and demanding change. Or it might be an experience so profound that we find it impossible to continue in our old ways. But for Roseanne, the key to awakening was her passion for motherhood, and her intuitive certainty of its value and sacredness.

My husband used to tell me I wasn't "a real woman." Whenever he said this, I would instantly collapse into the victim mentality. It was always, "If you were a real woman, you would have sex with me, scrub the floors better, travel with me," or whatever he wanted. I bought it. Outwardly, I would protest, "I have a vagina, and I have breasts—what else does it take to be a woman?" But inside, there was this doubt that I really *was* a woman.

But when Roseanne's husband started accusing her of being a lousy mother, she dug in her heels and began to fight back:

I *knew* I was a good mother. So I looked at him, and said, "What's your problem?" In this case, I knew my truth without a doubt. One day, I was sitting, thinking about this, and I realized I really was a woman, just as I really was a mother. I saw that it didn't matter what he thought of me. What mattered was what I thought about myself. So I started looking at what I felt about myself. I stepped out of the victim role, and I discovered my power as a woman.

For Roseanne, being a mother has been front and center in her life. Aglow with passion, she told me how much she loved having babies. "I truly adore children," she said with a sigh. "But you only had two?" I asked her. She nodded, and explained,

I always wanted to have lots of children. But then I became aware of the overpopulation of the earth, and I felt really strongly about not having more than two babies. Still, I have pined to have more children. The emotional aspect of having a baby is the most powerful thing in my life. Nothing has ever equaled it since.

I had my first child in Korea and the second in the United States. The difference was unbelievable. In Korea, I was very nurtured. The doctor spoke English very well, and we talked about everything for hours. At one point, the doctor wanted to do an IV. But I was terrified of needles, and said no. We went though a process of negotiating, and he was wonderful. I didn't have an IV. Every single moment, someone had their hands on me.

Having my second baby was very different. I was in an American hospital, in a totally sterile environment. The doctor would come, poke around, and run. I would say, "Hey, wait a minute, I want to talk to you." And he would say, "I'm delivering four babies right now, I don't have time." I was so upset that I couldn't relax and the birth was very painful.

The cultural stereotypes of motherhood as a "pure"—that is, asexual—experience never had much hold over Roseanne. "I always experienced giving birth and nursing a baby as profoundly sexual," she told me. Her babies evoked in her feelings not only of great love, but also of deep sexual pleasure.

When I held my baby I was just aching all over with love, total love for this little creature that had just been through this incredible journey with me. When I put him up to my breast for the first time I had an orgasm that was unbelievable. I thought, "Holy shit, am I a pervert?" It scared me to death. This happened in Korea, and after a few days, I got up the courage to talk to my Korean doctor. "I have these funny feelings in my stomach when the baby nurses," I said. He looked at me very seriously, and he said, "Oh, that's very good, very good. It's nature's way of getting your uterus back in place and ready to have another baby if you want." It was such a relief. All of a sudden, the whole relationship with the baby was okay. It was not perverted or dirty at all.

But about five years ago, I read in the newspaper about a woman who had experienced the same thing in this country, and had asked her doctor about it, and they took her baby away from her because they said it was a sign she was going to be a child molester. I just gasped when I read this. The whole relationship between a mother and a baby is so sexual, and so loving.

Later, we will hear from another woman who describes coming to orgasm while nursing her babies. "Impossible," declared her (male) doctor when she told him about it. The nature of women's sexuality has been defined by men for so long that a woman's simple act of saying, "This is my experience," can challenge long-standing assumptions. The fact that nursing can be a sexual turn-on offends the patriarchal ideal of the asexual Madonna, and has therefore been suppressed. Nonetheless, the experience is not nearly as unusual as much of the medical establishment would have us believe.

Unhappy though she was with her husband, Roseanne nonetheless stayed with him for twenty years. "I believed that once I had committed myself to the marriage, I should never leave," she recalled. But finally, she could no longer ignore her need for change.

I was having a lot of health problems. My heart was not beating regularly, just from stress. My oldest son was leaving home, and all of a sudden I could see that there was nothing left between myself and my husband but the kids. I was forty-six, and I felt totally devastated. The sense of failure and hurt and disappointment was awful. After we split up, I spent six months sitting in front of the television, smoking cigarettes, vomiting, and trying to stop from hurting so much. The pain was just unbearable.

Yet as time began to heal her broken heart, Roseanne took stock and realized that now, for the first time in her life, she was in a position to know what she really wanted, and strong enough to not settle for less. She knew she wanted to be loved in a far more intimate, passionate way than she had ever been, and she knew she was ready to receive sexual pleasure. "I think Jack and I found each other when we both were ready," Roseanne told me. "We would not have been ready earlier in our lives. Jack had to grow into himself, and I had to be ready to be loved in a complete way."

Today, Roseanne has shed her old, submissive identity and has redefined herself as a woman worthy of honor, respect, and love—including sexual love. When I asked her about her experience of making love with her current partner, Jack, a radiant smile lit up her face. Then, she said:

Sex has been so wonderful between us, and it keeps getting better. Jack and I can really talk about sex. One of us might say, "You want to try something?" And the other might say, "I don't know, I'm a little scared." Once, I wanted to experience having sex with a dildo, being pleasured with a dildo. I was really scared to ask him, but I decided to talk about it. It was fine with him and he thought it was really fun and interesting. Our relationship is very sexual even outside of lovemaking. We have such deep intimacy and respect for each other. When we work together in the garden, most of the time we don't even talk. We're just out there doing something we love together, feeling really connected.

Sometimes I'm not interested in sex, and Jack says, "There's a whole lifetime. Please don't feel pressured to have sex." He is the most confident man in his masculinity that I have ever met. He is totally comfortable with who he is as a human being, and as a man and a lover. I've told him how my former husband used to say that I owed him sex, and Jack is visibly hurt by that. He finds it inconceivable that a man would look at a woman in that way. This is the kind of relationship I always dreamed of. We have been partnered for fourteen years, but we have no intention of getting legally married. We don't need a marriage license. This is real commitment.

To me, the physical things you do are sort of irrelevant and boring to talk about. Sex is about being connected to something bigger than both of us. Any sense of duty or obligation blocks the way to that realm. You can't make it happen; in fact, trying to make it happen blocks it. There is a unitive energy where the two truly become one. And once in a while, you transcend even that, and you become one with the universe.

At times I have experienced that. It's like a great light, but that doesn't exactly describe it, either. It doesn't last very long. You can't force it, but you can open to it and be receptive. You open more and more. Then, you feel yourself becoming one with your partner, and that is just the doorway you pass through into something beyond, something transcendent.

These are the words of a woman who knows the power of her sexuality, as priestesses throughout the ages have known it, and who approaches lovemaking not just as an outer activity, but as a sacred inner journey. To Roseanne, both sex and giving birth are journeys that have taken her to the threshold between the worlds and have allowed her to touch upon the source of life itself.

Roseanne's perception of sex as an inner journey is universally shared by people who honor the sacred dimensions of sexual experience. Malidoma Some, a shaman from the Dagara tribe in western Africa, says that his people have no word for what we call "having sex," but instead use words that literally mean "going on a journey together."[5] Before making love, they create a ritual container and invoke the blessings of the ancestors, who determine where the souls of the lovers will journey during their lovemaking. To the Dagara, lovemaking is therefore always a sacred ritual journey.

Of course, none of the religious images Roseanne was raised with encouraged her to value her sexuality. Nonetheless, she speaks of sex and birth with a reverence as ancient as it is universal. Sex, Roseanne told me, is sacred to her:

Sex is where the life-force comes pouring into existence. There are other places I see it, too. I sense that sacredness when I look at my children, or when I look at a beautiful flower in my garden. Birthing babies was like that for me, too. Everything is aligned in that moment. You know you are exactly where you are supposed to be, and you understand everything without thinking about it. Life comes pouring in, and for just a second, you get a chance to look at it and see it happening.

Like most of the women I interviewed, Roseanne emphatically refused to equate sex with genital arousal. Such a narrow defini-

SEX AS A JOURNEY

In the paper this morning, I saw an ad for a whale-watching tour. You go out on a boat to where the whales like to hang out, and sometimes they come, and sometimes they don't. You never know. Making love is a lot like that. You take off with your lover and you ride the heaving waters out toward the horizon. You have a sense of where you might be headed, but you can never tell. Sometimes you see a whale, or even a whole family of whales, and sometimes you don't. Sometimes all you see is a fin or a giant tail slapping the water. Even then, you take a deep breath and you give thanks. It feels good to know that beneath the familiar ocean surface live huge primordial creatures that sing haunting songs to others of their kind hundreds of miles away. The first whales I ever saw were a mother with her baby, their two backs, side by side, breaking the surface like two shiny black submarines. Remembering them made me think about orgasm, the way it rises out of the black depths of the body like a swelling dark ecstasy.

SUZANNE

tion, she said, invalidates her experience of sex as a much vaster phenomenon. "What I call sexuality is an energetic interaction," she said. "It's not necessarily genital or even physical. It's creative energy. For example, when I write something I really like, it's a definite turn-on."

We can be "turned on" in this way because we are in fact electromagnetic fields. In our culture, we usually mistake sex for a physical energy. But sex is *not* a physical energy. When we experience sexual sensations in the body, this simply means that the formless life-force is charging through us. Spend time around highly enlightened beings, and you will probably find their presence to be a turn-on. Enlightened beings are like high-voltage electrical circuits. Their energetic field is charged and will in all likelihood stimulate the flow of your own creative energies. You may find yourself composing music, writing poetry, or making love all night. Most of

BEYOND THE BODY

When we make love, we bring our naked, unadorned essence to each other. That place of essence is most obvious when one is orgasmic, but it's beyond orgasm, beyond the body. It is framed and contained by the body, but the experience moves beyond that. And what we want is to be met there, and to be received by the other.   DONNA

For me, the most ecstatic, expanded sexual experiences have always come out of meditating together and invoking the higher energies. At times, I have actually seen these energies shining off our bodies like a very fine bubbly haze. When that ecstatic energy is present, I disappear into it and I move beyond gender and beyond my body. The ecstasy is so powerful that sometimes I think I am going to break. My body can't contain it, and it dissolves. I become the fire, the light. This kind of lovemaking leaves me with a lasting high, not merely energized or relaxed.   ANYA

us operate on a low charge, like five-watt lightbulbs. But when the wattage leaps up, our inner light brightens, and we realize that within us lie shining worlds as vast and unexplored as the spiraling galaxies of outer space. And while sex is not the only way of upping our internal wattage, it is an undeniably powerful, pleasurable, healthy and universally available way of "turning on."

Roseanne has come a long, long way from her Mormon roots and from her former role as repressed, victimized wife. Today, she is a staunch supporter of women's rights, and a woman whose words express her deep awareness of the beauty and sacredness of the feminine:

In this culture, there is no understanding of the feminine. Listen to anything Jesus said; he was talking about bringing the feminine into the world. And yet so many Christians hate the feminine. Both men and women are afraid of it. I think a shift

TURNING ON

The first time we kissed, there was this incredible explosion of light. I had never felt anything like it before. And when we made love, I entered a world that was filled with light and melting, brilliant love. NAOMI

With one of my lovers, I discovered an orgasmic state that just didn't end. It's not really an orgasm as much as a frequency level. Once you are on it, you just ride the wave and it does not have to stop. It's like plugging in a circuit, and you ride the wave as long as you want. It's already there, you just hook into it. MERCEDES

is occurring, but at the same time, an escalation of fear is causing a backlash. Our ability to form such loving, close relationships, let alone have a baby, is all very magical and mysterious. We really are magic, aren't we, when you think about it? Yes, we are. That is something I know from deep within me.

Roseanne emphasized repeatedly that for her, making love and giving birth have been the most important spiritual gateways in her life. "What about men?" I asked her. "Is sex a gateway for them, too?" She nodded, hesitating a little. "Yes," she said, "I am sure it is. But I think there is something about our nature as women and as potential mothers that makes us relate to sex in a way that men don't."

Among all the inscrutable processes of the human body, woman's sexuality is the most complex, the most mysterious, and the most miraculous. All the activities of our sexual body—menstruation, intercourse, conception, pregnancy, birth, and menopause—involve streamings and swellings and transformations we have little control over, even though they take place in the very core of our body. At puberty, our breasts grow and angles become curves. Blood streams from our vagina. Our moods soar and plummet, carried on strong, billowing waves of hormones. When we make love to a man, we are penetrated to the core, while a man remains more or less his compact, contained self. In pregnancy and birth, nature takes the ball entirely out of our hands. We swell like balloons. We are nauseated or ravenously hungry. In birth, we crack open like eggs, and that is just the beginning of decades spent in service to our offspring. Then, menopause hits, and again, we are buffeted by the winds of hormonal changes.

Life in a woman's body invites us to cultivate receptivity, openness, and surrender. The good news is that these are the very skills that help the contracted ego to relax and accept its place in the greater scheme of things. Though women all too often perceive their bodies as sources of discomfort, shame, and embarrassment, the body deserves to be honored as one of our primary spiritual teachers. Roseanne is typical of millions of women who have not spent years in deep meditation and intense spiritual practice, and yet, by heeding the teachings of their bodies, have achieved what are by any standards essential spiritual virtues—compassion, humility, kindness, and willingness to serve the greater whole of life.

2

MOTHER, HELP!

For the Aphroditic woman, her spiritual life, or, as Jung would say, her "individu- ation," might be linked to her sexual life. For this type of woman, sexual encounter is the most profound of human experiences, a revelation of her own depths. It is therefore not only a source of joy but also a path of inner knowledge.

Ginette Paris

Alexandra is a strong-looking, earthy woman in her mid-fifties, married, with a fourteen-year-old son. She looks like, and in many ways is, an average American housewife, and yet, she is also a sex- ual priestess and an outspoken advocate for the wisdom of the body. When I arrived in her quiet suburban house, she greeted me at the door wearing a T-shirt that said: "My body is my home and the door to my soul."

This was by no means a message her parents gave her. Alexandra summed up their sexual philosophy in one short sentence: you don't talk about sex and you don't express it. As a child, Alexandra wanted to be a "good" girl. And so she obediently disconnected from her sexuality and focused on the life of the intellect. She read a lot, excelled in school, and avoided intimacy with men. "In high school," she recalled, "I really enjoyed going out with boys and kissing in the parked car. But there was never any more than that. I had internalized the message that sex was a no-no that could get you in deep trouble. I did very little dating and become totally a 'head' person."

But Eros was merely biding his time. After college, Alexandra fell deeply, passionately in love. To her dismay, the man was interested but ambivalent. He wanted fun; she wanted commitment. Desperate to keep him in her life, Alexandra did what women have done for centuries. "I'll have sex with him," she decided, hoping that sex would make him love her and tie him down. As is often the case in such trade-offs, her body had no say in this decision, but was offered as the sacrificial lamb on the altar of her emotional needs. Alexandra's hands tightened their grip around her coffee cup as she described her first sexual encounter with harsh honesty:

It was self-inflicted rape. It wasn't my body's choice. I was using my sexuality, and I wasn't feeling sexual; I was feeling desperate. So my body was not opening, and it was just very painful. At one point, David was having so much trouble entering me that he asked me whether I really wanted him inside of me. Everything in me was screaming, "No!" But I said yes. From then on, my sexuality became something to be used, disconnected from my feelings and my body and my desire.

"And did your plan work?" I inquired gently. A frown creased her smooth forehead as she nodded. It worked, she said, insofar as she achieved what she had set out to achieve. She and David dated for five years, then got married. However, the pattern of sexual self-denial continued. Alexandra did not know her own likes and dislikes, or how to communicate her sexual needs. She had no idea of who she really was as a sexual being. Sex remained a painful and frustrating experience for her, a performance given for her husband's benefit. Like a pot that simmers yet never boils, she often felt aroused yet never satisfied:

As a good, red-blooded American girl, I was brought up to believe that the man had to give you sexual pleasure, and that if he didn't give it to you, there was no way to get it. I also believed that you never, never said anything about a man being sexually inadequate. That was bound to destroy his ego and leave him totally flattened. So I never talked about my sexual frustration.

Many women are terrified of offending their partners by honestly expressing their desires. To ask for what we want in bed is so essential, yet it can feel so difficult—even impossible—so deeply ingrained is the fear of being rejected, humiliated, and shamed for our wants. To say the words that must be said, if we want to achieve sexual intimacy, we need to know that we deserve to feel pleasure, and we have the right to ask for it. Without an inner foundation of self-love, the risk may feel too great, the sense of possible rejection unbearable.

Of course, men's social conditioning can make it difficult for them to listen without getting defensive. "I remember being seventeen, with my first girlfriend, and feeling like I was supposed to know what to do," a male friend told me. "I was too embarrassed to admit that I didn't have a clue." Another friend, a woman, told me how her husband would encourage her to talk about what she wanted sexually. "'Whatever you want, just tell me, I really want to please you,' he kept saying. But the first time I asked him to do something while we were making love, he stopped and said in an angry tone, 'Don't tell me what to do.'" My friend groaned in frustration and concluded, "You have to have this incredible creativity so you can teach a man without his feeling that he's learning something from you." We can hope that these patterns are finally changing. Men long for sacred union as much as women do, and sacred union is a flower that thrives in the soil of honest communication.

Consciously, Alexandra never dreamed of viewing her sexual frustration as a challenge to spiritual growth. Everything she had been taught led her to believe that sex and spirit were opposites, and that god disapproved of sex. Like many of us, she was raised to think of the body as something dirty, messy, potentially sinful, and definitely not spiritual. How could there be anything godlike about our crude physical habits of eating and shitting and copulating? The very idea of asking god for sexual pleasure seemed irreverent. Still, something in her unconscious knew better. Alexandra laughed as she remembered how, after ten years of unsatisfying sex, she was willing to try just about anything to relieve her intolerable sense of frustration. In her desperation, she turned to spirit as a last resort.

SPEAKING UP

In a culture that is so negative about sex there is no way for people not to have projections on black women. Once, I went to an event with my boyfriend, and we met an elderly white couple there. And as we were standing together in conversation, the man reached out and touched my breast while his wife and my boyfriend were standing right there. It was so outrageous that afterward we could hardly believe it had happened. And none of us said a word. It was such a clear example of the intersection of sexism and racism which led this man to believe he could touch me in this way. And the silence—nobody said anything. DONNA

I think that as women, we should take it on as our responsibility to enlighten the men we are with about what we really want sexually. If we don't do it, nobody else is going to. If we can communicate honestly, then we can grow together. Otherwise, we let everything get sucked down the drain. MERCEDES

Until fairly recently, I lived in a kind of muteness, where I had no words and never talked about my sexuality. Nothing was named, and everything was surrounded by a wall of shame that wasn't named either. Now I believe that being able to speak about everything, just everything, is indispensable for good lovemaking. That takes skill and commitment to exposing yourself. I like talking about what's happening while we are making love, and weaving words into the fabric of physical excitement and pleasure. NAOMI

Gradually, my frustration was overcoming the desire that would build up. I came to a complete dead end, an absolute brick wall dead end. I had no idea what to do. I knew I wasn't satisfied. I was desperate. At this point, I said the first genuine prayer I have ever said in my whole life. And it was to the Great Mother. I said, "Great Mother, *help!*" And that was all it was. Just: *"Help!"*

Alexandra's voice rose to a shrill pitch as she imitated her desperate cry. Then she grinned at me and said, "Six weeks later, a letter came in the mail." It was an invitation, addressed to her and her husband, to participate in an intensive weekend workshop on sexuality, the first in a series designed to assist people in embracing the wide range of human sexual behavior. So often, spirit's ways are more outrageous, joyful, and humorous than we might expect. Alexandra knew without a shred of doubt that her prayers had been answered, and her immediate response was sheer terror. She had asked, and the solution had been offered. Now, it was up to her to accept the opportunity. Sexual priestesses need a lot of courage, and in this moment, Alexandra's courage was being tested. "I was literally shaking with fear when I arrived at the workshop," she recalled. "We entered the building, and the hallway was lined with erotic pictures. I walked down that hall with my head bent—I just could not bear to look at them." Then, with a sparkle of satisfaction in her eyes, Alexandra described the impact the workshop had on her life:

It was the only time so far in my life that I have ever experienced an absolute transformation. Before then, I never even knew what transformation was. I had worked through problems in therapy and have done so since. But this was a different matter altogether. That weekend, I heard a message that I had never heard before in my life. The message was simple: "You can have sex the way you want it."

When I grew up, the message I heard was that you shouldn't have sex. In the sixties, it was the opposite: you were *supposed* to have sex. This was the first time I really got that I could have it any way I wanted to. It didn't matter whether I was celibate or whether I was into group sex every night, as long as I accepted my own sexuality and made my own choices. I suddenly understood, for the first time, that

TEACH YOUR LOVERS WELL

One of my lovers had been a Buddhist monk for many years. The first time we made love, it was the worst sex I've ever had in my life. I felt like I was with a kid who didn't know anything. It was slam-bam-thank-you-ma'am sex. He had been celibate for so long that he had not learned to control himself. He came right away, and there was no real exploration of each others' bodies. Afterward, I thought, "Well, isn't it a shame I'm in love with him, because he's such a terrible lover." I knew I couldn't live with this. He seemed to think things were fine, but they were not fine at all for me. I felt like I would blow his mind if I were really free with him. I'm used to touching and kissing and sucking and licking and exploring the body. So I thought about it and I finally decided that I was just going to be who I was sexually with him the next time, and if he couldn't handle it, then I needed to know that. The next time came around, and I thought, "Okay, I'll seduce him this time. I'll show him who I am." So I did. I got out my oil; he had never used oil before in his life, ever. I began teaching him how to be a lover. He reciprocated right away that night; he learned very fast. From a five-minute experience we went to a forty-five-minute experience. He was really open to learning, very open to the erotic experience and to my sexuality.

DIANE

whatever I wanted was okay, and that it was all right for me to want pleasure. The leaders of the workshop believed this so thoroughly that the message really got through to me.

All of a sudden it became absolutely clear to me that I had to ask for what I needed. My husband was extremely responsive and very glad to have me let him know. I myself didn't yet know exactly what I needed, but I started experimenting. I knew that what I *didn't* need was for things to hurt. All these years, I had not been telling David that he was coming on stronger and more forcefully than I liked. His touch was too hard. Suddenly I was able to say, "Stop doing that so hard. Move more slowly. Do it lighter." For the first time, I started talking, and our sex got a whole lot better.

Soon after, Alexandra and her husband participated in a second workshop:

They showed a film in which a woman was having multiple orgasms. So on the way home, I said to my husband, "Someday that will happen to me, too." And he said, "Why not tonight?" So that night, I let it happen. He slowed down, and after I had one orgasm he didn't stop but kept arousing me. There was so much energy running through my body that night. I stood up and this stuff just poured out from between my legs. I put my finger down and smelled it and I thought, "That isn't urine." Now I know that women can ejaculate, but at the time, I had no idea.

Whether we hear it in church, or in a sex workshop, the message that we are worthy of being loved exactly the way we want to be loved is always a profound spiritual teaching. Soon Alexandra realized that the sexual awakening she had invited with her simple two-word prayer was also a spiritual awakening. "Ask and ye shall receive," Jesus told us. What an amazing and radical claim! Yet this was indeed Alexandra's experience. When she sincerely prayed for guidance, it appeared. Life, she realized with amazement, *wanted* to use her and dance through her and had only been waiting for her invitation.

I had said this prayer when I was up against the wall with no answer and nowhere to turn, and my prayer had immediately been answered. After that, I would ask for help in many other areas as well, and I would get it. I began to trust that I could ask and receive guidance, and so I found that a spiritual opening was tied to the sexual opening. For the first time in my life, I felt a sense of spiritual support for my sexuality.

To think that god might approve of our sexuality and even participate in our pleasure requires a radical turnaround for those of us raised to equate sex with sin. Essentially, it means that we must replace a strict, punitive god with a generous, loving one. Joseph Campbell once said, "In choosing your god, you choose your way of looking at the universe. There are plenty of gods. Choose yours."[6] For Alexandra, choosing a sex-positive deity meant turning toward the sacred feminine. Not only did the patriarchal god seem an unlikely ally in her quest for sexual pleasure, but she needed a figure who could mirror her own feminine essence and validate her female body. As a daughter looks to her mother for guidance, so Alexandra, in her sexual and spiritual awakening, intuitively reached for the goddess.

I had never prayed to the Great Mother before. I think I said the prayer to her because there was no way I could pray to a masculine god for sexual help. Everything I knew about the masculine god said that sex was bad. I had been taught that it was better to marry than to burn, but better, much better, if you could go into a convent. So, in a sense, I prayed to the Great Mother because there was nobody else to pray to.

Once I found my prayer answered, I realized that I envisioned her as a deity who smiles joyfully on my sexuality. She gives her blessing to pleasure. As a Presbyterian, I had received no religious messages about any female deity at all, so she was a clean slate. When we made love, I began to deliberately bring in her image, and she was right there with her supportive, positive energy. I often conjure up the image of the Great Mother when I masturbate or make love, and I imagine being held and smiled on and blessed. Today, I hold my sexual response as a gift to her, as a tribute. I feel her saying to me, "Yes, this is good. Your pleasure is an affirmation of my universe." It is definitely through my body that I am accessing the spiritual. For me, my spiritual awakening had to come through sexuality. Through sexuality, I got the message that my needs were okay, that I could have the pleasure I wanted, the way I wanted it.

Alexandra also found that her sexual opening led to an unexpected blossoming of her creativity. "My mother always wanted me to be an artist," she told me.

All my life, my creativity was blocked by my guilt at not becoming an artist. Then, a few years ago, I suddenly realized that through all the difficult times of my life, the one thing I had always done was write. I realized I was a writer, and that I didn't have to try to be a visual artist. It felt like a huge weight lifted from me at that point. I saw that I could express myself in my own way, just like I could have sex the way I wanted. I understood that I could receive pleasure through simply being me, and that spirit would love me for that.

By putting what she learned at the workshop into practice, Alexandra discovered her true capacity for sexual pleasure. Slowly, her body began to reveal its true nature as a shimmering, radiant field of sacred energy. Suddenly, she realized that sex was an energetic phenomenon, and that she possessed energetic skills she had previously not even known existed. She found she was able to direct energy within her body, channeling it through her pelvis or her heart, and that she could visually perceive her energy body.

"What did it look like?" I asked her. She hesitated. "It looked like . . . like millions of points of light on a grid. Sort of like a blueprint." I nodded. This was not the first time I'd heard women describing their energy body as a grid of light. We tend to think of our bodies as solid, three-dimensional objects, but in fact, they are no more solid than the clouds that drift across the sky, dreamily shapeshifting as they ride the wind. If we dive deeply into our body, we will find nothing but energy, light, and consciousness dancing within vast expanses of space. Our body is a shimmering web of vibrating energy. Mystics have long known this, and Western science is catching on fast. Aphrodite, it is said, is a goddess of sex, a goddess of the flesh. This is true. But what is this flesh? Aphrodite touches us, and we explode into fireworks of light.

Once Alexandra had connected with the divine mother as a source of healing, she began to ask for help, not only in healing her marriage, but also in healing the sexual wounds of her past. When she was just twelve years old, she had undergone surgery for an ovarian cyst, in which her entire ovary had been removed, along with a tumor that she described as "the size of an orange." "I didn't even know what an ovary was," Alexandra lamented. "Nothing at all had ever been said about sexuality. It was all taboo." The experience was traumatic. The doctor was rough and insensitive to the feelings of a terrified twelve-year-old girl who had never had a pelvic exam. With a shudder, Alexandra said, "It hurt, and he made my mother hold my shoulders down. He spoke to my mother, but he never spoke to me."

Young as Alexandra was, her inner priestess knew exactly what she wanted and needed. However, as is so often the case, none of the adults around her understood her feelings or respected her wishes.

After the surgery, the doctor brought in the tumor and the ovary in a bottle of formaldehyde to show me. I was absolutely fascinated by it, and I wanted it in the worst way. "No," he said, "you can't take it, it belongs to the hospital." "It's mine!" I objected. But they refused to give it to me.

I felt very deeply that in the surgery, something had been taken away from me before I had really had a chance to claim it. Everybody was disgusted and thought my feelings were totally gross, but I really wanted that ovary. In recent years, I realized a part of me knew that both the ovary and the tumor were really mine. They were part of me, and I wanted to own them. As a result, I felt very damaged. I felt there was something wrong with me. I had nobody to talk to at all, and there was no permission to grieve. My parents pretended everything was fine, and after the operation, it was never again mentioned.

Here we see a young girl intuitively knowing her primal female nature and wanting to own her female organs. To others, her body parts appeared gross and disgusting, but in her eyes, they were precious and fascinating. Staring at the jar in which her ovary floated, Alexandra obviously felt that she was looking at something mysterious and powerful. As a child, she would not have used the word "sacred" to describe what she saw; nothing in her religious up-bringing had taught her to associate the organs and processes of her female body with sacredness. Today, however, she knows that she had recognized the sacredness of her own female body.

After claiming the Great Mother as her ally in healing, Alexandra knew she needed to attend to the wounded twelve-year-old girl within her psyche. Drawing upon her skills as priestess, she staged a simple yet powerful healing ritual on her own behalf. Her voice full of pride and wonder, she said:

> Recently, I built a Great Mother for myself and did a cere-mony around her. Let me tell you, it was an amazing experi-ence. For the first time, I realized that what you create takes on its own life. The Great Mother was there in our living room for about three days, and her presence just filled the en-tire room. All I had done was put her together from things I had around the house, such as towels and sheets and an old robe of mine. And there she was, extremely powerful, with an absolute life of her own. It gave me great respect for what can happen when you have the intention of investing something with power.
>
> I built her in our living room, and then I sat on her lap. I was trying to reclaim what I needed to reclaim around the ovary that was taken away from me. I couldn't have done it from my ego. It came from somewhere else. Sitting on the Mother's lap, I held an orange. The inside of the orange sym-bolized the ovary and the peel was the tumor. I peeled the or-ange, and then I burned the peeling, affirming that this tumor was gone, and I took the ashes outside and buried them. Then I ate the orange and prayed that whatever part of the lost ovary needed to return to me be returned. "Let it come back now," I said. It was a very strong ceremony.

Some women discover the sacredness of their own sexual nature without consciously connecting with the sacred feminine. However, many find, as Alexandra did, that as they begin to relate to their own femininity with greater reverence, they spontaneously open to the feminine principle in a new way. Some draw inspiration from specific female images. Others prefer not to personify the divine, yet nonetheless find themselves opening to the "motherly," benign, nurturing qualities of the universe.

Most likely, you were not raised with feminine images of god, and to suggest that you might want to work with them may seem like asking you to convert to a new religion. But in fact, every world religion, even the most patriarchal, has a mystical branch that honors the feminine face of god. In Judaism, she is called Shekhinah. In Christianity, she is Sophia.

A goddess is simply an embodiment of an archetypal feminine energy that exists within us all. Many women feel drawn to certain visual images of the sacred feminine, such as the graceful form of Kuan Yin, the Chinese goddess of compassion, the mysterious Black Madonna of Christianity, or Changing Woman, a goddess dear to many Native American tribes. Such images remind us that we need not transcend the world to meet the divine. Spirit is present within our world of duality. It embraces the limitations of this world and enters into specific forms, male and female, light and dark, loving and wrathful. Instead of relating to goddess images as statements of religious belief or as literal representations of a deity, we can use them as reminders of the infinite forms spirit assumes in our world. The very multiplicity of these forms assures us that no matter who we are or what we look like, we carry the divine spark within us and have the potential to become embodiments of divinity.

In Tibetan Buddhism, a teacher will often instruct a student to meditate on a specific deity. The teacher will describe the deity in detail, along with all the surrounding colors, symbols, and attendants. Among hundreds of images, the teacher selects a particular one, not because it is superior to all others but because of its beneficial effects on the psyche of the meditator. Thus the focus lies very much upon the healing quality of the relationship that unfolds between the individual and the deity. To the Tibetan, the idea that everyone should meditate on the same deity is as ludicrous as the idea that all sick people should be given the same medicine. Obviously, the medicine must be suited to the particular nature of the ailment. Our images of the divine are best used as medicine, as tools for healing. Female images can be extremely helpful to us—not because spirit is female, but because at certain times, such images contain the appropriate medicine for what ails us. We can easily sense how the thought of a beautiful, compassionate mother evokes a different energy within our body and mind than does the thought of a just and wise father. To recognize the medicinal nature of all our sacred images frees us to see that these images are not meant to enslave us, but to assist us in realizing our own divinity. What effect does a particular image of the divine have upon us? Does it help us to live our lives in a more peaceful, balanced way, or does it cause us to feel unworthy, guilty, and inadequate to the challenges we face? Does it make us happy or miserable? Does it give us courage, or does it stifle and hold us back? Does it support us as priestesses? Does it teach us to value the earth, to value animals, to value our sexuality?

By meditating on the Great Mother, Alexandra was preparing to recognize the sacred presence within her own self, as well as in others. When she speaks of the fruits of her journey, she emphasizes that the image of the divine feminine has given her the courage to relax, to trust, and to open to life in ways she never knew were possible. Initially, her intention was simply to embrace sexual pleasure. However, in the process, she discovered herself opening to life itself and to spirit.

Ever since my first prayer was answered, I have always felt the support of the Great Mother. I have studied Zen Buddhism and found a lot of things in it very attractive and useful. But I needed to have some personification of spirit. My transformation required enormous trust, and in order to trust, I had to have somebody to trust in. To me, the Great Mother was and is that personification of pure Being.

The greatest challenge has been to give up the need to know what the consequences of my actions will be. I have had to let go of control. This is not easy for me, given that I was brought up to believe that control and repression were the solution to all difficult emotions and feelings. I have been able to let go this much only because of my trust in the Great Mother and in the process she has initiated in my life.

The transformation I have experienced is quite incredible. I am so much stronger a person than I was five years ago. Even now, my sexuality keeps changing and transforming. Initially, it was just about experiencing sexual feelings in my body and being able to relax and enjoy them. Then I started looking at the energy patterns and finding that I could guide and direct the energy. Now something in me doesn't want to let the energy manifest genitally. It is pushing up into the heart chakra. It's like the energy is nudging me gently and saying, "Come a little more over this way." I am connecting more from the heart level in general. I pick up on the opportunities to run heart energy with people, whether or not they know it. When my husband and I are together, I run the energy back and forth between our hearts. I figure, it can't do any harm. I stop and talk to the cat who is sitting on the sidewalk.

Alexandra fell silent for a minute. Then she said, "I see now that it's all the same energy. I see that so clearly. It's not just genital, it's the dance of the life-force."

I just need to pay attention to where it wants to go and what it wants to do. My ego can't guide it. It doesn't have a clue. Having so many years behind me as a control freak, a part of me still freezes every time something shifts. "What's this?" it says. "What's happening? What's going on? I thought I had everything in place." But I am letting go. I am learning to follow and trust the changes, and to be present with whatever arises.

I have decided to do a ritual in which I will take a vow. The vow is this: "With immense gratitude toward the Great Mother for all that She has given me, I vow to try to walk in her ways and to live with compassion and discernment in all that I do." I am not quite ready to take this vow yet. It's a very scary vow to take. I know that if I make it, I will take it very seriously. I have no idea what it will bring, and I can't put conditions on it. It will take me wherever it takes me. But within me, I know this is going to happen. It is what I need to do.

3

ELDER SISTER'S STORY

How shall I begin my song
In the blue night that is settling?
In the great night my heart will go out,
Toward me the darkness comes rattling.
In the great night my heart will go out.
                    Papago Medicine Woman Chant

During my interviews with women, a strange thing would occur. After having talked about sexuality and spirituality, about marriage and motherhood, and about love and lust, women would suddenly, out of the blue, start talking about death, specifically about the death of close relatives or loved ones. This happened so frequently that I began to anticipate it. For a long time I puzzled over this phenomenon.

One evening, I started thinking about India and Nepal. I pulled out an old box of photographs that had sat untouched in the back of my closet for years, and began to look at them. There were the beautiful mirror-smooth lakes of Nepal; there were the monkeys chattering from the rooftops; there were the children of India flashing their wide grins at me. And there—I drew in my breath, startled. I was looking at a small, somewhat blurry image of the old devadasi I had met in Mysore, sitting straight as an arrow while her hands danced. What startled me was the faint outline of a prone body in the background of the picture. I had quite forgotten that as I sat with the old priestess, her even older sister had been resting on a cot in the far corner of the room. The sister was more than ninety years old, and my teacher told me in a whisper that the old woman was dying. By then, I had come to appreciate the fact that in India, death does not occur behind the closed doors of hospitals and nursing homes, but out in the open. The sick and the old die surrounded by their families, attended to by the younger ones. And so the presence of a dying woman in our midst was nothing unusual. Life went on as usual.

During our visit, the dying woman lay silently, sometimes softly moaning. But suddenly, she spoke. My teacher turned to me and said, "She is calling you." It seemed the most natural thing in the world for me to go over, sit down with the dying woman. and hold her hand while we looked at each other with the deepest, most tender love. Though she was a complete stranger to me, we shared a moment of total intimacy, our souls touching in silent communion.

Now, as I carefully returned the photographs to their box, I saw that the juxtaposition of the priestess and the dying woman was no coincidence. Both were participants in the extraordinary initiation I had received that day. Suddenly, I understood why so many women were telling me stories about death. Intuitively, they perceived sex, birth, and death as three kindred mysteries in which the body itself leads the way into other-dimensional realities. I imagine that in the old days, before reliable forms of birth control were available, the possibility of giving birth, but also of dying in childbirth, must have been very much on a woman's mind when she made love. Even today, nearly 600,000 women a year—roughly 1,600 women every day—die giving birth.[7] No matter how we try to shield ourselves, the dark goddess of death always appears during moments of passionate love. As one woman said, "When we make love, I always feel the connection of love and death, creation and destruction. I feel myself melting, dissolving, dying."

It is therefore only natural that the sexual priestess would act both as midwife into life and as midwife into death. As a go-between who herself moves back and forth between the worlds, she can also assist others in their passages. Alexandra, who told her story in the preceding chapter, told me how she served as a guide for her father as he was dying. "Before my sexual awakening, I could never have been there for him in the way I was," she declared. Quietly, her voice resonant with emotion, she explained:

I could not trust the natural process of dying until I had learned to be present in my body. I had to be at home in my body; I had to be *here*. For a long time, there was nobody home in my body. And until somebody was home, there was no chance of having a spiritual life. It's impossible to get that basic trust in spirit until you have come into your body, because that's where you experience it. I realize that sounds contradictory, because the body is the part of us that is going to get sick and die and disintegrate. But I believe that the body is okay with that. It's perfectly natural, and it's exactly what should happen. Its only the ego that has a problem with it.

I received a great gift by being able to be with my father through his death. I once heard Stephen Levine [a popular meditation teacher] say that death is what makes life safe. That is so true. We count on our death. We never would have taken birth if we weren't absolutely certain that death would allow relief if the agony became too great.

Evelyn is another priestess who has been learning through first-hand experience how to stand on the threshold of the Great Gateway and assist others in their passages. She is a striking woman who, with her dark hair and eyes, her tall, slender body, and her combination of powerful feminine sensuality and boyish grace, looks as if she just stepped out of an ancient Egyptian painting. I had met Evelyn several times at social occasions, but when I ran into her one night at a concert, I knew right away that something was different, that she had changed. She seemed to be moving through the mass of laughing voices and jostling bodies like a sleepwalker, like someone who is present in body yet whose spirit is caught up in another world.

I recognized that look. I had seen it in a close friend after she had lost one of her children to cancer, and I had seen it in clients who had ventured dangerously far into the land of death and were struggling to find their way back to life. Without wanting to be intrusive, I asked Evelyn how she was. The story that she poured out to me was the story of a woman who chose to serve as a priestess to a dying man in his time of need, and to guide him, both sexually and spiritually, into the arms of love.

"Would you be willing to share your story with other women?" I asked her. Without hesitation, she agreed. Hers is a contemporary story about a contemporary priestess, and yet, it is also a story that might have happened one, five, or ten thousand years ago.

I met Jason six years ago in a spiritual group I belong to. At the first meeting, I looked around the circle and when I got to Jason, an inner voice said to me, "He will be your partner, your mate." "Oh no, he won't," I thought, "not with a body like that." He was a little short and thick at the waist with sweatpants that came up really high. He looked like Humpty Dumpty. Oh, my god, why didn't I follow that voice? If only I had followed that voice. Looking back, I regret that I was so attached to physical looks. We didn't get involved till five years later, just before his death. He really yearned for a relationship. In his journals, he once wrote that life was not worth living without a mate. I read that two days after he died, and it just broke my heart. If only I had listened earlier.

We became very, very close friends. He made people feel special. He was the only man I ever knew who totally respected women in the most sacred way. He lived in the temple of the goddess. We understood each other totally, and we shared the same spiritual path. We were priest and priestess together. When I heard that Jason had been diagnosed with cancer, I prayed, "Mother, of all men, don't take this one. We need this brother." And I offered myself in service. "Mother, whatever I can do to help him stay around, I will do it. Use me." I moved in as close as I could right away. It was metastasized colon cancer and he had to have surgery. He thought he might be rendered impotent, and he knew that at the very best, he would have to have a colostomy.

There was a place Jason loved to go to in Hawaii. He would rent a condominium that faced east, where you could watch the sun rise over the ocean every morning. Jason wanted to go there, and he invited me to go with him, as a platonic friend. After his surgery, as soon as he was strong enough to go, we went there together for ten days.

Early the first morning, I woke up. It was still dark, and I saw that Jason had lit candles. There was something so beautiful about it, so sacred. He had lit the candles in the temple. We sat together, drank our coffee, and watched the sunrise. And we prayed. Here we were, priest and priestess in a state of prayer, watching the sun rise. We had the most glorious sunrises every day, with peach and crimson clouds. Occasionally he or I would share some thought with each other. It felt like a consummation of spirit. I asked him, "Do I interrupt your meditation?" "No," he said, "you deepen it." God, that was so delicious. One morning the sun rose behind a cloud, and it sent out rays like a huge golden crown. I turned to Jason and I said, "This is your crown." And in that moment, he looked like royalty to me.

I now know that part of the work I showed up to do with Jason was to help him make peace with the feminine before his death. I was there to assist this man's passage into the Light, in a sacred way. He needed to heal his relationship with women before he left his body. There was a side of him that never trusted women, and I can see why. His mother had been a real witch, really mean and controlling. And for years, he had been hooked on this woman who would seduce him, and when he opened up to her, she would reject him. This happened over and over. When we flew to Hawaii, he said one of his regrets was that she would be the last woman he slept with. "Hm," I thought to myself. This was when I started thinking about sleeping with him.

But we were so used to just being friends, I didn't know how to cross that boundary. We both had been so proper with each other for years. One night we were lying next to each other, and he said, "It's so nice to be lying next to a compatible vibrating unit." I still crack up over that. It was really cute. And it was also very true. We were both vessels for very powerful energies, sacred energies that vibrated in harmony. So I knew exactly what he meant. It *was* really nice to be lying next to a compatible vibrating unit.

One night, after we had been there about five days, we were lying next to each other. For the first time I was really attracted to him, and I also wanted to satisfy his desire to not have Tina be the last lover of his life. We were lying in front of the ocean, and there was nothing to stop us. "Why not?" I thought. It was a simple doorway, and at the same time a huge doorway. He was a very skilled lover. He started licking me. My legs were spread to my lover and to the ocean, and I started having an orgasm—I felt such ecstasy and joy and sensual passion. We had sex twice in Hawaii. After this night, my being with him was almost beyond choice. It was like plunging over a waterfall. There was no going back.

I had these two black scarves with me. At one point, he said he wanted to tie his colostomy bag to his body to keep it secure, and I handed him one of these black scarves. But he took it and hung it around his neck. Instantly, I saw him as the Priest of Death. I didn't like seeing that, and part of me wanted to take the black scarf back. But yes, he was the Priest of Death. This *was* a death walk. He wore that scarf constantly, for the rest of his life, so I wore mine constantly, too. It became a symbol of our union and our death walk together.

After we came back from Hawaii we both knew we were in love. We were hooked on each other. We had a couple of ecstatic weeks. He was elated because he thought his cancer was in remission. He just loved and honored and adored me. At one point I was on the floor, stretching and moving, working out in front of my altar. And he just attacked me. It was so delicious. We made love right there on the floor in front of the altar. Everything was so ecstatic and beautiful. That was when I started realizing how high we were getting off each other. Once, Jason said to me, "Our love will change the DNA structure of humanity." "What do you mean?" I asked. "Well," he said, "our love is so strong that it can be felt by others and it will change them forever." I really took that in. We inseminated something. We brought a love into the earth plane that may affect people who didn't even know us.

When we made love, we were wild like cats. We were just bursting with excitement and joy. "Do you feel me in you? Do you feel my fire?" he would ask. It was so sexy. I didn't know what an incredible, sensuous, passionate animal he was, and what a great lover. Our sex was so primal. To have that good fucking with my priest. . . . It wasn't just about breathing together, or about being spiritual. Our lovemaking brought spirit all the way through to the animal in us. I just adored it. Oh, I loved his shoulders, his arms. I was in adoration of his body. It was amazing how I had switched from not liking his body to adoring it. Everything went so fast. We bonded so deeply that we felt ourselves to be in a sacred marriage.

Jason was very nervous about his colostomy. It embarrassed him, but he dealt with it really well. One time, the colostomy bag got pulled off while we were making love. I smelled it and I said to him, "Jason, I think you have initiated me." It was something we both feared. He was mortified. He didn't say anything. He just got up and went straight to the bathroom. He came back to bed absolutely devastated. I just felt total compassion for him. But other than that, it didn't get in the way that much. It wasn't that big of a deal for me.

Several weeks after we got back from Hawaii, the pain in Jason's body just exploded. He was yelling with pain and shivering with agony. And it was so strange because my own body felt fine. I wanted to share his pain and I couldn't. Then I knew that all I could do was drop down into the peace inside of me and hold him from that place. That's what I did. And slowly, he was able to let go. Suddenly I knew he would die, and that our lovemaking was over. And we had just started. We had just discovered each other. It was true; we never made love again. We both grieved so deeply over that. We had wanted this all our lives, and we had two, three weeks of good lovemaking, at most.

The next night, he needed to be alone with his pain. Later, he told me that all that night he had yelled and cried, "God, all my life I have been calling for this woman, and you send her to me in the last moments of my life. Why?" When he started taking morphine, I called it Mother Morphine, and I thanked her. The Mother came through to take care of his pain. Losing a part of him to morphine was the first step of my turning him over to the Mother. It was out of my control. We both had to keep dying, surrendering.

Our union served a very high purpose. He told me that his

whole relationship to women was reframed. He had a new sense not just of what a lover was, but of Mother, because he allowed me to mother him in a sacred way. During this time, until his death, I felt a sense of being fully guided in every moment. I knew what to do in every moment. Spiritually, I felt completely supported in this journey.

Right around the time I was realizing Jason and I would never have sex again, I went to an exhibit of sacred Chinese art, and there were several images of Kuan Yin, the goddess of compassion. In one image, she was wearing white gossamer and was barefoot. I learned that she was also a goddess of sensuality, an aspect of Kuan Yin I had never heard of. Apparently, men on the verge of attaining enlightenment and becoming Bodhisattvas would come to her for a final sexual communion, to go beyond desire of the physical. "Oh," I thought, "what I am doing with Jason is part of the spiritual path. I am being Kuan Yin to him." It was a consoling thought.

Jason had so much faith there would be a miracle, but there wasn't. Another CAT scan revealed that the cancer was still growing. After hearing the results, he crawled up on the couch and imagined he was putting his head on the lap of the Mother. He had a strong connection with the Mother and she consoled him and gave him comfort. He knew he was returning to the lap of the Mother, and he really felt her holding him. Jason meditated like this for hours, and by the time I called him, he was ecstatic. Some part of him was laughing.

Just one week before Jason's death, I had an visionary experience of seeing a labyrinth over his head. I saw a dark shadow coming down one of the passages and I said, "Who are you? Are you of the Light?" And it said, "I am Death, and I have come to interview Jason." And I said with great strength, "He's not ready yet. He still has some work to do. Back off." I saw all the different passages of the labyrinth and I saw that death was very close. It was coming. I could use my will to keep it at bay for a little while longer. That was all I could do. The following Wednesday night I saw the labyrinth again. This time all the passages were filling up with darkness and I knew death was close. And by then, there was no reason to resist. Jason had completed his work. "Thy will be done," I prayed. "May it be a peaceful passage."

We had candles going the whole time, and sacred music. By Thursday night it started getting hard. "I'm so grateful that you are here," he said to me. "It gives me great comfort." That night, I left and he had a long visit with his teenage son. When I came back his son was sitting in the light of the full moon and his face was full of holiness. Friday night, in the throes of all his pain, somewhere between peeing and throwing up, Jason turned to me and said, "I love you so much, and I wanted to take you so many places." That night, his daughter lay down with him, and so did his son, and he became very peaceful.

He died Sunday morning. Saturday night, he would moan softly with every exhale. I watched him and I saw a little tear come out of his eye, and I kissed it. And another. That night, I got out the prayer arrow that he used in his spiritual practice, and I started guiding his spirit up, wafting his soul out, showing him the way through the top of his head. I was talking to him, and even though he could no longer talk, I believe he heard me. The owl was one of his power animals, and in my mind I could see the owl. "Jason, do you see the owl circling overhead? Let the owl take you through the doorway," I said. I could see him let go. Around five in the morning I remembered how he loved to imagine putting his head on the Mother's lap. So I said to him, "Jason, put your head on the Mother's lap and surrender to her. She is holding you." I could feel his whole being letting go and saying yes. It was so palpable. "Mother, take him," I prayed.

Then the dawn came. "It's a beautiful sunrise," I said to Jason. "May this be your last sunrise." It became a beautiful clear day and the church bells started ringing. And then he stopped breathing. It was eight-thirty in the morning. It was so awesome to see him moving into the vastness of the infinite Light, light years from this place.

I saw very clearly that dying was not a moment in time. It was a long process. At some point, his soul had simply moved over to the other side of the great divide, that's all. Jason had taught me a Celtic blessing: "I've known you before, I'll know you again; our bond is eternal." I said it to him now. When the night came, I felt like staying with his body, so I did. I slept right there next to his body, and that felt very wonderful. It was very peaceful. I felt so happy that he was free, and there was a deep softness in me.

The day after his death, I wanted to check in and see where he was, so I went into meditation. Immediately, I saw that he was being held by the Mother, and that in that state, he could hold me. And for the first time, I could be in the fullness of my grief. Until then, I had held back my tears to protect him. Now, I felt him holding my sorrow. I sobbed and sobbed, and it felt very sacred. But god, it hurt. When the time came for me to go back to my own home, I knew I needed some sisters to welcome me back to my altar and into my sacred space. So I put out the word, and my women friends came with flowers and food, and we sat in circle in my house. It was really beautiful to feel such support.

But my grief kept increasing. By about four days after he died, it hurt so badly that for the first time I started questioning: Was it worth it? It shocked me to ask that question. But this hurt, oh it hurt. I was not prepared for how much it hurt. I really hope I never have to help a lover die again. I was really shocked at how incapacitated I was. I could barely drive. I stopped eating. It took weeks before I could prepare my own food. A lot of friends brought me food. I know now that people who are grieving need huge amounts of care. Fortunately, I had a strong community, but still, I needed even more than I received.

One night, three weeks after he died, I felt like in my sleep I spent the whole night in conversation with him. In one dream, he told me he felt good about his death, and about the ceremonies we had done for him. Most of all, he felt really good about how we were letting him go. I woke up about five in the morning, and I heard an owl hooting in the tree right outside the window. I had never, ever heard an owl around the house before, and here was Jason's soul animal calling me awake. Then, inside of me, I heard Jason saying to me, "I have to ascend now. It might feel a little cool." I had the image of a spiral moving up through the clouds. I just said, "Thy will be done. Go." Then I felt a breeze, and he was gone.

I had always protected my heart. But with the experience of losing Jason I was blasted wide open. There was no protection left. I feel like a neutron bomb went off in my heart and I exploded. Particles of my old ego are still flying around. My self as I knew it got blasted apart and I am just this cloud of energy. The dust is settling, but where, into what? I am not the same person. There is a huge empty space. What do I attach onto as real, as having meaning, as the ground of being? Part of me wants to grab the armor back, to hide from this pain. But no, no.

Recently, I realized who I am. I am an Elder Sister. I like those words. They're not grandiose, like the "High Priestess," not lofty. The Mother has said to me, "Become an Elder Sister." I never had a spiritual Elder Sister myself, but I am becoming one for others. I showed up at the threshold and walked as far as I could into the labyrinth with Jason's soul, and I knew how to find my way back. I did that, and that knowledge is now becoming part of my being. And I feel Jason is right here, available to console and to counsel me. I am closer to the realm of spirit than before his passing. I have a friend on the other side.

4

THE REFINER'S FIRE

But who can endure the day of his coming, and who can stand when He appears?
For He is like a refiner's fire that purifies the silver and the gold.

Malachi 3:2

Having heard many people speak of Hannah with great love and respect, I was looking forward to finally meeting her one rainy morning when I knocked on the door of a large house in rural Maine. The door opened, and a middle-aged woman appeared, dressed in old baggy sweatpants, a couple of warm sweaters, and big woolly slippers. "Hannah?" I asked, unsure whether I had come to the right place. She nodded, beaming, and welcomed me into the spacious old house she shares with her husband, Raymond. In her face, framed by masses of dark curls, I read integrity, caring, and kindness. As I soon discovered, Hannah also possesses a kind of ruthless honesty that does not flinch from facing difficult truths.

Soon we were nestled in with mugs of steaming hot tea. While the rain drummed gently on the roof, Hannah plunged into her story. "The most difficult challenge of my journey," she began, "has been to integrate two conflicting attitudes towards sexuality."

For most of my life, I have felt that my sexual consciousness inhabited a different room from my normal consciousness. These rooms were quite separate and didn't even know about each other. One room belonged to the Controller. He believed you had to cut off your feelings in order to be safe and make your way in the world. In another room entirely lived my passion and my sexuality—the part of me that just wanted to dissolve in the bliss and ecstasy of making love. Here were tender, exciting, mysterious feelings which I never talked to anybody about. I knew how to be in one room or the other, but there was nothing in between. I was either in the room of passion or in the room of control.

For children of a control-based society, it may be helpful to understand that an obsession with control is always a sure sign that the ego is frightened and is trying to bolster its fragile sense of security. "Hold on, stay strong, don't let go," fear whispers, as it latches onto us like an insidious parasite. "Whatever you do, don't lose control." Fear warns the ego to resist its own death at all costs. And yet, without ego death, sacred union, whether with god or with a lover, is impossible.

A healthy ego is no more afraid of sacred union than a raindrop is of merging into the ocean. Flexible, fluid, and infinitely sensitive to the needs of the soul, it welcomes pleasure and willingly allows its own dissolution.

Or we might compare the healthy ego to a loyal, protective watchdog who warns us of danger but lies down quietly when our lover arrives. In contrast, the Controller is more like a crazed pit bull who keeps us imprisoned in our own house. Love, passion, and ecstasy had better watch out. If they dare show up at our door, they are liable to be chased away in no time, with much snarling and gnashing of teeth. As we shall see, Hannah's Controller effectively chased away one of her most exciting lovers.

Here, I will follow Hannah's lead and speak of the Controller in the masculine gender. Of course, women can be just as controlling as men, and if you were raised with a critical, controlling mother, your inner Controller may well have a female voice.

No matter how we envision the Controller, in a culture where success depends on control, and loss of control equals failure, the woman who does not internalize his repressive voice is rare indeed. You may recall Alexandra's claim that the greatest challenge in both her sexual and spiritual journeys has been to let go of control. Like several women I interviewed, she told me how much her first powerful orgasm frightened her:

> I tried out a vibrator and suddenly I found my clitoris, which I had never discovered before. After using the vibrator several times, I had a really cosmic orgasm and I ended up in the center of the universe, absolutely at peace. And it terrified me. I flipped myself right out of it, and for many years, I could never get back to that place again. I think what really scared me was losing control. I was swept away.

This fear of being swept away sits deep within our guts, and no wonder, given that patriarchy has conveniently placed the burden of sexual self-control upon women. When a man loses control, he is called passionate. A woman, on the other hand, is called a slut or worse. According to Anaïs Nin, Emile Zola courted the novelist George Sand "and obtained a night of lovemaking. Because she revealed herself as completely unleashed sensually, he placed money on the night table when he left, implying that a passionate woman was a prostitute."[8]

In defense of her Controller, Hannah admitted that his mistrust of her passion-seeking side was not totally unfounded. Sexual passion can bring out the best in us, but also the worst—greed, obsession, arrogance, and selfishness. There is probably no society on earth that does not place certain restrictions on the expression of passion. Like any natural power, raw, unrefined passion can harm as well as heal. Hannah told me how in her younger years, she lightheartedly made love to a number of married men without giving much thought to the matter. As we shall see, she was later forced to acknowledge the suffering she had mindlessly caused.

Most of us experience some degree of internal tension between the Controller and the free-spirited Passion-seeker. "My psyche is a war zone," one client told me. "There are hidden minefields, there are temporary cease-fires, and sometimes, there are battles that leave me exhausted for days." During the sixties and seventies, these battles erupted into public view as the flower children and the rebels began to openly confront the Controller. "You are uptight, repressed, authoritarian," they cried. Furious, the Controller retorted, "And you with your dreams of free love—you are immature, ungrateful, immoral, and irresponsible."

Is it possible to reconcile the warring opposites and achieve a true state of peace? I believe it is, for Hannah has done so. However, as we shall see, she has succeeded only because of her unwavering commitment to the spiritual journey and her willingness to let the fires of life totally transform her.

I asked Hannah when she first noticed that a war was being waged in her psyche. "It was in my late teens," she said. At this point, she had already made love to quite a few men. "I thought I was stopping the war in Vietnam," she said with a laugh. One would think that her Controller would have risen up in arms in the face of such free-spirited hedonism. Not so. What threatened him, far more than casual sex, were the moments in which Hannah's ego boundaries evaporated like ice in the hot midday sun. In our sexually liberal society, many people find that casual sex allows them to satiate their physical needs while steering clear of true passion. Hannah, too, found her Controller to be quite tolerant as long as passion was not part of the picture. She looked at me and grinned. "Then," she said, "I met Steve."

"Yes?" I said eagerly.

Hannah took a deep breath. "Well," she went on,

Steve was a man from India who was about twenty years older than I. This guy must have studied the Kama-sutra for a long time. I never even knew this kind of lovemaking existed. It was as if someone had disconnected my brain and turned me into a totally sensual woman. He lived about seven hundred miles away, but every weekend, we would get together and spend the entire weekend making love. I don't think we even left the house.

Steve had learned how to sustain an erection for hours without coming. Even when he came, he wouldn't lose interest. I had anal sex for the first time in my life and discovered I loved it; it felt wonderful. There was nothing that he wouldn't think of or do; he was totally creative and sensual. He unlocked all my doors and was totally uninhibited. It gave him immense pleasure to pleasure me, unlike the other men I had been with. He just loved to play and have fun and be sensual, staying in bed all day. I never even knew that was possible.

Then, after about six months, I woke up one morning and couldn't stand him. I felt utterly revolted. After feeling so passionate and surrendered, I suddenly couldn't bear to be around him. So I told him I didn't want to see him anymore. Of course he was terribly hurt. I think that the revulsion was linked to a sense of panic because my controlling side had been locked away for too long. The Controller feared the power of my feelings, so in order to come into that surrendered and utterly sensual and deep place, I had closed the door on my more fearful, prohibitive side. But at some point, the Controller reasserted himself and came back with a vengeance.

Hannah was twenty years old at this point. Soon after, her Controller selected a husband for her, a decision in which passion had no say whatsoever. We throw up our hands in horror when we hear of arranged marriages in other parts of the world. But who arranges our own marriages? It seems a good number of them are arranged by unconscious—and not always wise or benevolent—forces, which sabotage our conscious intention like guerrilla rebels. Her brow furrowed in puzzlement, Hannah told me that from the onset, she felt little desire for her first husband, but married him anyway because he struck her as a good person. "All my feelings for my father were tangled up in my feelings for my husband," she said. "I felt like I had to be a good girl with him. Our sex life was never that great from the beginning, and gradually, sex became more and more aversive to me."

Around the same time, Hannah became involved with a particularly austere branch of Tibetan Buddhism. "My Buddhist teachers taught me to cultivate detachment," Hannah said. "Desire was considered the worst thing, the very worst thing." The Controller clapped his hands and rejoiced. As far as he could see, he had won the battle on all fronts: Hannah's sexual and spiritual life were now both under his firm control, and passion was securely locked away.

The Controller has always valued patriarchal religion as one his most effective instruments of repression. Every Sunday, his wrathful voice echoes through thousands of churches, calling us to sexual abstinence, decrying Aphrodite's supposedly evil influence, and threatening the pleasure-seeker with spiritual damnation. The controversial priest and teacher Matthew Fox remarks:

> I believe that the Western church, following in the spirit of St. Augustine, basically regrets the fact that we are sexual, sensual creatures. "If only sexuality would go away," the message goes, "we could get on with important issues of faith."[9]

But the problem is not unique to Christianity. You will find the Controller firmly ensconced in Buddhist temples and Hindu ashrams as well as in Christian monasteries. He loves the challenge of austere asceticism and harsh discipline, and wherever mortification of the flesh is on the religious menu, he is sure to show up. Invariably, he is a perfectionist who believes that life should be mastered through personal effort. Nobody can meet his standards or is ever quite good enough for him. He will whip us until we drop dead from exhaustion, and then he will shrug and say, "Too bad. She could have made it had she not been so undisciplined." It's like the race of the turtle and the hare. We are the hares who race to the goal, only to find, with dismay, that the Controller is already there, waiting for us, waving his stick and telling us we are spiritual failures. "You should try harder," he yells. "Meditate more! Purify yourself! Give up your attachments!"

Often, the women most vulnerable to self-abuse in the name of religion are those whose spiritual hunger is greatest. The very urgency of their longing can blind them to the dark side of the teachings to which they give themselves, body and soul, in their fervent quest for sacred communion.

Hannah became an avid student, practitioner, and teacher of Buddhism, and for several years she remained unaware of the dangerous undertow of self-hatred that contaminated her practice. Like an innocent, gullible child, she had accepted the Controller's pretense of being a wise mentor. In the meantime, she silenced the voice of a far more trustworthy spiritual guide—her own body. But finally, after years of self-abuse in the name of spiritual purification, her body shook her awake by literally rubbing her face in the truth.

I did a three-month retreat. I just practiced and meditated, doing five hundred prostrations a day. As I did all these prostrations, I kept pushing my forehead against the pillow. Finally, I had a sore on my forehead, which I decided to ignore. I did nothing about it until a dermatologist friend of mind said, "That looks bad. You absolutely must go to a doctor right away." And it turned out to be skin cancer.

That cancer was really symbolic for me. What I see now, but didn't realize then, was that I was really cut off from my body. Every way that I knew to be good meant saying no to my sensuality and my aliveness. It meant sitting still and disciplining myself. This form of spiritual practice definitely appealed to my Controller, and there was no place in it for passion or desire. I had firmly closed the door to my sensuality.

There's a terrible Buddhist story about a woman who really longs to do spiritual practice, but her beauty is distracting all the monks. So she takes a hot iron and puts it on the side of her face. Then she's so scarred she can go anywhere without arousing their desire. I felt like I had done this to myself by ignoring the skin cancer for so long. I feel differently now, but at that time, a part of me felt liberated by the thought of having my face destroyed. I was denying my body and my beauty and aliveness.

Where is the fine line between self-indulgence and self-repression? When is discipline healthy, and when does it become a form of abuse? When are we nurturing ourselves, and when are we simply feeding our addictions? There are no general answers to such questions. All we can do is sit with them in the most honest, open way we are capable of. The spiritual path *does* require discipline. At the same time, discipline has no value on its own. If you have ever been around an anorexic, you know the enormous discipline with which an anorexic can starve herself to death.

Nonetheless, Hannah knew better than to throw out the baby with the bathwater. The problem was not discipline itself, but the fact that she had been using it in the service of self-hatred, rather than in the service of love. "When did you first experience sexual self-control as a positive, life-affirming force?" I asked her. She considered for a minute, and then told me the following story.

Eventually, I became one of my Buddhist master's main teachers. One of his other students was a monk named Arnie. Arnie and I fell deeply in love. Outwardly, I was still a good, proper wife, but the truth was that I was on fire over Arnie. But Arnie had taken a vow of celibacy. At one point, my teacher and five of his students, including myself and Arnie, took a trip around the world, teaching and giving initiations everywhere. We were all supposed to go to Romania. But then, because of political issues, they wouldn't allow my master into the country. So he said, "Okay. Arnie and Hannah, you go to Romania for me and do the teachings there." So here we were, just Arnie and me, traveling together through Romania. We knew that to talk about our feelings would just fire us up even more, so we didn't.

At one center, over a hundred people had squeezed into one small room. The house had only one other room, a tiny space which our hosts, out of their kindness, offered us to sleep in. That night, neither of us slept a wink. All night, I thought, "I don't give a damn about him. I just want to fuck." Another voice said, "But Hannah, you will make him break his vows." "Who cares?" said my lust. I had never experienced lust in such a powerful way. I was just sweating all night. I was shaking with desire. But I did nothing. This night remains as one of my deepest experiences of sexuality. Even though we never touched, every cell in my body was trembling.

The next day, we gave the initiations, very powerful rituals, which include taking vows. I could feel the centuries and centuries of people who had taken these vows before us. One of the five vows is to abstain from lust. Well, this was the vow all the Romanian students were most interested in, and they insisted that Arnie and I both give our dharma talk on the subject of lust. What a joke!

"Did you ever regret not having made love with Arnie?" I asked Hannah. She shook her head.

No. I didn't regret it at all. So often, I had not cared about the consequences of my passion for other people. I just wanted what I wanted when I wanted it. Now, I clearly saw that what I was feeling was lust and not love, and I also saw that my lust didn't care one bit about Arnie or his vows. I couldn't pretend to myself that this was love. I don't believe that sex and love necessarily have to go together, but in this case, they were in conflict, and I chose love. I was shocked at the strength of my lust, but there was such power in not acting on it.

As Hannah's story shows, sexual self-denial need not spell repression. In this instance, she denied herself sexual pleasure without rejecting or judging her desire. Where passion was poised to grab the goodies and run with them, compassion forced Hannah to consider the wider implications of her actions and insisted that she subordinate her lust to the higher power of love. In making a choice—not so much *against* lust as *for* love—Hannah began to reclaim the power of self-control as a moral agent in her life. At this point in Hannah's story, we see her Controller, with all his righteous zeal, beginning to change into a true servant of the soul.

Thomas Moore defines morality "as the imagination for channeling Eros into workable human forms. Above all, it is a positive force, not a negative one."[10] Instead of repressing our sexuality, true morality seeks creative and practical ways of helping us live a full sexual life. Ultimately, such morality is rooted in a very pragmatic, practical understanding of what works and what doesn't, what brings peace and what causes suffering.

The old redwood trees that grow in northern California are a powerful symbol of such morality. Sometimes they stand far apart, yet their roots travel long distances underground, reaching out toward the roots of fellow redwoods. When they meet, they entwine their root systems and form communities that support each other. Morality, at its best, functions in the same way. We begin to grow moral roots when we become aware of our far-reaching interconnection with many other beings who share our desire for happiness. As a healing force dedicated to sustaining peace, true morality considers the whole interconnected web of life and honors the role and purpose of each part within the whole.

Years passed, and Hannah stayed with her husband, even though the marriage had become like a dead tree that will burst into flame when lightning strikes. And finally, in the fifteenth year of her marriage, lightning *did* strike. At a conference, Hannah met a man who evoked such powerful feelings in her that she fled in confusion. "The rest of the summer," she told me, shaking her head at the memory, "I felt totally out of control. I started having sex with some other guy I met who was married, in my house, in my marriage bed, which I thought was terrible, but I couldn't help it. All the old restraints were cracked open."

Six months later, Raymond visited Hannah's hometown on a business trip and asked her out to dinner. Listen to the story of this encounter, and you will see Eros at work—not the innocent, baby-faced cherub of our Valentine's Day cards, but the formidable, ruthless god whose arrow strikes deep into the human heart.

I told my husband I was going to meet someone for dinner, and would be back at nine-thirty. Instantly, Raymond and I fell madly in love. We couldn't eat a bite. We were just hopelessly, passionately in love. Raymond said he knew I was the woman he was meant to be with, and my feelings were similar. Raymond was married, and he told me he was going to leave his wife. I was supposed to go to Europe with my husband next week. "Well, you can't go, can you?" Raymond asked, and I agreed, "No, I can't." We found a churchyard and sat there together. Raymond would say something, and then we would just sit in this very deep, quiet space. Then I would say something, and we would wait. And what we were doing was making vows. "I vow to be your partner and to love you all my life. I vow to support you on your spiritual path." We were making marriage vows. Sitting in that churchyard, he and I were marrying one another.

At nine o'clock I told Raymond I had to go home. When I got home, I said nothing to my husband; I just didn't know what to say. The next morning around seven the phone rang. It was Raymond. "Did you tell him yet?" Raymond asked. "No," I said. "You better tell him," Raymond insisted. I just said, "Good-bye," and hung up.

"Who the hell is that, calling you at seven in the morning?" my husband demanded. So I told him. I said, "Something happened last night with this guy. I don't know how to tell you what's going on, but the way I feel about him, I just don't feel married to you anymore." He told me I was crazy, out of my mind. "Maybe," I said, "but that's how I feel, and I'm going to move out." So I did, and that was the end of our fifteen-year marriage.

"Without warning," wrote the Greek poet Sappho two and a half millennia ago, "as a whirlwind swoops on an oak, love shakes my heart."[11] Exhilarating, terrifying, and unpredictable, passion descends out of the clear blue sky and sweeps us up and away like autumn leaves. The ego may tremble as love spins us around, turns us upside down and inside out, but the soul rejoices as it tumbles into the arms of the golden goddess. And so, when Eros called, Hannah offered no resistance, but descended willingly into Aphrodite's deep ocean waters.

For the next six months Raymond commuted five hundred miles every weekend to be with me. We made love maybe four times a day for a year and a half or so. In those days, my breasts grew, and I had orgasms just from being so utterly surrendered. I could not believe that at the age of forty, having made love with maybe fifty men in my life, the sexuality and love I experienced with Raymond could come as a total revelation. When we made love, I would experience my body dissolving, and there would just be flowers, thousands of flowers. Sometimes we seemed to be under the ocean, swimming like fishes. Everything would drop away except this consciousness of unfolding and melting and dissolving and flowing.

In opening her heart to love, Hannah had entered the refiner's fire, a fire that would expose her humanity, her vulnerability, and her limitations in ways her spiritual practice never had. Where religion had given her an illusion of control, love immediately started to blast apart all the mechanisms she had used to protect herself

MERMAID MEDITATION

You are a mermaid, one of Aphrodite's gentle daughters. Diving deep into the ocean, you breathe easily, and a flick of your shimmering tail sends you gliding on a long, arched curve through the warm, blue-green waters. You close your eyes and drift, letting the currents rock you gently back and forth. Resting in the embrace of the ocean, you feel peaceful and safe, and your heart begins to glow with deep happiness. Your body is completely at ease, relaxed, and as the waters playfully nudge you, you surrender to their gentle pressure. As you drift weightlessly, an arm floats out. Gently, the waters turn you over and over, playing with you as with a piece of driftwood. Your old shape, your old boundaries are melting away. You have become a golden body of light, a luminous orb drifting gently across the ocean floor, a galaxy floating in the Milky Way. As you let go into the delicious, velvet-soft sensations, the light within you intensifies and brightens. You are filled with a spreading joy you could never contain, were you still trapped in your old body. You are a sparkling field of blissful, ecstatic pleasure, a joyful, pulsing dance of light. You know, as a baby in the mother's womb, that you are held in love. Your heart is content, and the arms of your soul are opened wide to the embrace of life. All the old wounds, the bruises, the hurts, and the pains are soothed by the sweet balm of deep, healing pleasure. You have come home to yourself, and all is well.

and keep life at arm's length. Step by step, Hannah began to descend from her spiritual ivory tower into the messy, ever shifting morass of worldly life. The first step was leaving the Buddhist center.

Raymond thought his path to the sacred was with me and through me. This was a whole new idea to me. He felt that personal love was a way to divine love. I had always thought of personal love as a hindrance on the path. Through my meditations, I would close down and drop into what I called the ground of being, a very deep, austere, silent reality. One day, Raymond and I went for a walk, and he said to me, "You're open to the sky and the birds but you're closing down to me." I realized this was true, and I thought, "No, no, no. I will not do this." I saw that I had been using my spiritual practice as a way to wall off true intimacy. That was the end of my life at the Buddhist center.

It is a strange irony that after having struggled to humble our egos through years of spiritual austerities, we often discover that our very discipline has fostered a false sense of pride in us. Now, Hannah began to develop true humility, a word that derives from the Latin *humus,* meaning "earth" or "soil." Humility teaches us to stand in right relationship to the earth and to the earthy parts of our own being, so that we can be comfortable with the ways our body eats and shits, with its imperfections and its decay. Only when we lack such humility do we perceive our body as a source of humiliation.

Raymond and I had just gotten together when I had to have surgery for the cancer. Here I was, newly in love, with this huge bandage on my forehead. I went to stay with him, and I was really scared about how he would greet me when I got off the bus. Every day, I would go into the bathroom and lock the door to change the dressings; the wound looked really gross. Around the third or fourth day, Raymond asked me whether he could see it. I let him, and there was something about him being with me and looking at it that just melted my heart. He was able to be with me in these intimate, vulnerable places where I had never let anybody in before.

Hannah laughed as she remembered the first months of her new marriage. "With Raymond," she told me, "every way in which I wanted to be really perfect for him didn't work. One thing that happened is that the toilet would always overflow. I would shit, and the toilet would flood, and he would have to help me with a plunger.

Here was this exquisitely wonderful love, yet it seemed really important that we were being forced to look at all these basic physical realities, the blood and the shit and the wounds."

However, these initial challenges were minor compared to the far greater and more painful ordeal that was to follow. Hannah and Raymond got married, but the first four years of their marriage were extremely difficult for many reasons, including financial strain. As can happen when people long to escape a heavy burden of insecurity, self-doubt, and worry, Raymond entered into a brief but passionate affair with a much younger woman. "I was really, really devastated," Hannah told me. "The sense of betrayal was overwhelming." She sighed and fell silent for a minute, her face darkened with sadness. Feeling deeply betrayed, Hannah separated from Raymond, and for two long years, she lived in the midst of the refiner's fire, undergoing what she now views as a profound inner cleansing. During this period, her humility and compassion would deepen immeasurably. All this Hannah sees, in hindsight. But when one is sitting in the midst of a fire, all one feels is intolerable heat.

I clearly recognized the karmic nature of what was happening. I remembered saying, when I left my first husband, "I never, ever want to cause this kind of pain again. Next time, let it be me who feels the pain." Well, now I was. The suffering I had caused was returning to me. I had never really experienced jealousy before.

I went down to the ocean every evening and chanted. As I kept chanting, the pain would eventually turn to ecstasy. By the next morning, I would wake up with this shattering pain again. I would go out and run and sing and yell. Then I began to feel my anger. I felt such rage at Raymond and his lover, Angi. I would sing and yell my anger to the ocean, and I would kick and punch. This went on for about two years.

Like a rock tossed into an corrosive acid bath, Hannah found herself immersed in that slimy, vomit-green, bitter-tasting brew that only jealousy can concoct. Jealousy makes us feel small, ugly, and vengeful. A swarm of angry bees is let loose in our belly; snails crawl over our heart and coat it with noxious slime; and a dull green cloud descends over our mind. Like it or not, jealousy often comes with the territory of sacred marriage. All the years of Hannah's first marriage, her husband's infidelities had barely ruffled her feathers: "All I thought was, 'Great, less strain on me,'" she remembers. Freedom from jealousy comes easily to those who are not deeply in love. Now, any illusions Hannah might have harbored about her own capacity for resentment, anger, and hatred vanished overnight.

If you were part of the sexual revolution, you, too, probably learned to think of jealousy as a no-no, a troublesome expression of personal insecurity. Some couples are, in fact, able to overcome jealousy entirely. But in our culture, such relationships are rare indeed. Most of us are as likely to overcome jealousy as we are to climb Mount Everest. Moreover, like all the dark emotions, jealousy does have its purpose. Why else would it be attributed to Hera, one of the most powerful goddesses among the Olympians? Hera, the goddess of marriage, treasures monogamy as a sacred container within which intimacy can deepen endlessly. She represents the part of our own psyche that senses the promise of monogamy and cries out in pain and protest when the container is shattered by infidelity or betrayal. Jealousy, then, is Hera's guardian angel, who stands, sword in hand, at the door of the marriage chamber.

Sexual betrayal can initiate a dark night of the soul, a bleak and lonely time in which we feel our life is bereft of meaning and joy. We, who once felt beautiful and cherished like Aphrodite herself, now feel old, ugly, and gray, useless like a rag that has been tossed onto the garbage heap. All our physical insecurities rise to the surface. "Angi was much younger than I, and I felt very old and fat next to her," Hannah recalls. Knowing that betrayal happens to the best of us, to the most lovable and the most beautiful, does not help. We still feel broken and shattered.

Nonetheless, these can be spiritually rich times. They are times of descent, of returning to the rock-bottom foundation of our lives, and of rediscovering ourselves as independent individuals. Often, they are times of healing very old wounds, for wounds are like strings on a harp: when one is plucked, others resonate and hum in response. So the wound of one loss may evoke memories of earlier losses, earlier betrayals. This is a time to hold ourselves with all the gentleness, compassion, and kindness we can muster. It is a time to nurture ourselves, to rock and cradle ourselves, and to give ourselves deep, undivided attention. Looking back, Hannah says, "Those two years that I spent by myself were a dark and difficult period. I took a lot of comfort from the land and the trees and the ocean. It was also a really deep time, and I miss it, in an odd way."

In the process of stumbling through the fires of her personal purgatory, Hannah developed deep compassion for the pain of the sexually betrayed, and equally deep respect for the sanctity of marriage. Her innate honesty forced her to admit that she herself had in the past often violated the sanctity of other people's marriages. "An Aphrodite woman may be mistrusted by other women, especially by Hera women," says Jean Bolen in her book *Goddesses in Every Woman*.[12] Aphrodite is not a vulnerable goddess, nor does she have much compassion for the vulnerability of others. But since all deities live within us, the Aphrodite woman may find, at some point in her life, that she has herself become a jealous Hera. As Hannah opened to her own vulnerability, she began feeling compassion for others. Courageously, she now faced the dark shadow of her sexual passion—lust and ignorance.

Raymond's lover Angi was a Zen priest. When her teacher heard of her affair, he told her she was screwing up and causing suffering. So she wrote me a letter and asked whether I was ready to forgive her yet. It was a very snippy letter. The tone was: "Are you evolved enough to let go of your anger?" I realized that quite honestly, not only was I *not* ready to forgive her, but I hated her. So my answer was clearly no. It was embarrassing but true. I wrote her that I was not ready to forgive her, that I felt extremely hurt, and that she had no idea how deeply she had hurt me. After sending this letter, I kept writing her letters that I didn't send, in which I told her how much I hated her, how she didn't understand what love was, what was possible between a husband and a wife, and how sacred marriage was.

But as I worked on this letter I started to remember all the married men with whom I had had love affairs. One by one, I actually saw them coming into my living room. The first one entered; I didn't know his wife. Then I remembered the next one, and I thought, "Oh yes, him . . . I forgot about him. He was married too, wasn't he?" And then there was another one, and another one. . . . I think there were thirteen in all. In some cases, I had known their wives, and in others not. I had most of these affairs in my twenties, when I was Angi's age. I remembered how I had felt that this was between me and the man, and that it had nothing to do with the wife. After all these men had come into the room with their ghostly wives, I understood where Angi was coming from, and I didn't feel angry at her anymore. Instead, I felt a sense of compassion. It was nothing elevated, but an extremely practical realization. "Oh, yes," I thought, "I know just what that was like; I did it again and again and again. I had no idea what was possible in marriage, and I didn't care."

So a month or two after the first letter, I wrote Angi a second letter. I told her how devastated I had been by what had happened, and I also told her what I had seen and felt about these married men in my own life. I told her that I did forgive her, although I had no desire to see her again. However, several years later, she asked if she could come and see me. I said yes, and we had a very good talk.

For more than two years, Hannah struggled through the billowing waves of rage, grief, and jealousy. As the contractions of birth soften a woman's cervix, these years softened her ego, leaving her deeply humbled and aware of her vulnerability. Then, after she had completely lost hope of salvaging her marriage, she and Raymond began to reconnect. Crushed and brokenhearted though she was, something within her demanded that she once again open her heart to him. "Slowly, slowly we started seeing each other," Hannah told me, and then added with her characteristically blunt honesty,

I don't really know why I chose to return to him. For a long time, my body was like rock; it had no trust in him at all. But a number of things had shown me that in my deeper consciousness, I still loved him despite my anger and my pain. Our time together began to become quite enjoyable. But I still felt that I wasn't attractive enough, that I just wasn't *enough*. It was painful to feel so vulnerable and to care so much. I had done so much in my life to avoid caring and getting hurt, and the very thing I had feared most had happened. At one point, we went for a walk and saw these two old redwood trees that had been burned out. I said to Raymond, "I feel like that." He said, "So do I." We both felt burned out and empty.

Now, we have been living together for three years. I was fearful, but things have been very good with us. When we make love, I feel a deep generosity and appreciation for the journey we have traveled together. We are amazed at the love we feel for each other. I am experiencing a depth I never felt before in a relationship, and I am seeing how over time, with commitment and caring, love can deepen and deepen.

I feel really, really ordinary these days. I don't feel special at all. But I finally feel that who I am is enough. Many things I'm not good at and don't know, but I know enough, and I can tell women the truth about my life. My love and caring for people is all that matters. My capacity to see and value them. That's all I need, and that's all I have anyway.

By now, Hannah and I had emptied many cups of tea and still, the rain was dancing on the roof. Quietly, we sat together, grateful to have shared this time in sacred space. Her journey, I thought to myself, has been the journey of a modern alchemist. As C. G. Jung recognized, the medieval alchemists were not just eccentrics obsessed with transmuting lead into gold, but mystics who couched their quest for the enduring gold of enlightened consciousness in alchemical terminology. According to alchemical lore, a marriage of opposites had to occur before lead would turn to gold. Water had to be wedded to fire, the sun to the moon, and the masculine to the feminine. Similarly, Hannah has struggled to reconcile the inner polarities of passion and discipline, control and abandon. As the alchemists labored over their great cauldrons, so she has labored over the sacred vessel of her psyche.

The alchemists also believed that before the opposites could unite, they had to be reduced to their purest essences by a lengthy process of distillation, purification, and refinement. In Hannah's story, we see the truth of this claim. Again and again, her journey has led her into the white-hot blaze of the great Refiner's fire, where the elements of her psyche have been melted down and purified. The Controller's harshness has softened, and he has learned to place his powers in service of the heart. Her Passion-seeker, too, has been broken open in the fires of suffering, and ignorance has given way to a deep, tender awareness of human vulnerability. Hannah has indeed achieved the inner marriage so many of us are seeking; ecstasy has joined hands with morality, passion with compassion.

Compassion, I realize as my eyes meet her peaceful gaze, is the gold Hannah has sought and found—deep, loving compassion for herself and others. We do not usually think of sexual love as a means of developing compassion, humility, and kindness, the ultimate and most precious fruits of spiritual evolution. And yet, as Hannah has found, love can melt down the impurities of our ego in ways that meditation and prayer cannot. In a sense, Hannah's years of spiritual discipline were only preliminary steps that prepared her to follow Aphrodite's call into the white-hot blaze of passionate love.

5

APHRODITE'S REBELLION

Even though she was awake
even though the sky jewel was up
even though her friends were at the door
even though her unlawful lover serpent
had loosened his embrace she
did not move

East Indian, undated

Tall, fair-skinned, in her early forties, Irene radiates the vibrancy and self-confidence of a woman well loved by family, friends, and lovers. The graceful strength and ease of her movements, her sensuality, and her lighthearted laughter all evoke the image of Aphrodite, whom the Greeks called the laughter-loving goddess. In this chapter, we will hear the story of her marriage.

Marriage need not and should not exclude sexual fulfillment, but for many women of previous generations, including Irene's mother, it did. Unconsciously, Irene absorbed her mother's unspoken belief that a good wife should be willing to sacrifice her own sexual and creative needs for her family's sake. Before marriage, Irene was a joyously sensual, sexual, pleasure-loving woman. But once she married, something shifted. Unwittingly, she began to follow in her mother's footsteps. Irene frowned as she remembered the insidious patterns of denial and avoidance that were present from the very onset of her marriage:

Aside from sex, everything was going great. I never said no to sex overtly, but I made it clear I wasn't interested. We got along well, and we felt committed to each other. We were both incredibly busy and had little energy left, which certainly contributed to our lackluster sex life. We had a strong bond in terms of running a home and operating in partnership, and somehow that didn't include being sexual. I was acutely aware that on the night we got married we didn't make love. We were tired, and we just didn't.

Of all the men I have made love with, my husband was one of the few who physically fit me so well that I had orgasms while he was inside me very easily. That was rare. So we could make love with very little foreplay and I would find it quite satisfying, and so would he. But we didn't like to kiss the same way. I kept telling myself, "This doesn't really matter." Now I think it *does* matter. I say to my friends, "Kiss the man and think about it." At least for me, it was very important. At first, I asked him to kiss me the way I liked, but he didn't like doing it.

Also, he never did oral sex on me; I only did it for him. We had had oral sex at first, but it slowly stopped. I started feeling shame, like there was something wrong with me or I was dirty. A few times I asked for it, and he said, "I just don't feel like doing it." That was his right, but it was so hard for me to ask for it that it felt like a crushing blow. It seemed to prove all my fears were true. I think a woman's vulva can be scary to men. A woman's vulva is really amazing. It gives birth and it totally transforms.

Gradually, we stopped talking about sex; it became one of those things that felt too difficult to dredge up again. We had our routines, and we didn't want to mess them up. So why bring up one more time that I didn't like the way he kissed, or that I wanted something else too? We did this dance around the hot spots. And the very things that became too hard to talk about, that didn't seem worth the trouble, were the ones that blew us apart in the end.

At some point in these years, something indefinable happened to me. I tuned out my sexuality, shut it off. I couldn't talk about it, I couldn't articulate it, because I didn't even identify it in my mind as something I had better talk to someone about or seek help for. It was too far down in my consciousness. The truth was that I had dropped into my mother's patterns, and they seemed so normal and familiar that I didn't even recognize them as a problem. I saw marriage as a partnership agreement. Not quite a business agreement, but a partnership, just like Mom and Dad had had. It felt so normal. But every once in a while I would wonder. I still believed that I was this wild, sexual woman. "Now if that's who I am, why don't I ever make love?" I would wonder. Then I would shrug it off. "I don't know. Oh, well . . ." This continued for the next ten years.

Over these years, Irene's husband had several affairs, both short and long. What little Irene discovered about them shocked and hurt her, deepening the emotional rift between the couple. The birth of their son complicated the situation and intensified their growing alienation. Eventually both Irene and her husband acknowledged that their marriage was in trouble, and they decided to go to couples counseling. "We worked with our therapist for about half a year," Irene recalled, "and in that time she never brought up the topic of sex, and neither did we. It was just not mentioned. Isn't that something?" It is indeed, especially given the importance the founding fathers of Western psychotherapy placed on sexuality, and given the fact that Irene's marital problems were rooted in sexual problems. Unfortunately, it is not uncommon for people to undergo years of psychotherapy without ever touching on sexual matters. Alexandra recounted a similar experience:

Even in therapy, where you are supposed to be able to talk about everything, I never, ever, talked about sexuality. Never. I was in therapy for years and years. I had fantasies about my therapist, but I would have been scared to death to express them. I was well trained to keep quiet, so that was easy enough. My therapist never brought it up, and neither has my gynecologist. I realize I have responsibility for that too, but there is a collusion of silence.

Finding no way to communicate or relieve her sexual frustration, Irene did her best to ignore it. But a woman as passionate and sensual as Irene could hardly suppress her erotic life indefinitely. As a tiny spark in the summer forest suddenly explodes into a huge wildfire, so Irene's desire finally burst forth in a wild blaze:

> I wanted to go to a dance class to learn this very sexy couples dance, and I needed a partner. My husband said he had to work, but that it was fine if I went with someone else. So I called some male friends, and lo and behold, one of them called back and wanted to go with me. His name was Brian, and he was a good friend of my husband's. He had a girlfriend called Sonya, and Sonya didn't mind either.
>
> Well, as soon as Brian and I started dancing together, we were lost. You could have knocked me over with a feather. I just couldn't believe what I was feeling in my body. All my sexuality came flooding back at once, for the first time in over ten years. I felt so attracted to Brian. It was like an irresistible magnetic pull. I just wanted to smell him and be close to him. It was like being a parched person in the desert, who crawls along and then finds a lake. Except that until that moment, I had had no concept of what I had been missing. I had forgotten. I had written it off.
>
> That very first night, I kissed Brian. I sat in his lap and he touched my breast, and I hadn't felt anyone touch my breast like that as long as I could remember. I had thought no one would ever touch me that way again, and I had accepted it. It had seemed okay. But suddenly, it was not okay anymore. I felt so desperately that this might never happen again. I remember thinking, "I may never feel this again. I am *not* willing to repress this." After Brian left, I just stood looking out over the rooftops. I had been given this amazing gift, and I felt an overwhelming sense of joy. Nothing was a problem. I had my femaleness back.

Irene looked at me and sighed with a look of puzzlement. "I had no sense of my marriage being in trouble," she said as she remembered tumbling headlong into what was to become an all-consuming passion. Such blindness to the fragility of marriage is typical of Aphrodite, the best-known adulteress in Western mythology. Aphrodite does not intentionally set out to break marriages, any more than a hurricane intends to wreck havoc. Her paradoxical nature is such that though she brings beauty, harmony, proportion, and many other gifts of civilization, she also crashes through the established order, leaving chaos and confusion in her wake. Like all deities in a polytheistic mythology, Aphrodite represents what *is*, not what we think *should* be. When Aphrodite's husband catches her in bed with her lover Ares, the myth neither applauds adultery nor condemns Aphrodite. It simply points out that those who think they can totally control a woman's sexuality are fools. Aphrodite is an aspect of every woman, and as a goddess, she will find ways of slipping free of all social restrictions. We may not approve of her faithless ways, yet our disapproval will not change them. "Like it or not," she tells us, "I am part of you. If you would create strong, resilient marriages, you had better include my worship."

Aphrodite's myths describe her as a jealous goddess who does not take neglect lightly. Those who deny her power had better watch out for her revenge. When she means business, she usually proves herself stronger than all our moral principles. And here is Aphrodite, reclaiming her errant priestess with a vengeance:

The dance class went on, and we were really shy with each other. We kissed again, and both of us were just floating away on romance and ecstasy and passion. It was such an awakening. For the next months, we would go dancing together, and it was obvious that we were in love. We made no attempt to hide it, either. I started hanging out with Brian and Sonya. I was in love with him, and I loved her too. I was so happy; life just seemed terrific.

At first, we weren't making love. Then we made love once, and then avoided each other for a couple of weeks. I thought we wouldn't go any further because it was too dangerous. What mattered to me was the rebirth of my passion. But soon, we started sleeping together regularly. We had wild sex, anal and oral and every which way. I was never into bondage, but anything that was safe and worshipful of the body I would do. Brian was a great lover, much better than any other lover I had had. I had been so hurt by my husband's dislike of oral

NEGOTIATIONS WITH
THE GODDESS

Aphrodite is very strong in me. I have had to say to her, "We have to negotiate, because you are trouble." When I was eighteen, I had a baby and gave her up for adoption. I felt so much shame about that. For years, I felt that I walked around with a scarlet letter on my forehead. And it was Aphrodite who got me in trouble. She has gotten me in trouble a lot. Still, I don't want to shove her away. So I said to her, "I don't want to banish you, but we need to negotiate."   NINA

sex. But Brian loved it, and it was such a healing. I started feeling, "Oh, my genitals are beautiful things. They are wonderful, and I love them." I realized how much shame I had been holding there. That whole part of me had not felt okay.

Brian and I had many mystical sexual experiences. We would breathe together, and this hypnotic feeling of expansion would happen. It felt like pure life-force, very powerful. We weren't trying to make it happen, it just did.

As a child, I had believed deeply in the magical quality of life. I would go out and sing to the fairies. I knew there were beings and spirits in the world. I would go for midnight walks down the street in the moonlight and feel them all around me. I wasn't afraid of them. I would talk to them and befriend them. But for so many years, I had put all that away. I had lost my belief in the magical side of life, and I had become cynical and pragmatic. Now, I came full circle. I remembered that miracles were possible and that life could be easy and pleasurable and fun.

Like Irene, many women remember having been natural priestesses as children. Their senses were alert, their small bodies bursting with vitality and joy and wordless knowing. They describe spontaneous acts of worship and celebration—moments of pas-

THE SEX MASS

There was this girl called Tanya who lived on our block. Her family was Catholic—very Catholic. Tanya was about fourteen, and I was five or so. Tanya would arrange these rituals in her backyard, where there was an old chicken yard and a chicken house that had been cleaned out to function as a playhouse. She would have all the little boys and girls over, and then she would stage something like a Catholic mass. I remember it very clearly because it happened not just once but quite a few times. The girls would wear old curtains and get all dressed up. Afterwards, they would have sex, really and truly, almost like an orgy. The little kids weren't supposed to get into it, but we were definitely there and watched. The little ones were like the congregation. The joke is that Tanya became a nun in later life.

Well, this little boy and I got the idea that we were going to do it, too, but we didn't exactly know what to do. We went into the basement and crawled way into the back where it got really narrow. We took off our clothes but when we got that far, we didn't have the least idea what to do. So we just sat there looking at one another, and then we just crawled back out, and that was it. But the fact that I had that impulse and that I was the one who initiated it has always struck me as a redeeming factor. I remember it as a point in my life when I wasn't repressed yet; I was still very healthy and normal and open.   EVA

sionate communion with a tree, naked dances in the rain, whispered conversations with angels, secret acts of magic, innocent songs of praise, and heartfelt prayers.

But eventually, we closed down. Seeing the dangers of disapproval and judgment, we slowly but surely dampened our exuberant aliveness and went numb. There is not one among us who was not forced to sacrifice her essence at the altar of survival and to submit to values that were not her own. Later, we may realize that what we left behind were not merely "childish" ways, but natural forms of spiritual communion. Falling in love can be such a remarkable experience because it dissolves the rigid, hardened crusts of age and restores to us the innocent openness we once had. "It was not just sex," Irene said of her love for Brian.

It was a complete spiritual, sexual experience. I suddenly realized that in denying my sexuality, I had also denied my spirituality, and I began having a total spiritual rebirth. Suddenly, my sexuality and my spirituality began moving as one. Brian was embracing the woman that I was and the spirit that I was.

He was never a man I would have wanted to marry. He was a fluffhead in many ways, weak and indecisive. But as a lover, he was none of those things. He was totally in his element, attentive and loving, sweet, thoughtful. Physically, he worshipped me. It was a complete healing for my body, for having a female form. I lost weight and felt beautiful. We shared this worship of bodies. We loved each other from head to toe, touching and kissing and holding and massaging. Everything was erotic, and everything was worship.

Those possessed by Aphrodite are notoriously self-absorbed, prone to transgressing against rules, sanctions, and prohibitions, and to offending social propriety. Given that Irene and Brian were hardly attempting to hide their passion, I asked Irene how her husband reacted. She sighed and seemed to wilt before my eyes like an unwatered plant. "At one point," she said, "my husband asked me about Brian. But I denied we were in love."

Irene's dishonesty colluded with a lack of maturity in Sonya, Brian's girlfriend, to create one of those complex tangles for which Aphrodite is well known. Lost in a fatal idealism, Sonya professed to have transcended jealousy and possessiveness and indicated to Irene that she was quite willing to share her lover. "She sent me mixed messages," Irene recalled. But when the truth struck home, Sonya felt utterly devastated.

Sonya and I spent a lot of time together, and I admired her tremendously. I was convinced that Brian would never leave her, and I was repressing the awareness of hurting her. Sonya kept talking about how she believed people could have multiple lovers. So in my mind, I took that to mean I had her permission. "I don't care what you all do," she said to me once. "Just don't tell me about it." She said that, but she didn't really mean it. But I just didn't get it. The ante was up: I wanted to keep my lover, and I didn't want my marriage to be wrecked. I believed that what I was learning from my lover I could take to my husband. I thought maybe my husband and I could heal our sexuality. But in the end, that wasn't possible. We had done so much to close the doors between us. Now, I believe in monogamy. I believe you must bring all of yourself into the relationship. You need to give it all you have. But I didn't believe that at the time.

Sonya was interested in paganism, and she started teaching me about it. She introduced me to a class on feminist spirituality, and we took it together. In this class, we talked a lot about the sacredness of sex and the body. It was really more of a women's circle than a class. And with a kind of hopeless naive idealism, I believed it was okay for me to be in this group with Sonya while having an affair with her boyfriend.

Of course, it wasn't at all okay. When Sonya found out, she was absolutely devastated. She hates me to this day and has never talked to me since. She refuses to admit I even exist. That is one of the most painful experiences I have ever had. I can't blame her. That's just how she had to do it. But it was horrible. I had to face that I had really hurt this woman. My affair broke up the class. When the truth came out, Sonya left the group. Another woman was so uncomfortable that she left, too. A third woman totally freaked out because it turned out her marriage was on the rocks for the same reason.

Irene could no more deny her passion than an erupting volcano can choose to press the red glowing torrent back into its depths. Nonetheless, some readers are likely to react to Irene's story with anger and judgment. The subject of sexual betrayal raises strong, volatile feelings, and how could it not? In marriage, we hope to find the stability and security we once sought from our parents. Any threat to that security is bound to evoke primal fears of rejection and abandonment. Unable to control those we love, helpless in the face of betrayal and loss, we use our judgments as barricades against pain. It is, after all, easier to feel righteous anger than to feel helpless vulnerability. Still, the most valuable gift we can give each other is to honestly share our confusions, our rough edges, and our failures.

Irene agreed. "I am trying not to be judgmental of myself," she said, acknowledging that her actions did hurt several people she cared deeply for. Compassion and the intention to avoid harming others are basic tenets of any spiritual path, yet human nature is such that we often do hurt others. "I have told my story," Irene emphasized, "because I believe that the more we break the codes of silence that surround our sexuality, the more we as women will benefit. It's so important to tell our stories. It's not about smut. It's about ordinary lives, the lives of women."

A few minutes later, Irene mentioned that her belly was hurting. Suspecting a connection between her pain and the process of telling her story, I suggested that she might take a moment to close her eyes and listen into her body. She did so, and then said:

> This tension and holding in my belly, this pain in my second chakra—it seems to relate to agreements I have entered into with men, nonverbal agreements that sex was not to be spoken of. To tell my story, I have had to break these agreements. It comes up not as a thought, but as a fear in my heart and a confused vibration in my body, a trembling. The pain in my belly is resistance, a holding in, a sense of tightening and compression. I feel a striving, a desire to be good enough and for my story to be good enough. I want it to be the story of a woman who is good enough. When I feel whole, my story is just my story, and it's fine. But at other times, I judge myself. I see that the judge is internal, though I might project it on others.

Morality, with its clear-cut answers, tells us that adultery is wrong. But no matter how much we try, the mysterious ways of the soul will not always conform to the narrow confines of moral judgments. Spiritual awakenings can occur under any circumstances. Though it may seem strange to look at an act of adultery as a moment of spiritual breakthrough, in Irene's case it undoubtedly was.

Responsibility is the ability to respond, with whatever wisdom and compassion we can muster, to the challenges life places in our path. Whenever we face a true moral dilemma, there are no prefabricated solutions. There is only the process of carefully listening inward for guidance and groping forward in the dark, step by step. And later, there comes the bittersweet moment of looking back upon our own struggles, our victories, and our failures with greater wisdom. Musing on Irene's story, I ask her how she would have responded to temptation, had she been a Buddha or an enlightened being. Irene hesitated. Then she said,

> I doubt whether I could have reclaimed my life-force without getting involved with Brian. I believe that was necessary. The pull was so insistent. But the most enlightened way would have been a lot more honest. It was the dishonesty that betrayed the trust in my marriage. I lied to my husband, instead of telling him the truth. The dishonesty supported a fragmentation where each one of us would take parts of ourselves out of the marriage.

Dishonesty rarely works—not, at least, if our goal is a deeply intimate and passionate sexual partnership. Psychically, it drives a wedge between the partners and stunts their intimacy. And when the toxic truth eventually leaks out, as it tends to do, the mess is much greater than it would have been had we had the courage to be honest in the first place.

"Amazingly," Irene said, "my husband was willing to forgive me." The couple stayed together another six months.

> But finally, I realized I needed to leave. My husband was convinced I was leaving to be with Brian, but that was not true. I had lived with a man for fifteen years and I was dying to be by myself. Brian triggered it, but I was really leaving to claim myself as a whole person and a woman, and I felt I needed to do this alone.

And I have. I really own my femaleness now. I have set aside one night every month to celebrate my womanhood, and this is a real bond with myself. I also feel much more able to relate to other women, to let them have their beauty without feeling threatened or in competition.

Today, my ex-husband and I have a good relationship, and we are releasing the past. I see that I can let the past go and live life with a freshness, out of the moment. I can really let what I have done be done and move forward. I feel really simple right now, and clear. I feel like the sea, both full and in motion. I don't see everything as perfect, but I can let things be. I was a woman who hardly had sex for ten years and could hardly talk about it. Now my friends think of me as their sexual sage; they call me and ask me questions. They see me as open. I have always been open at some level, but for so long, my life did not reflect that. Now, it does.

6

THE DEMON LOVER

Shawn was the most incredible lover. I didn't have to teach him anything or say anything—he just took my breath away. He knew just where to touch me. He knew how to tease me just the right way, and then he'd back off. He knew how to make sex breathe. He would work me like a piece of clay, shaping me. He knew when to stop and when to start, when to change and when to move. That guy had me screaming like a wild animal. It didn't matter where we were, I just couldn't help it. I had no shame at all with him. We did it in every position and every way. Everything else seemed inferior to the sensations I had with him. It was ecstasy beyond description.

Shawn was also a dark, dark man, an alcoholic and a drug addict. As for me, I channeled every addiction I ever had into our sex. I didn't need anything else. I stopped smoking, just like that, and never touched a cigarette again, but I became a total sexaholic. I just could not get enough of this guy. At the same time, we really didn't have a relationship. We weren't friends. Our relationship was sex, and that's how we communed. Gradually, I started realizing that there was no closeness between us, and I started feeling ashamed. I would feel depressed after orgasms. After I left him, he started harassing me and giving me trouble. But I wanted no more to do with him.

Pamina

Remember the Controller? Now, meet his archenemy, his dark twin, his opposite—the Demon Lover, immortalized by Mozart in his opera *Don Giovanni*. Where the Controller fears sexual ecstasy, the Demon Lover is an all-out sex addict. Where the Controller worships discipline, the Demon Lover wants to blast free of all restrictions. Like a military dictator and a guerrilla rebel, like point and counterpoint, the Demon Lover and the Controller emerge together, both products of a wounded culture that teaches us to sever heart and genitals, love and pleasure, sex and spirit. Like the Controller, the Demon Lover can be either male or female. Traditionally, however, men have had more permission than women to explore the extremes of unbridled sexual license.

The Demon Lover initially looks like an erotic fantasy come true. But though he sweeps us away to a sweet erotic paradise, he ultimately leaves us drained, with empty hands and hearts. A sexual connoisseur, he is also a very disturbed human being. Old fairy tales claim that the Demon Lover has sold his soul to the devil. What this means is that, like Lucifer, he has chosen power over love. The pleasure he feels never reaches his heart, which remains numb, starved, and barren. When the heart goes hungry, the soul goes hungry too, and the Demon Lover's ravenous soul hunger manifests as an insatiable sexual appetite.

Like all addicts, the Demon Lover is an escapist who wants life to be an extended peak experience without any valleys or "down" times. Love is willing to share the suffering of the world as well as its pleasures. This the Demon Lover refuses to do. "No," he says defiantly, "I will not surrender to love." Thus, he blocks his access to sacred union and tosses away his key to the spirit worlds. And yet he is consumed by longing for spiritual communion and for contact with the source of life. Unable to open the heavenly gates himself, he seeks out men or women who will allow him, like a vampire, to devour the marrow of their soul in return for the sexual pleasure he gives them. He is a sex addict, then, not merely because he loves sex, but because sex is the only way he knows to feed his spiritual hunger. Often, the Demon Lover is addicted to alcohol or drugs, as well as sex, and often he expresses his frustrated rage at god by abusing his lovers. One woman described her Demon Lover as follows:

> The basic problem was his deep hatred of women, his desire to degrade the feminine. He had broken the trust of every woman he had ever been with, either by taking her money or by betraying her sexually—there was always something. His ex-wife hated him, his daughters hated him, his ex-lovers hated him. It was all about dominance, power struggle, struggle for energy. And he never faced his own shadow. During

our final breakup, I remember shouting at him, "Patrick, I was your last chance. I was your last true love. I was your last Shakti." I really knew this was so. It was his last chance to surrender to love. And in my mind, I heard him slam the door and say no. No to love, no to enlightenment, no to the feminine.

Ironically, this man, with his deep-seated hatred of the feminine, was a well-known "Tantric master" who supposedly transmitted the wisdom of a tradition that begins and ends with worship of the feminine. Several other women have also told me of so-called Tantric masters who turned out to be full-fledged Demon Lovers. Such men may be masters of the erotic arts who know how to lead their partners into highly ecstatic states, but they do not walk the path of love. They have acquired their erotic power only in order to manipulate others in self-serving ways. If we define a priest as a servant of the divine, then they certainly are not priests.

One of the misconceptions that plagues Western Tantra is the view of ecstasy as a the final goal of spiritual practice. Ecstasy is an extraordinarily healing state for body and mind, and a sign that we have entered into an expanded state of consciousness. But moments of ecstasy are merely a by-product of the spiritual journey, never the goal. Usually, they are followed by some degree of contraction, because our energy body is not yet prepared to maintain the expanded state for very long. When people make ecstasy their primary goal, they become addicted to whatever substances or activities they use to get high. To repeatedly force the body into states of ecstasy against its natural inclination is as harmful as natural ecstasy is beneficial. Those who abuse their chemistry in this way do so because they reject the sobriety of their "normal" state of being. But the body resents being forced and will eventually resist. Then the highs will no longer be quite as high, and the ecstasies will become more elusive.

Diane, now in her mid-forties, not only became involved with a Demon Lover but married him. She's slender, blond, and blue-eyed; her long-legged, full-breasted beauty can still catch a man's eye and turn his head. Reminiscing about her parents, Diane described the

typical patriarchal combination of a gentle, long-suffering, repressed mother and a Demon Lover father.

> My father never really gave me anything, but he was a very
> exciting man. He was not really nice and caring, but more
> shadowy and dark. He was a gambler and a big risk-taker. He
> was attractive to women, a Casanova type, arrogant. As much
> as I didn't like him, there was a part of me that felt that my
> mother was too accommodating, and if I had to pick someone
> to resemble, I would rather be like him than like her. She was
> not happy. All she had was us, while he had the world as well
> as her. He got a good deal.

Even as Diane judged her father, she also absorbed the belief that
exciting men are irresponsible and untrustworthy. As an adult, she
would turn to "good" men for security and love; her first husband
was one of them. Like her mother, he was gentle and kind, but not
exciting. "Sex between us was horrible," Diane groaned.

> I began to grieve at the thought of living my whole life with-
> out sexual passion. But I had been taught that if my marriage
> failed, this meant I was no good as a person. My mother
> stayed in her marriage, even though she wasn't happy. She
> sacrificed herself by having sex when she didn't want to, tol-
> erating affairs and abuse—all sorts of stuff. But her life didn't
> count as a failure because she stayed in the marriage. These
> were the values I inherited.
>
> At one point, I talked to my mom about my husband. "I'm
> really worried," I said. "I just don't feel anything for him."
> And she said, "It's your duty to give him sex. He provides for
> you and your children, he's a wonderful husband, and this is
> what you have to do." I was sickened by that, and I remem-
> ber thinking to myself, "Maybe it's what *you* had to do." And
> then I knew she did. She never owned her own sexual passion.

Like Irene (Chapter 5), Diane refused to follow in her mother's
footsteps and settle for a passionless life. But to her, a passionate re-

lationship meant a relationship with a man like her father. Diane laughed as she identified the pattern:

> The bad, the sweet, the bad, the sweet—now that I tell my story, I see the pattern so clearly. I have alternated between sexy but seedy guys and nice guys who took care of me but weren't so exciting. Unconsciously, I always believed I could either have a nice but dull guy who would be totally mine or a guy like my dad who would be exciting but not fully there for me.

Thus, Diane's Controller-dominated mother and her Demon Lover father took up residence within her being. Sexuality became the Demon Lover's domain; being sexual meant escaping the Controller's grasp. "My life was very boxed and confined," Diane reflected. "Sexuality was one of the few ways I knew to relinquish control. In sex, I could just blast out and let go. The edge was the out-of-control space." Making a motion of slicing herself in half at the waist, she continued, "The split was physical as well as psychological. For many years I was out of touch with the lower half of my body. I didn't know anything below my waist. Even though I was a very sexual woman, there was some way in which I would cut off my upper-body consciousness to go into my sexuality. I disconnected heart and sex." The "good girl" who lived in Diane's upper body and did as the Controller told her to do was at war with the rebellious "bad girl" who lived in her genitals and sided with the Demon Lover.

The most important thing to understand, when a Demon Lover shows up in our life, is that he or she is holding up a dark mirror to our own addictive tendencies and our self-hatred, for like the Controller, the Demon Lover is first and foremost an inner figure, and only secondarily an outer person. Eventually, Diane was bound to attract a man who would reflect her own ecstasy addict, the part of her that longed to shake off every shred of self-control and blast free of all restrictions. His name was Stanley, and Stanley was in every way a typical example of the Demon Lover species.

> Stanley was tall, dark, and handsome—dark in every sense, archetypally so. Everyone he met fell in love with him. He was

as smooth and manipulative and charismatic as anyone I've ever met. In my whole network of friends only two people saw through him, both men, and they were both scared for me. They told me straight out: "Don't do this, Diane. Please don't do it." Of course, I wouldn't listen to them. My parents were horrified, and my father used every possible force he had to get me to leave this relationship. And I know that my mother did not want me to tap into this kind of passion, which she herself had never had.

But the sex was just unbelievable. I had never had a lover like this. He had no constraints, no barriers. Nothing was bad or forbidden to him. So for the first time I could just blast free. It was wonderful, and it was what bonded me to him and kept me there when I should have let go. Every possible red flag went up, but I ignored them. He was a sociopath, but I didn't realize it at first.

This relationship was my true initiation into darkness. Stanley would take me to ratty bars where he played pool with his friends, all of them crooks. It was so exciting to me. I was like an angel to them. They saw the light in me, and I saw the dark in them. It was the princess and the hoodlum. His parents were a classic blue-collar working family, but also hard-drinking people. He was physically abused very horribly and made into a bad kid very young. He had been involved in all sorts of seedy activity, spent time in jail, and had supposedly come clean. He was extremely attracted to my money and my higher class and prestige, to my blond beauty, to all that was not part of his background.

Though Diane spoke about her shame at having succumbed to the seduction of a Demon Lover, she also admitted that the experience had all the impact of a spiritual initiation. As her former illusions of control cracked and crumbled, she was forced to acknowledge her immense hunger for sacred union, a hunger that continues to motivate her spiritual quest to this day.

Meeting Stanley was without question the beginning of my spiritual awakening. Why? Because when you awaken to that level of primal desire you touch the place where you are no longer in control. We all have that uncontrolled part in us, but we are so afraid of it. This guy's whole being and his life was totally out of control and had been from the time of his birth.

In our lovemaking, we entered a field of energy which was bigger than either of us. And it allowed for such passion to come forth, a burning, consuming, primal passion. There was as much animal in the room as human being. There was no sense of any part of us holding back or observing, nothing but the meeting of passion and the exploration of the limits of passion. Just how far can we go? It was physical and emotional and spiritual. It was like being taken out of this small self into something much brighter and bigger.

If I can separate the lovemaking from all the judgments I have about Stanley as a person, I see that it was an extremely spiritual experience. Both he and I felt totally loved in that realm, though we could never match it in our daily lives. There was no way to match that level of passion in normal life. It wasn't Diane and Stanley; we were mirroring something archetypal for each other, something much bigger and more ancient and powerful. It was a feeling of being goddess or Everywoman or just Woman. It wasn't anything I ever knew existed, certainly nothing I had ever seen in my mother. It was part of the feminine that was so real and powerful, and also devouring. And he was the devouring masculine—the two powerful archetypes matched.

The feeling reminded me of ancient statues of the goddess with full breasts and hips and a big belly. In the fullness of the experience, I felt like a goddess, brimming with feminine power. It was the first time I felt the power of the sacred feminine. Until then, I had known that being female could be powerful, but I had never experienced it in myself before. And I knew it was not about Stanley; I knew the power was within me, and I have never lost that knowledge since.

To this day, the most compelling aspect of making love is that somewhere in the process of arousal and connecting body to body, there is a total dissolution of any boundary. I'm no longer aware of who is doing what to whom. I'm hardly aware of the outer physical level at all but just of merging. It feels like the momentary fulfillment of the deepest longing of my soul to not be separate, but to merge with the Beloved. In that moment, the longing of my soul is satisfied. When a relationship is just perfect, the longing is temporarily abated, but the minute something is imperfect, it returns, as deep as ever.

Every priestess has felt this insatiable longing for a state of union that always eludes her grasp. "Who is it that we spend our entire life loving?" asks the Indian mystical poet Kabir. Often, we are pushed onto the spiritual path when we realize the immensity of our soul's longing and are forced to acknowledge our inability to satisfy that longing through our own efforts. Here, Diane contemplates the roots of her addictions which drove her to involvement with a Demon Lover:

At the deepest level, my need for sex is about filling a very deep hole. That's why being alone is so scary. Not being in a relationship means being with the hole that can't be filled. I can't cover it up anymore like I used to. Now I have no choice but to face it. The distractions don't work any more. There is emptiness and longing. It's a psychological hole from lack of good parenting, but at an even deeper level, it's a spiritual longing for god. The yearning really is spiritual, though it can be interpreted as sexual or emotional. This longing of mine has never been satisfied. In the last few years, I've finally accepted that nothing external will fill the hole, and that I have to turn inward to be with it and trust that in doing so, I will find a space beyond it. I'm still struggling to tolerate the longing without using addictions to avoid it. I have used so many addictions—running, marijuana, MDMA [Ecstasy], food, and sex.

Rumi, the thirteenth-century Sufi poet, called those who have embraced this insatiable longing within themselves "Lovers." We usually think of a lover as one who makes love, and in doing so satisfies his or her desire. But we do not begin to be Lovers, in Rumi's sense, until we learn to burn with love, knowing full well that nothing in the world will satisfy this longing. Listen to popular love songs, and you will see that what many of them are really about is people's deep yearning for an otherworldly joy that even the best love relationship can never fully satisfy. When we fall in love, we think we have found what we want. Then things change, as they will, and we are left with empty hands once again. Thus, the quest for love forces us to go further and further, riding that pure stream of yearning which has no worldly goal but shoots upward and heavenward.

To the ancient Greeks, Aphrodite embodied the ultimate, unobtainable object of desire. They had a special name for the insatiable love-longing Aphrodite inspired in them: *pothos*. Psychologist James Hillman defines *pothos* as a yearning for that which cannot be possessed. He explains:

> *Pothos* would refer to the spiritual component of love or the erotic component of spirit. When *pothos* is presented on a vase painting . . . as drawing Aphrodite's chariot, we see that *pothos* is the motive force that drives desire ever onward, as the portion of love that is never satisfied by actual loving and actual possession of the object.[13]

Pothos is that sacred love sickness that gnaws at our insides, bruises our hearts, and sticks like a thorn in the flesh of the soul. But when pothos is misunderstood, as it often is in our spiritually bereft society, we fall into addictions in our desperate attempts to fill a hole that cannot be filled except through the inflow of spiritual grace. When we lack the strength to feel our hunger for love all the way to its white-hot core, we grasp at quick, short-term fixes—fast food to fill the belly, soap operas and Hollywood movies to keep the mind entertained, casual sex for an illusion of love, alcohol to numb our despair, drugs for fake ecstasy.

The concept of a love-longing that is meant not to be satiated but to be *experienced* is difficult for our goal-oriented, control-loving Western minds to accept. In E. M. Forster's novel *A Passage to India,* an Indian man sings a love song in which his (feminine) soul expresses her longing for the divine lover, Krishna. But, as the singer explains to his English friend Mrs. Moore, Krishna does not come. Mrs. Moore is disturbed:

> "But he comes in some other song, I hope," said Mrs. Moore gently.
> "Oh, no, he refuses to come," repeated Godbole, perhaps not understanding her question. "I say to him, come, come, come, come, come, come. He neglects to come."[14]

In this passage, Forster brilliantly captures one of the core differences between the Indian and the modern Western mind. Mrs. Moore thinks of desire as a question which calls for an answer. Desire, she assumes, is meant to be satisfied. Unfulfilled desire strikes her as tragic, and the idea of valuing desire as something complete in itself is alien to her. Thus, she fails to understand that Godbole's song celebrates the intensity of longing itself. The singer becomes one with his longing, his entire being suffused with passionate desire for the Beloved. Krishna does not come, because it is the very intensity of the singer's yearning that is meaningful.

Sinister though he is, the Demon Lover still reflects something of Krishna's ecstatic sexuality and of a wildness that the Christian god lost when he became the god of virtue and celibacy.[15] Like the Demon Lover, Krishna is free, untrammelled by social rules, and non-monogamous. He is a thief, an adulterer, and an extraordinary lover who, in a feat of Tantric mastery, makes love endlessly without ever ejaculating. Tantalizing and paradoxical, he embodies the epitome of male sexual attractiveness. Just as Aphrodite eludes any man who tries to possess or control her, so Krishna reflects the free, wild, unsocialized quality of the god who inspires our deepest desire, and who grants true sexual fulfillment, yet cannot be pinned down or possessed. One glance at his face, the stories say, will make us his love slave in this and all future lives. The songs of the Indian saint Mirabai are, without exception, songs of love for Krishna, but they are also songs of deep suffering, because the god she loves loves a million others and torments her with his careless comings and goings:

O friends, I am mad
with love, and no one sees.

My mattress is a sword-point,
how can I sleep
when the bed of my Beloved
is spread open elsewhere?

Only those who have felt the knife
can understand the wound.[16]

Like other sexual gods, Krishna embodies god's irresistible allure, his power to inspire a love too vast, too wild, and too bound-
less to be contained. However, a god is not a man, and a man
should not mistake himself for the god. Any archetype becomes demonic when the ego tries to claim the powers of the deity for itself
and to possess what cannot be possessed. Sexual deities like
Aphrodite, Dionysus, and Krishna are well known for their capacity to drive insane those unfortunate men and women who relate to
them carelessly or arrogantly. The Demon Lover is possessed by the
god's erotic passion, yet lacks the humility and integrity with which
a god must be approached.

In the latter part of Diane's marriage, her husband's destructive
and self-destructive tendencies became more and more apparent.
When I asked her whether she was still in touch with Stanley, she
shook her head slowly and said, "I feel like he's dead. I have the
feeling that he wasn't long for this world, and that he was going to
meet his match pretty soon. He lived so on the edge."

What began to undo us was that although he told me he was
no longer dealing drugs, I could see that he was using them
heavily, and I believed he *was* dealing, and neither of these
two things was okay with me. I started to feel afraid of him,
because I could feel that on the other side of the passion was
rage, tremendous rage. He didn't show me any overt signs of
it, but I started feeling it when he was angry with me.

He quit his job for some stupid reason, so I quit, too. We
moved to Georgia, a stupid move. Almost immediately, I
thought, "What have I done? What am I doing here?" Any-

how, I got a job, and he started pressuring me to marry him. Finally I agreed. I think that on my part, it was the ultimate rebellion against my background. It was the ultimate way of saying to my family, "Fuck you." My father cut me out of his will. I said, "Fine, see if I care."

We got married, and within a year, it was clear that our marriage was not going to work. By then, I had met another man, a really sweet man, true to my pattern of alternating the sweet and the bad. He became a very important friend and ally. I thank god for him because he helped me find the courage to leave. Stanley was getting wackier and crazier and meaner, more violent in his rages. He didn't hit me, but he would hit the wall. I was scared of what would happen if I left. For the first time I was with someone really unpredictable. I knew anything was possible, and he had a gun. What first seemed attractive and exciting now looked seedy and unattractive. I used to worry that I might get AIDS from him. We were still having good sex to a certain extent. We would fight and then have passionate makeups. We could still tap into that wonderfully passionate place, but it came more from having fights than from our normal interactions.

Finally, I told Stanley I was leaving. He seemed pretty calm about it—too calm. But I felt too relieved to question it. He moved out. A few days later, I went out in the evening and, when I came back, he had destroyed my house. Of course, I had no proof it was him. He had done all the classic things people do when they really want to hurt you. He had stolen all the things that meant anything to me. He went into my underwear drawers and cut up all my underwear. The whole experience felt like a rape. My friend Wayne stayed with me that night; I was too scared to stay alone. Wayne put his arm around me and I just shook all night long. It was really a blast in the face for me and an awakening to what passion will do. I began to think, "Oh my god, I'm so fucked up. What is going on here? Why did I get into this?"

For the next ten years, I was always afraid Stanley would find me. I never told anyone about this marriage. I hated him more than anyone else, but I also felt more passion for him than anyone else. Both sides were there. Looking back, I see that this was all inevitable. I married the secure, acceptable guy and then I just had to go and marry the shadow figure. It's embarrassing, but true.

In my family, everybody pretends this never happened. All the years of not talking about it have just deepened the shame and the feeling of falsehood. I myself have made this marriage a secret. Even to this day, unless I force myself to be truthful, I don't tell people I was married three times. I just tell them I was married twice. I never wanted to own this part of me. I wonder whether I will ever not feel ashamed of this marriage. It's okay to be addicted to money and security, but it's not okay to fall into an addiction to passion, especially not for a woman. We are not supposed to lose control like that.

It is easy to feel ashamed when one has allowed oneself to be demeaned. But we must also acknowledge the enormous courage it takes to explore the territory of sexual passion all the way down to its primordial and sacred depths. Diane's story is not only a story of sexual obsession, but also the story of a very courageous woman who dared to open to a passion so intense that it became a spiritual initiation. It is the story of a woman in search of the glittering, shimmering, seductive side of the sacred masculine.

Through the Demon Lover's unhappy, distorted form, we catch a glimpse of the ancient sexual god who, though exiled from Western religion, remains a powerful presence within our collective consciousness. Reviled and eventually ignored, the sexual god had no choice but to take refuge in the dark corners of society, in its mentally unstable members, its psychopaths and criminals. The Demon Lover is an extremely important figure in women's spiritual awakening, because he brings them face to face, not only with the addict they would prefer to avoid, but also with the sexual god they long to meet. "I have to acknowledge that Stanley awakened the goddess in me," Diane admitted with a sigh. "In a sense, it was more appropriate to marry him than either of my other two husbands. There was a sacred union in our sexual connection that was lacking in both my other marriages."

It is perhaps inevitable that the Demon Lover should leave us with such ambivalent feelings. He possesses the power of Eros, the power to inflame a woman's passion, to ignite her desire, to fan the white-hot blaze in which all human identity is burned to ashes until only god and goddess remain, fused by the heat of passion into a single brilliant light. However, since he is unable to relate to his own gift with humility, it consumes him like an uncontrollable, destructive genie. He is a sad figure, disconnected from his soul, twisted and entangled in darkness—and yet he challenges us to remember one of god's most beautiful forgotten faces.

7

THE SACRED MASCULINE

In many tribal cultures, it was said that if the boys were not initiated into manhood, if they were not shaped by the skills and love of elders, then they would destroy the culture. If the fires that innately burn inside youths are not intentionally and lovingly added to the hearth of community, they will burn down the structures of culture, just to feel the warmth.   Michael Meade

As we all know, our planet is in crisis. Every day, we hear news of worsening environmental pollution, crime, warfare, overpopulation, poverty, and hunger. What parents have no fear for the future of their children? Poisons leaking out of canisters carelessly abandoned burn into the earth's flesh. Her aura, the air we breathe, has turned a dull, noxious gray. Huge cities multiply like cancer growths upon her body. Her shining green-forested skin has been flayed in many places, leaving her flesh raw and open to infection. Her babies lie dying of starvation and neglect. And we who are women know this not only as an intellectual metaphor, but as an anguish that screams through the cells of our bodies. Men know it too, though perhaps in a more muted way, a way they can more easily push aside. Something about the feminine way does not support us in denying earth's illness even though we, too, might welcome the relief of ignorance. Like great vampires, we have sucked nature's lifeblood to feed our insatiable greed, and have become Demon Lovers to the earth.

As a woman, I look at every major political crisis, be it in Bosnia, in Rwanda, or in the Middle East, and I see men who have lost touch with the spiritual foundations of their life, men who deny their vulnerability, and who equate tenderness, gentleness, and forgiveness with weakness. Rape is a commonplace weapon that this false, perverted masculinity employs to assert itself while trampling down the nobility of both the feminine *and* the true masculine. The god within men seems to have forgotten his god-self. Disoriented and bloated with self-importance, he staggers this way and that like a drunk. Any minute now, he may stumble and fall into the ditch. And since the sickness of the god is also the sickness of the goddess, she too has forgotten her own magnificence and has become small, sad, tight, harsh, and fearful of pleasure.

As women begin to reclaim their feminine pride, they often feel great swells of anger against men. Bitterness in her voice, a woman tells me, "Men have been taught to have a very rapacious attitude toward sex. It's all about conquest, domination, rape. How can you experience anything sacred when the dominant paradigm is rape? It makes the penis demonic. Men in this culture are taught that the worst thing they can do is surrender, especially to women."

The true nature and the beauty of the masculine and the feminine reveals itself only when their equality is honored. The patriarchal concept of masculinity is inherently perverse, based as it is on the degradation and denial of the feminine. The ideals of this perverse masculinity are toughness, independence, personal survival, invulnerability, competition, ambition, control, and success. War provides men with the perfect environment within which to hone these attributes, and those who master the game become warlords. In the meantime, everyone suffers, most of all the earth. When we look to the corporate world, we see a similar, equally insidious type of warfare going on. There, the battlefield is big business, and victory brings control over financial rather than physical territory. But the effects on the earth and the earth's people are just as devastating as the effects of physical warfare.

It is only through the experience of the sacred masculine and feminine that healing of the estrangement between the genders can occur. When I asked women whether they had ever encountered the sacred masculine, many shook their heads or shrugged. Sadly, they had not experienced masculine energy as safe or nurturing. One woman commented, "I think that the sacred masculine is able to meet the feminine whole, unafraid, with honor, and to know itself

MEN AND WOMEN

I have heard that the Hopi believe that the survival of the planet depends on the union of men and women. That is something I, too, believe. As long as men and women live in a state of imbalance, there will be no peace on earth.

FRANCESCA

I have become a powerful protectress of love. I used to be a spiritualist who wanted to transcend the body. Now, I believe that god lives in us, and that we must learn how to love each other as men and women. It's a radical change for me.

OLGA

as complementary to the feminine. But I don't think I have ever met a man who carried that." Tara spoke for many women when she said:

> I don't really know the sacred masculine. I have experienced the masculine as tight and hot and something to be wary of. When I think about men as a collective, I feel fear. In my experience, men see everything as there to be possessed or conquered.

Other women, however, told me that they *had* experienced the sacred masculine. For some, it happened in the context of an intimate relationship. But more often, they recalled moments when they experienced the masculine in a less personal way, as a quality of vibration. Irene's story is a good example:

> I didn't connect with the sacred masculine through my lover. I don't think he fully owned his own masculine energy. But I had a powerful experience that transformed my awareness of masculine energy. It happened while I was singing in a large choir where men and women were equally balanced, half and half. We would sing sacred music, spiritual music that had a deep earthiness—hymns to the Mother, and to the earth. It was beautiful. I would stand there and feel the sound of those men's voices and the presence of their bodies and their male-

COMING CLEAN

I have a teenage daughter, and I have been watching how teenagers deal with their sexuality. Both girls and boys come to talk to me. I don't know the rules myself, so we are discovering things together. One boy has a massive crush on my daughter. He really wants in her pants. My daughter is only thirteen, and the guy, who is fifteen, has already been in a lot of pants since he was ten years old. Still, I really like the kid. I think he is really something.

One day I said to him, "Nick, do you think you are attracted to my daughter because she is a virgin?" And he said, "Yeah . . ." "Well," I said to him, "have you looked to see whether that is sacred?" He thought about it, he really did. And then, he came back to me later and said, "You know, Mrs. Roberts, after I thought about that, I felt kind of dirty." "You did?" I said. Then he said to me, "Just look at my dad. My dad's dirty." He told me that all day long, he had been looking at men. "Most of us are really dirty inside," he said. "Well," I said, "what do you think you ought to do about it?" "I think I'll tell your daughter," he said. And he did. "I want to go to bed with you," he told her, "but it also makes me feel dirty because I don't know any reason other than that you are a virgin." And she answered, "That's why I haven't let you touch me, because you make me feel dirty, too."

A few days later, I was talking about how some people do ritual and connect with spirit before they make love or make a baby. "What's ritual?" Nick asked. I told him that ritual was used to cleanse your body, your thoughts, your emotions, and your mind. Nick sat there for a minute. Then his face lit up and he said, "Could I use it too? Could I make myself clean?" He was really excited. "Yeah," I said, "you could."

FRANCESCA

ness. It gave me a profound vision of male strength and beauty. And then there was the female energy, and the blending together of the male and female voices. Those sounds would pass all the way through me and merge into me. It was a deep awakening to the male god and his power, a power I could approach without fear.

Jungian psychology tells us that there is a feminine aspect of every man and a masculine side to every woman. By emphasizing the need to integrate the masculine and feminine polarities within our psyche, the Jungian school has helped us appreciate our inner landscapes and the ways we recreate them in the outer world. Yet much of Jungian literature blithely accepts traditional definitions of masculinity and femininity, and so reproduces the limiting gender stereotypes of a diseased culture. Describing a nurturing man as having integrated his "feminine side" denies the full scope of the masculine. Similarly, I doubt whether it really serves women to hear their outgoing, active side described as a "phallic thrust." Such language subtly drives a wedge between a woman and her dynamism—or a man and his nurturing energy—by implying a gender-based polarity where, in my opinion, no such polarity exists.[17] I would prefer to say that when women own their analytic intelligence and their assertiveness, or men their erotic sensitivity, they are simply manifesting their wholeness as human beings.

This is an important point because to reconnect with the sacred masculine, we must break ancient cultural habits of automatically identifying the feminine with matter, the earth, nurturance, and passivity, while linking the masculine with spirit, the sky, assertiveness, and activity. If, as Irene's story would suggest, the masculine and the feminine are first and foremost fields of vibrating energy, this means that we can never define them verbally or conceptually, any more than words can convey the taste of a banana to someone who has never eaten one. To know the sacred masculine and feminine, we must directly experience their vibrational essence.

It is, of course, true that on one level, our cultural association of woman, earth, and nurturance makes perfect sense. As babies come from women's bodies, so the earth gives birth and nurtures plants, animals, and humans. Accordingly, the reawakening of goddess spirituality in the West has come hand in hand with a valuable and necessary call to reverence for nature, the body, and the earth. For women, it seems easy and natural to think of the earth as mother, thus affirming our kinship with her. But in the act of projecting all procreative and nurturing power onto the feminine, the seeds of patriarchal estrangement from the earth and from women are sown. We must remember that we are dealing with metaphors, not reality. In truth, the earth is no more feminine than spirit is masculine. Unless we relate carefully and consciously to such gender-based projections, they are bound to imprison us in outdated concepts. It only serves men to think of the earth as mother if they feel equal permission to conceive of earth as father, as the German poet Rainer Maria Rilke does in his prayer to a dark, earthy god:

> Whom shall I call upon, if not him,
> who is dark and more of night than night itself.
> The only one who wakes without a light
> yet has no fear; the deep one, as yet
> unspoiled by the light, the one of whom I know
> because in trees he bursts forth from the earth
> and because as fragrance
> he rises softly from the soil
> into my down-bent face.[18]

This is the sacred masculine whom we have forgotten, who not only reveres the earth but is *of* the earth, and who not only respects nature but manifests *through* nature. This is the divine flute player whom the Greeks called Pan, whom the Native American Hopi know as Kokopelli, and whom the Hindus call Krishna—the one who sings to the soul through the hollow reed. Christianity has told us that his cloven hoof and his horns are emblems of evil, when in fact they are marks of his affinity with nature. He is the original "good shepherd" whom Christ echoes, the earthy god who lives with his animals and protects them. He, and not the sexless patriarch, is the lover of the goddess. Together they enact the sacred marriage, and in their union form the Great Gateway through which new creation enters the world.

This is a truth that comes across very beautifully in the following story, told by Naomi, a woman whose story we shall hear in Chapter 21. Deeply wounded by male violence, Naomi has worked hard not only to heal herself, but also to heal her broken relationship with men. When I asked her whether she had any experience of the sacred masculine, she initially responded: "I don't know much yet about men's sacred sexual energy. I think that whatever men may have is different than what women have. I assume they have something equal, but I don't know about it yet." Then, reconsidering, she told me the following story:

Actually, I think I *have* experienced the sacred masculine, though only very recently. I took a course that teaches people to defend themselves against assailants with weapons—guns, knives, and clubs. I had taken other self-defense courses that were only for women, but this one was for men and women. Knowing that men would participate made me a little nervous, but I saw it as an opportunity for healing some of my issues with men.

There was one man there, a tall, slim, strong young guy who was physically very beautiful. It turned out he was a boxer. With great dignity, but also with shyness and pain, he said, "I gotta lay it out, I gotta be frank with you. I'm scared. I'm here because my parents came after me with everything you can think of. They beat me with everything they could get their hands on." I just felt my heart open to him, and I felt so moved by his dignity and his pain.

At the end of the class, we all sat in a circle. This man was crying. He was trying to be manly about it, but he was allowing himself to cry nonetheless. I felt so connected to him. When his turn to speak came, he said, "I'm in a lot of pain about this. I just can't tell you about all the violence; the violence that was done to me, the violence that I'm capable of doing. . . . I'm sad. It makes me really sad. I just hope that my going through this will help me not to do this to my kids. That's the only hope I have." I went up to him after the class and said, "I just want to tell you how much I respect you. I was really moved by what you said." And he said, "Well, Naomi, I feel the same way about you."

Afterward, I was driving along in my car, and I felt a gathering of sacred energy. In my mind, I could see this man, and I saw the healing energy of the divine Mother gathering around him. So I asked him internally whether I had his permission to enter into a visualization involving him. He was completely willing. I saw myself with two other women bathing him in healing energy. I saw him screaming and shaking and his body going through spasms as the terror that his mother had instilled in him was being driven out of his body. I was crying while this was happening. I was still driving along, and at the same time, I was in another realm where this healing was taking place.

I thought that was the end of it. But then, in my inner vision, I saw him turn to me and say, "I have something to give you." This really surprised me. Even though I felt very loving toward him, I thought he couldn't possibly have anything to give me. But he turned to me, and radiated onto me a nurturing male energy which was so beautiful, so beautiful . . . I cry when I think about it. He did for me what I was doing for him; his energy permeated the places where I still believe in the cruelty of men and in the destructiveness of male energy, places where I'm totally convinced that nothing else is possible. There was a purity of nurturing energy that was protective, but in a completely different way than a mother's energy. It was moving and also very humbling, because I realized my willingness to offer my feminine energy to men does not mean I have overcome my hatred and my condescension toward them. To believe that men have something equally healing, nourishing, and validating to give me in return feels very new.

Hearing this story from a woman herself so deeply abused by men should give us hope—hope that men are taking steps to acknowledge their wounds and initiate their healing, paving the way for a true partnership between men and women. Hope that the god is returning—not the old bearded patriarch, but Pan, the lover of life, the lover of women, the goatherd with his flute and his earth magic. This much is certain: women are eagerly waiting. We have missed his joyful presence too long.

MEN AS HEALERS

There was one lover whom I called the frog man, or perhaps lizard man would be more appropriate. He was all body. He loved making love, and he was a nature spirit. He was a natural force, something without ego or personality, pure body and instinct. Making love to him was like making love to a serpent. I would come to him fresh off some television show, all made up and completely artificial, with my high heels and miniskirt, and totally disconnected. I would take off all the trappings, climb into bed with him and feel myself returning to the natural world as our skin touched. It was really healing. ANYA

Like most Jewish women, I always thought I was too fat, and I criticized my body. I took diet pills from the time I was fourteen; I always wanted to be a smaller size. One of my lovers had told me my breasts were too droopy, and forever after I didn't like my breasts. But my husband takes such delight in my body that all this has disappeared. I have never again worried about being fat—never! It's amazing to me. His love has been so healing in so many ways. His support for the feminine kept allowing me to let my patriarchal judgments go. HANNAH

With some hesitation, I went to see a male therapist. As an African-American woman, I was not happy that he was white, or that he was male. But he was good. In one session, I had a extremely powerful experience of healing the abuse that my mother inflicted on me, and of knowing my essence as light. My therapist was right there with me and he cried. I believe that this experience had something to do with his maleness. Later, I dreamed that he and I lay together in bed and talked. We were naked, but there was no sex between us. When I woke up, I realized that psychically, we really had been completely naked. We created something together as male and female but not in a genital way. To me, that was a moment of sexual healing. DONNA

8

SEX AND RITUAL

In my culture, the culture of the Dagara, the whole concept of the intimate relates to ritual. Outside of ritual, nothing can be truly intimate . . . Any close, intimate relationship is impossible without ritual space. Anything beyond the normal, day to day issues like how to plow the field, how to plant millet or dig yam, touches upon the spiritual world, the ancestral world, and therefore, belongs in ritual space.

Malidoma·Some

Most people in our culture believe one should have sex only with a person one loves, or at least has a close personal relationship with. Otherwise, we disdainfully call it promiscuity or prostitution. But look back through history, and you will find that other cultures thought very differently. In medieval Europe, brides and grooms were not expected to be in love; in many cases, they hardly even knew each other. Sex was valued not so much as an expression of personal love, but rather as nature's way of ensuring survival. Most ancient cultures had special festivals that celebrated sexuality in ways that would probably shock many of us. Here is a poem from ancient India that conveys the powerful feelings of fear and ecstasy these sacred sexual rites evoked:

> Holy sixth day
> in the woods they worship the
> trees then
> then my heart beat hard
> at how far I was going into
> the woods
> a snake appeared in front of me

125

and I fell down
I started writhing and rolling
this way and that
my dress fell off
my hair burned along
my back
thorns scratched me
everywhere
suddenly who am I
who was I
how I
love those celebrations[19]

Thus, in ancient times, men and women would make love (the snake here refers to a lover), abandoning themselves to the power of the life-force, letting it move them and use them and wash them clean of their selfhood, until they were left stammering, "Who am I? Who was I?" This poem scintillates with the glint of an ecstasy long exiled from our own religious traditions, but also with a clear consciousness that such ecstasy leads deep into a primeval wilderness where fires burn out of control, thorns pierce the flesh, and all the protections of civilization fall away like the poet's clothing, leaving one naked and defenseless in the face of a cosmic power. Such passion is a sacrament in which danger and ecstasy are perfectly balanced, and which, like all true mysteries, has the power to completely undo one's boundaries and defenses. When lovers meet on this level, they meet as participants in an ancient rite in which the couple's personal relationship is secondary to the rite itself. Giving themselves over, they become the sacrifice, the burnt offering, two fused into one by the creative fire.

"Love is blind," we say, and that is true in some respects. But love can also give us true vision, true insight. When Irene and Brian fell in love, they found the archetypal dimensions appearing clearly before their astonished eyes:

Sometimes Brian would look like a completely different person during our lovemaking. His face would transform, and he would look like someone I had seen in another life. He saw the same in me. Once he looked like the face of death, but it wasn't scary. The archetypes would pass through as I witnessed them. I would feel like a beautiful, celebrated lover, glowing and radiant.

Presumably, the ancient sacred sexual rites transported lovers to the same archetypal depths Irene describes here. However, there was one important difference: the ceremonial union of male and female, god and goddess was usually enacted by men and women who were *not* lovers in daily life and related sexually only within the context of the ritual. In some societies, *every* woman was expected to step out of the realm of personal relationship at least once in her life in order to serve as a sexual priestess. In the fifth century B.C.E., Herodotus described the customs of Babylonian women:

> Babylonian custom . . . compels every woman of the land once in her life to sit in the temple of love and have intercourse with some stranger. . . . The men pass and make their choice. It matters not what be the sum of money; the woman will never refuse, for that were a sin, the money being by this act made sacred. After their intercourse she has made herself holy in the sight of the goddess and goes away to her home; and thereafter there is no bribe however great that will get her.[20]

Many women remember a time in which they made love to a stranger and reenacted a ritual reminiscent of the Babylonian women's. When I asked one woman about her fondest sexual memories, she told me the following story:

> Once, at a big party, I started dancing with a guy. I didn't know him at all but we danced together for hours and we were practically making love right there. After the party, we went upstairs and made love like wild. It was so beautiful and so earthy and so completely uninhibited. Then we fell asleep. In the morning, he got up and left. I felt so great. Neither of us wanted to see each other again. It wasn't a personal thing, it was pure life energy. I never did anything like that again,

but I am so glad I allowed myself to do it just that once. It helped me find myself. It showed me what it meant to be female and move in my body and be completely free in my sexuality.

This story brings to mind the raucous yet sacred spring rites of pre-Christian Europe, in which men and women would make love in the furrows of the earth to celebrate the rising sap of nature. Even during the Christian era, these spring celebrations survived in the form of Carnival. In the Black Forest in southern Germany, where Carnival still has a strong pagan flavor, the last remnants of the ancient fertility festival still linger. I will never forget climbing up the steep stairs to the cavernous, dark attic of an old village farmhouse where the family of my friend Anke had lived for many generations. Sneezing as I breathed the musty attic dust, I watched Anke open the creaky old doors of a huge wooden closet. Out spilled the most amazing costumes—bear costumes and queen costumes, fools and skeletons, leopards and leopard tamers, each outfit complete with its own gloves and masks. The drawers held tangles of lacy lingerie, hair clips, pins, strands of false pearls and glittering diamond brooches, scarves, shawls, and belts.

During the height of Carnival, Anke confided, her mother would get dressed up in one of these costumes and go out to play. "With your father?" I asked. "Oh, no." Anke shook her head, grinning. "This was her time to party, and he would be out doing his own thing. But it was important to stay incognito. If my mother thought someone might have recognized her, she would come home and change. Some nights, she changed costumes three or four times." Anke never knew what exactly her mother, a good Catholic housewife, did during those wild nights. Some things are best left to the imagination. But such holidays are increasingly rare, and are fast dying out entirely or deteriorating into drunken parties where the energies of the transpersonal realm are never acknowledged, let alone placed in a ceremonial context.

In the sixties and seventies, the long-locked doors to the transpersonal dimensions were flung wide open. Once again, men and women gave themselves permission to make love to relative strangers, and in doing so, many rediscovered the joy and the playful wisdom of their animal bodies. Most people just wanted to let loose and have a good time. But some, like Donna, an African-American woman in her fifties whose story we shall hear in Chapter 25, felt that they were being trained as sexual priests or priestesses. During this period, Donna awakened to the sacredness of her sexuality and its healing potential.

> I began to realize that in many cases, the men were not there to be my lovers, but that we had come together to do some kind of sexual healing. I started hearing stories from men whose mothers had sexually abused them, and I began to see how much healing men needed, and how important it was to listen to their stories. I began learning about energy, too. I began to realize that I knew how to perceive a man's auric field, and that men would respond to mine. With a certain lover, I found that if I just put my hand over his lower back while we made love, even without touching him, he would come. I started exploring energy fields, without having any guidelines for what I was doing. So many understandings came to me during this time, a period of openness and insight.

We would be wrong to think that when sex occurs outside a personal relationship, it must be impersonal, casual, or promiscuous. This is not necessarily so. Our manhood or womanhood contains the unique essence of our soul, and those who meet on that level sometimes meet more fully than many a husband and a wife who have shared the same bed for decades but have never surrendered to Aphrodite's whirling currents. Donna continued:

> Sometimes the sex was anonymous. And yet there is a very special way one can know a person through being sexual with them that does not require the container of a relationship. What is essential, though, is that the man really honor that sacred space. People would like to own that sacredness but it can't be owned. You must respect the energy and not try to claim it as a personal possession. What happens in that sacred space is not meant to feed the ego. It is a worship of the divine.

Today, we tend to view sexual love as a purely personal phenomenon. The sexual god has been demonized while the priestess, Aphrodite's daughter, has been called a slut, a whore, or a prostitute. When, several years ago, the surviving temple priestesses of Eastern India attempted to stage a public dance performance, they were pelted with rotten tomatoes. Such was the disrespect into which they had fallen, who were once revered as holy women.[21] We no longer acknowledge what the ancient Indian poem so clearly recognizes, namely that our sexual energy does not belong to us in a personal sense, but links us with the greater energies of creation. The rituals that once allowed men and women to meet as channels of the gods and goddesses have all been banned. All nonmedical consciousness-altering drugs have been made illegal, even though they are time-honored tools for connecting with spirit.

Where, then, do we stand, having blocked so many of our access roads to the realm of the gods? How do we connect with the vast transpersonal forces that govern our life? Today, in the age of AIDS, one can hardly recommend making love to strangers. So where do we take our longing to experience the power of the god and the goddess, without all the personal entanglements of a relationship?

I believe that much of our confusion around the sacred feminine and masculine stems from a lack of ritual. Most Tantric teachers suggest that couples enter into ritual space before making love. All ancient traditions surrounded sex with ritual and ceremony. But even more important than rituals for lovers are group rituals, which might or might not be overtly sexual but nonetheless lay the groundwork for sexual union by evoking and amplifying sacred masculine and feminine energies. Our modern world provides few such group rituals, and yet stories like Irene's account of singing in a choir show how deeply the remaining fragments can still affect us. As the temple dancers of former times needed their temples, so we too need sanctuary spaces. We need to recreate our temples not through physical structures, but through the power of our intention. Centering ourselves in sacred space not only helps us heal old wounds but also reconnects us with the usually veiled depths of our own nature.

When women hold the intention of creating a sacred ritual space, and spend time immersed in such a vortex of feminine en-

ECHOES OF THE GODDESS

Once, I went to a sex show with a lover. I remember watching one woman dance on a table. And even in that demeaning situation, you could see beyond, or through, to the face of the goddess. You could see that this was an echo of what had once been a sacred act. Even in this place where the men looked pathetic, as if they were ashamed to be there, something holy and magnificent was still shining through.

DONNA

ergy, they begin to connect with the sacred feminine in a new way. Simply by consciously gathering in a circle, feminine energy can be amplified and heightened until everyone feels its presence. This sacred feminine energy then mirrors her own essence back to every woman. "Oh, this is what I am," she feels. "This is where I belong." Through such experiences, we come to know ourselves as embodiments of the sacred feminine, and from this knowledge we derive an invaluable sense of reassurance and strength which has nothing to do with our individual qualities or personality traits, but everything to do with our essential female vibration.

Members of men's groups report the same thing in regard to the sacred masculine. When a group of men gathers in ritual space, their masculine vibrations unite and intensify, thus forming a strong energetic field of masculine energy that is easy to perceive.

Without such immersion in a field of same-sex energy, we lose an important connection to our soul. Malidoma Some's wife, Sobonfu, says that among her people, women sleep only among women, and men only among men. She explains that when we sleep, we are energetically open and vulnerable to being nurtured or depleted by the surrounding energy field. By sleeping among women, a woman recharges her feminine energy, so that when she moves out into the world, she will do so from the fullness of her feminine power. Though most of us would not go so far as to sleep only among women, it is true that we are not ready to meet the opposite gender until we have deeply bonded with our own. Only then can we encounter the other from a position of clarity and inner strength. For this reason, all tribal cultures have separate rituals for women and men, as well as rituals in which the sexes come together.

Group rituals that celebrate the coming together of male and female almost always include music and dance. Music harmonizes the rhythms of male and female energies; dance, because of its affinity with lovemaking, is a natural means of raising sexual energy. Typically, modern Western dancing focuses on the individual couple. In contrast, tribal dances commonly have the men dancing in one group, the women in another, like the plus and minus poles of a magnet. This generates a strong vibrational force field, which causes elemental sexual energy to pulsate back and forth between the men and the women. Such ritual dances channel creative juice into the community as a whole, as well as into its individual members. Men then know the sacred feminine as the collective energetic radiance of women, while women know the sacred masculine as the collective energetic radiance of men. Each experiences the other as carrier of a sacred energy.

Though our culture does not provide traditional rituals to honor and evoke the sacred essence of each gender, we do have the capacity to create new rituals of our own, both with our own and with the opposite sex. Several years ago, four friends and I decided to honor the sacred feminine within each other in a ritual way. We spent several days together cradled by trees, rocked by the sound of the ocean, and caressed by the summer winds. On our last evening, we put on our favorite clothing, lit candles and incense, and meditated together. Then, one by one, each woman stood up while the others gazed at her. Opening our inner eye, we began to name what we saw:

I honor you as the protectress of animals.
I honor you as the daughter of the mountain, wild, untamed, and free.
I honor you as White Buffalo woman.
I bow down to the eternal light of your being.

As we did this, an amazing shift occurred. What we had begun playfully, as an experiment, became a profoundly sacred initiation.

Each woman transformed before our eyes. One became tall as a tree, so that we had to stretch our necks to look at her shining face. Another began to glow with a sweet, soft radiance. Many beings seemed to float through us—aboriginal Australian shamans, Chinese wisewomen, and African hunters. In this experience, there was no place for arrogance to enter. On the contrary, we all felt deeply awed, humbled, and blessed. When we finished, we knew that a true healing had occurred. We had recognized, honored, and reclaimed the sacred feminine within.

Jungian analyst Marion Woodman describes her own experience of a traditional group ritual in which she participated during a visit to India. When her taxi driver told her that it was the birthday of Krishna (it also happened to be her own) and asked her if she would like to go see the celebrations, she spontaneously agreed and was ushered into a deeply sacred initiatory ritual.

Instantly he swung the taxi into the ditch and through the fields, singing all the way. Then he stopped. Immediately the car was surrounded by men. Someone opened the door and motioned me out. I stepped onto the ground and four pairs of hands took my sandals, my purse, my camera, and my belt. The driver was nowhere in sight. I stood looking into the impenetrable faces of at least twenty men who looked back at me as intently as I looked at them.

I had been told there was still human sacrifice in India and it passed through my mind that I never thought I would die this way. Suddenly the men all bowed in a low salaam and straightened; green eyes met fiery black ones in silent concentration. In spite of my concern, I felt their reverence, not for me but for Someone I represented. "If I'm going to die, I'm going to die," I thought. "This is certainly an interesting situation. I am going to stay with it. I am not going to faint."

They picked me up, raised me above their heads, and chanting, carried me to an altar and gently laid me prone on the ground. Convinced that I was about to be sacrificed, I was simultaneously dead and fiercely alive, quite beyond fear. I was receiving powerful energy from the men, a commingling of love and praise and awe. A man who seemed to be a priest put grass in my mouth, chanting with the others. He prayed over me. He took the grass and divided it among the men who ate it as if it were holy grass. They picked me up, put me on the altar and, again chanting, did a slow dance around me.

Vulnerable and alone, infinitely at the mercy of whatever was to happen, I knew it was not my will, not my love, but Her will, Her love, that there was some meaning to my life infinitely beyond anything I had ever imagined, and that my delicate body—in all its ugliness and all its beauty—was the temple through which I had come to know Her on this earth. Through the dark arms of those strangers in that dusty Indian field, Sophia reached out to me. In that moment, that eternal moment, I heard Her great I AM.

Again they salaamed. They carried me off the holy ground and returned my leather sandals, camera, purse, and belt. The taxi driver reappeared, smiling his nonchalant smile, and we bounced back across the fields.[22]

Here, we witness a group of men recognizing, invoking, and worshipping the goddess within a woman. Though nothing overtly sexual takes place, the entire ritual is an act of sexual homage, offered by the sacred masculine to the sacred feminine.

Both the modern women's ritual that my friends and I conducted, and this presumably quite ancient Indian ritual, centered around the worship of woman as goddess. And yet the relationship among the participants of the ritual was not hierarchical but equal, for the deity was equally present in all participants. In the Hindu *Gandharva Tantra* we read:

One should worship a divinity by becoming oneself a divinity. One who has not become a divinity should not worship a divinity. Anyone worshipping a divinity without becoming a divinity will not reap the fruits of that worship.[23]

Worship, in this sense, is a dance that awakens sacred awareness in both the worshipper and the worshipped. Both are transformed, united in a circle of enlightened perception, which evokes the ecstatic recognition of who we really are, behind the veils of illusion. If we would stand in right relationship to our sexuality, we must re-create such opportunities to re-encounter ourselves and each other in this way as embodiments of sacred energies. This is a gift we can easily give each other—it requires no more than willingness, intention, and reverence.

9

LINGAM, YONI, AND SERPENT

I, Lalla, entered the jasmine garden,
Where Shiva and Shakti were making love.

I dissolved into them,
and what is this
to me, now?

I seem to be here,
but really I'm walking
in the jasmine garden.
                    Lalla, fourteenth century C.E.

"Thank god we're finally taking a break," I thought as I gazed up the steep expanse of rock ahead of me. At an altitude of 14,000 feet, my heart was pounding hard as I walked. Along with a group of Western pilgrims, I was struggling through the high mountains of Kashmir in northern India, accompanied by several Kashmiri guides, men as hardy as their mules and goats and totally at ease in the thin mountain air. While we collapsed in exhaustion, panting like dogs in the midday sun, they all squatted around a tall water pipe to enjoy a smoke of marijuana. Grinning mischievously, one of them, a dark, swarthy man with eyes like black embers, turned to me and beckoned for me to join them. I grinned back without moving; we both knew full well that if I accepted, his herbs would flatten my already shaky body.

All over the planet, certain sites are held sacred as thresholds to the spirit worlds. Our destination was one such place, a cave known as Amarnath, which means "Abode of the Lord of Immortality." Here, according to an ancient myth, the god Shiva and his consort Shakti spent a night of passionate lovemaking. Afterward, Shiva thanked the cave that had so graciously sheltered them, and as a token of his blessing, he left behind a phallic pillar of ice—a *lingam,* as it is called in Sanskrit. Eleven months of the year, snow and ice block all human access to the cave, as if the divine lovers had returned and were protective of their privacy. And even when the path is open, the journey is risky. A week after my own visit to Amarnath, fifty unfortunate pilgrims were killed by a landslide.

Worship of the lingam, as is practiced at Amarnath, is by no means unique to Hinduism. The ancient Celts, too, worshipped phallic stones, as did the Greeks. Once in a while, I bring a polished black stone lingam to my women's workshops. As the lingam passes around the circle, some hold it with a sense of reverence and delight, cradling its heavy black weight in their cupped hands. Others take one look at it and pass it on, as if it were contaminated with smallpox. After centuries of enforced submissiveness, not everyone feels affection for a symbol that reminds them of rape, abuse, and male dominance. But, as I explain to them, the lingam is *not* a penis. Rather, it symbolizes the universal principle of firmness, substantiality, and positive Being within every atom of creation. A penis might be revered as a lingam, but then, so might a mountain, a tree, a pillar, or a staff.

Moreover, in Tantric ritual, the lingam is never worshipped alone, but always in conjunction with the *yoni,* the cosmic vulva. Complementing the lingam, the yoni represents the principle of receptivity, containment, and space, which may be worshipped in wells, lakes, and valleys, as well as in a woman's vulva. In every temple dedicated to the god Shiva and his consort Shakti, one will find a stone resting within a bowl, symbol of lingam and yoni in sacred union. In India, one also comes across "yoni temples," womblike spaces used as sites for initiation into the mysteries of the goddess. At Amarnath, where the god's phallus has taken the form of an ice pillar, the cave itself is the yoni of the goddess. Amarnath is a sanctuary dedicated to the transpersonal essence of the sacred masculine and feminine; to this day, the cave remains steeped in an aura of holiness and creative ecstasy.

As our group inched up the Himalayan slopes, the green shrubs and trees gave way to barren rocks baking in the summer heat, and we fell silent, concentrating on the long climb. Hours passed. Struggling to put one foot in front of the other, we felt the burning sun, the altitude, and the barrenness of the landscape conspiring to induce a dreamlike, hypnotic state. In the early afternoon, we finally caught our first glimpse of the cave. At first, all we saw was a vast hole in the side of the mountain. Then I realized that the little specks in front of the cave were the tents of pilgrims and vendors selling trinkets and offerings. People disappeared into the cave like tiny insects flying into the open jaws of a giant.

Half an hour later, we had arrived at the mouth of the cave. A priest indicated we should leave our shoes at the entrance. Barefoot and exhausted, we entered the dark interior. With a slight shock, I realized I was walking on a smooth sheet of ice that paved the entire floor. Another priest gestured us to follow him to the back of this vast cavern, where the Shivalingam stood, the phallus of the Lord of Immortality.

The lingam was a perfect phallic shape formed of white-blue ice about eight feet tall. Blinking as my eyes adjusted to the dim light, shuffling my freezing feet, I stood in silence, stunned by the strangeness of the scene—the great white pillar, the priest's voice echoing through the cave as he chanted the ancient incantations in praise of the god, the offerings of flowers and colored powder that the pillar had absorbed into its base. Entering this cave, I was aware of having entered the womb of the goddess, the place of my own origins. Here, the union of sacred masculine and feminine energies had been honored for untold centuries, perhaps millennia.

As I stood lost in thought, I suddenly became aware that for several minutes now, the pillar of ice had appeared to glow with a silent, subtle blue light. "It must be the exhaustion," I told myself. "You are imagining this." Fortunately, I was too tired for analysis. Real or not, as far as I could see, the pillar was glowing. For a moment, I remembered my dream of being taken to a temple where I was told I would marry the god who resided there in the form of a black rock. "Shiva," I murmured, "lord of the mountain." I began to shiver with cold—and with something else that trembled inside my body. As time passed, the presence of mystery became more and more intense. I was engulfed by a deep and subtle presence. From within the pillar, the blue light appeared to pulsate, penetrating my body and silencing my thoughts. The lingam radiated an almost hallucinatory quality of pure Being, of the world's innermost essence appearing in a vision which, at any moment, could melt away before my very eyes. Time dissolved and I felt that I had stood here, a tiny human being, for thousands of years. I trembled, no longer with cold but with awe. Slowly, silence descended within me—deep, unmoving silence.

The effect of any true initiation is revealed gradually, in its aftermath. In the weeks and months after my pilgrimage to Amarnath, I began noticing an ice-blue light that seemed to radiate out from the core of my being. Shiva's shining pillar had established itself within my body, and its light was pulsing through my cells. Any activity that heightened my energetic awareness, such as dance or meditation, would also intensify the inner light, until it expanded into a shining tube or pillar that fluctuated in size, sometimes growing beyond the boundaries of my physical body.

But nothing brought the inner light alive the way sex did. When I made love, the sensation of my lover's penis would merge with this inner pillar of light. Swirling mandalas would appear, and sometimes deities would dance before my inner eye and then merge into me. The physical pleasure and the surface sensations of lovemaking, which had in the past seemed all-important, now interested me far less than this inner dance of energy and light, this meeting and merging of essential male and female energies. Making love had become a worship of lingam and yoni in union. Any sense of hurry or pressure would obstruct this blossoming into the inner light, this dissolution into a luscious, delicious streaming, this sense of being washed clean, this delighted rediscovery of my own radiance.

In the course of talking to women about their sexual journey, I heard many stories that echoed my own. Sighing with pleasure, Jennifer told me about a very special encounter she had with her husband.

It felt like my vagina went up all through my body and out the top of my head, like a stream of liquid light. My husband said he felt the same thing in his body. I found that with my eyes

> *I have an enormous*
> *and long lingam*
> *erect.*
> *I have also*
> *my yoni.*
> *I am whole.*
>
> JANET ADLER[24]

closed, I could actually see an image of us both as these two long channels or pillars of light. Then they merged into this exquisite egg-shaped form that shimmered and pulsated. All the while, we were having sex, but I wasn't really aware of my body in the normal sense at all.

Every person, regardless of gender or sexual preference, is like a battery that contains both a plus pole (the lingam) and a minus pole (the yoni). Together, the lingam and the yoni constitute our energetic and sexual totality. Sexual union is at its best when both partners are in touch with both poles of their energy, so that energetically each can both penetrate and receive the other.

When women do not enjoy physical penetration, even with a skillful partner, a lack of energetic connection is often at fault. Julie Henderson, author of *The Lover Within,* mentions that when she began to awaken to her energy body, she started feeling sexually frustrated. Something was missing. Finally, she was able to articulate the problem: "I noticed that when my lover penetrated me physically, he didn't penetrate me energetically. The current of his excitement and aliveness remained within him. I felt untouched."[25] Unfortunately, our culture leaves us so uneducated in the sexual arts that lovers are rarely able even to articulate their energetic perceptions, let alone consciously move energy or dissolve blockages. But when lovers *do* connect energetically as well as physically, the man's penis will nourish and recharge the pillar of light within the woman. In return, her yoni awakens the receptive, enfolding energy within him. With this cyclical flow of energy, sexual union becomes healing, rejuvenating, and deeply satisfying. My friend Kyoko calls it "going home." "I think of my husband's penis as a kind of medicine," she says. "It's like his penis reminds me where I belong, and that I can go there. Something in me says, 'Oh, yes, there's my center, I forgot. Now I remember.' Afterward, I'm back home. I'm in myself."

Out of this union of male and female energies arises a rhythmic pulsation that can be as obvious as orgasm or as subtle as a fine vibration or hum. Throughout the ages, this primeval, pulsating wave of life-force has been symbolized as a serpent. All around the planet, one finds both religious and sexual rituals that honor the serpentine power. Cross-culturally, serpents also feature largely in creation myths as symbols of primordial creative energy.

Freud, who believed serpents to be phallic symbols, had it wrong. The serpent represents neither penis nor vagina, but rather the energy released by their union. As the sound of a bell is not heard until the mallet meets the metal, so the sinuous, undulating serpent appears only where the opposites unite. Therefore, in Hindu sacred art, both god and goddess are accompanied by serpents who twine lazily around their bodies like living necklaces, bracelets, and belts.

Sexuality is one of the most powerful means we possess of arousing and intensifying the serpentine movement within our bodies, until its undulating, primal rhythms take us over completely. Here, a man describes his experience of the serpentine energy moving through his lover's body:

> It feels like the vagina does a number on its own, tightening in different places that I don't think are in her control. . . . It takes an extreme level of excitement to get to, past all the barriers a woman has, all the training, all the psychology, I mean everything, every layer that's laid on top by society, all the way down to the base animal. It's a rare experience. . . . It's a pulsating effect that runs up through the cervix and through the limbs.[26]

Since we are naturally androgynous beings, we do not necessarily require a sexual partner to awaken the inner serpent. In fact, many women become aware of their serpentine energy long before they discover sexuality as a complex dance of self and other, lingam and yoni. Robert Bly calls Eros "the humming in the beehive that keeps the whole thing together."[27] Tara, an African-American lesbian now in her early fifties, remembers feeling this "humming in the beehive" long before she had words to talk about it:

> When I think about my sexuality it feels like a rhythm. It goes back as far as I can remember. It goes back to where I remember no incidents, but I do remember feeling. I remember feeling this same core that has always been a hum, a rhythm in a very deep place inside of me. It seems I was aware of that before I was aware of language. It came before any intellectual constructs. As I have grown up I have tried to make sense out of it. I have had to find my own language for it, in order to celebrate what has been my constant visceral connection with spirit.

The serpent represents both male and female sexuality. Nonetheless, serpents have consistently been associated with women. It was, after all, Eve whom the serpent persuaded to take the apple, not Adam. In many Semitic languages, the name "Eve" actually means "Serpent."[28] Women are, in fact, agents of the serpentine energy in a different way from men. Because a woman's body is designed to give birth, her intimacy with the workings of the serpentine energy is more profound than a man's. Every month, women in the childbearing years feel the serpent coiling and uncoiling within their body, releasing a single egg. And should that egg be fertilized, it is the serpent who presides over the mysterious process of reproduction. Shortly after the birth of her son, a young mother told the following story:

> About two weeks before my baby was born, I started having strong contractions. They were unlike anything else I had ever felt. I felt as if I were a boa constrictor swallowing a rat. There was this peristaltic movement that had absolutely nothing to do with anything I thought about it. It was completely biological, and it was extraordinary to feel this immense power at work within me. I had never given birth before, and I had

been concerned about not knowing how to do it. Now I realized that didn't matter. It had nothing to do with me personally. It was a biological event which would happen in its own time. I could either relax and go along with it, or I could fight it. It was like realizing you're going to die even though you don't know how to do it. It was deeply reassuring.

Because of the bias of Christian mythology, Eve's affinity with the serpent has not served her well. Perhaps we can now begin to reclaim a sense of pride in our own nature. Perhaps we can remember that our intimate knowledge of the serpentine mysteries is a gift, not a curse. Instinctively, we know how to call forth the serpent, how to invite it, how to entice it to bless our lovemaking with its healing presence. All traditions that worship the life-force also have great respect for serpents. Biblical mythology, however, reviles the serpent. "You belong to earth, to evil," the serpent has been told. "You have no knowledge of spirit. God has cursed you." The serpent merely blinks its eye at the gathered assembly of bishops and popes, and slithers off to safer ground. It has seen thousands of religions come and go with all their pomp and glory, but few that have so thoroughly misunderstood the mysteries of the serpentine way.

10

THE JOURNEY OF A TANTRICA

They try to say what you are, spiritual or sexual?
They wonder about Solomon and all his wives.
In the body of the world, they say, there is a Soul and you are that.
But we have ways within each other
that will never be said by anyone.

Rumi, thirteenth century C.E.

Theresa is a confident woman in her early fifties with clear blue eyes that meet your gaze straight on, expressive gestures, and a shock of blazing red hair that matches her fiery nature. There is a bigness, a boldness, and a sense of determination about her. Her loves are passionate and consuming, her rages are immense and explosive, and her pleasure skyrockets her to the stars.

One of the first things Theresa told me about herself is that she is a Tantrica, a practitioner and teacher of Tantra. A mystical branch of Hinduism and Buddhism, Tantra describes creation as the fruit of sacred union between god and goddess, honoring sexuality as a means of aligning human consciousness with the divine. The basic Tantric scriptures are the Tantras, many of which consist of dialogues between Shiva and Shakti, god and goddess, on the nature of cosmic reality. The cave of Amarnath is one site where the divine lovers are said to have transmitted such Tantras to the human race.

As the cross is the primary symbol of Christianity, so sacred sexual union is the primary metaphor through which Tantra views reality.[29] Tantra defines god as formless, unmoving spirit, and goddess as spirit in motion. He is the essence within all things, while she is energy and matter. She is the form-giver, the creator, the birth mother of us all. All that moves manifests her energy, and whatever has form receives that form from her. She is the life-force that animates us all; we exist only because she vibrates, dances, pulsates, throbs, and hums through every cell in our body.

According to Tantric teachings, all the gods and goddesses are internal as well as external realities. Therefore, the potential for sacred union exists internally as well as externally. Within our body, the goddess lies coiled and dormant at the base of the spine as the serpentine energy or Kundalini (literally, "the Coiled One"). Just a tiny fraction of her immense power suffices to control all the body's basic, involuntary functions—the rhythm of the heart and the flow of blood, the peristaltic movement of digestion and elimination, the orgasmic pulsation, and the contractions that expel a baby from the womb. When the serpentine goddess awakens more fully, she dances upward through the body, attracted toward the seventh or crown chakra, where her lover resides as pure, unmoving consciousness. Touched by the serpentine energy, each energy center or chakra of the body blossoms,[30] and a wide range of ecstatic states, mystical visions, and sublime states of enlightenment can occur. When the Kundalini reaches the crown, the inner lovers unite, and one experiences union with the cosmos.

We should not let the Sanskrit terminology mislead us—Kundalini is no Hindu invention, but an energy that has been experienced universally and described by spiritual adepts of all traditions. For example, the Kung people of the African Kalahari Desert call it *num*. They, too, say that *num* resides at the base of the spine. In dances and ceremonies that last all night long, they seek to awaken *num* and to channel it up their spine. When their *num* awakens, they move into states of trance and perform healings upon each other.[31]

It is difficult to pinpoint exactly what causes the awakening of the Kundalini. Spiritual energy is contagious, and sometimes contact with an enlightened being can trigger a Kundalini awakening. Other typical triggers are dance, meditation, and sexual stimulation. One woman described a Kundalini awakening that occurred during a period of intense spiritual practice: "I would be walking out in the street with my dog. Suddenly, I would feel lit up with

KUNDALINI AWAKENINGS THROUGH SEX

I did not have sex until I was in my forties. When I was first touched, the Kundalini was so awake within my body that I was orgasmic all the time. There was a flooding, a tremendous experience of lights and visions, which was very positive in some ways but also overwhelming and shocking. It was a spiritual breakthrough, a breaking through of all kinds of energies.

EVA

Recently, my husband and I were kissing and fooling around. It was nice, but not great. Then, we started having intercourse. And all of a sudden, I started feeling this incredible pleasure unlike anything I had ever felt before. "What is this?" I thought. The intensity of the pleasure was orgasmic, but it was located deeper inside of me, deeper even than my body. It took me to an-

all the light in the universe, and the sky would become a thousand times brighter. I would feel the hand of god coming down and touching my heart."

Not all Kundalini awakenings are so blissful, however. The Kundalini is pictured as a cobra for good reason. Sometimes it awakens with a hiss and a sharp sting, as if displeased at being roused from its deep sleep. Certain methods of intentionally arousing the sleeping cobra are risky, and people have been known to frizzle up, electrocuted by jolts of energy too strong for their systems. It is also quite common for the Kundalini to awaken spontaneously. Sometimes, this causes unusual or painful physical and mental symptoms that make people wonder whether they are seriously ill or going insane.

Some spiritual teachings ignore the Kundalini entirely or consider it spiritually irrelevant. Loving intention, purity of heart, and compassion are all we need, they say. Others believe that, on the

other dimension. Then it became so ecstatic I had to stop. I just couldn't handle any more. I knew something very major was happening. After some time, we started having intercourse again, and suddenly, my whole pelvic area opened up and this huge burst of white light exploded in me. "Whoa!" I said to Richard. He told me he felt something like an electric charge move through his body, out through his penis and into me. We call it "the day the light passed through us." All day long, my pelvis was tingling and full of sensation. But for Richard, it was different. "I gave that energy," he said, "and then it was gone." It came through him and went into me.

For the next three days after that, I had incredible cramps. It was the opposite of the pleasure. I am not sure what was going on, but I think old levels of tension were being burned off. It definitely felt electromagnetic. It felt like a gift, an affirmation of the power we have together. It made me feel excited about growing more, and expanding further. I think you need to be very strong and healthy on all levels to open to these energies. You have to be strong to experience life in its fullness. PAMINA

contrary, the awakening of the Kundalini is an absolutely essential prerequisite for true spiritual progress, and that all our actions will remain weak and ineffectual until the Kundalini begins to flow. Perhaps the truth lies somewhere in between. The Kundalini does indeed hold the secrets of embodied vibrational transformation. If we are concerned not merely with transcendence but with the enlightenment of physical matter and of the body, then we cannot ignore the great serpentine deity that resides within us. At the same time, the serpentine energy often awakens in people who are spiritually quite unevolved, so its waking should by no means be taken as a sure sign of spiritual maturity. The Kundalini is pure life-force, neither good nor bad, neither beneficial or harmful. It is like electricity or nuclear energy; depending on how one uses its immense power, it can make one a saint, or a monster. The stronger the energetic current we run through our systems, the more firmly we need to be anchored in purity, integrity, and compassion.

In contrast to orthodox (patriarchal) Hinduism and Buddhism, which despise the body and consider sex impure, Tantra affirms the inherent purity of all bodily experiences, including sex. Nonetheless, many Eastern Tantricas rarely utilize sexual practices. Instead, they seek to awaken enlightened perception primarily through breathing exercises, visualizations, and other internal disciplines. In the West, however, Tantra has been interpreted as the art, not merely of sacred union, but specifically of sacred *sexual* union. Therefore, the emphasis of Western Tantra lies on exercises and practices that enhance sexual pleasure.

Critics justly point out that most of what passes for Tantra in the West has little or nothing in common with Eastern Tantra. But spiritual traditions have always been transformed in passing from one culture to another. Moreover, most Western Tantrics honestly acknowledge that what they teach is not Eastern Tantra, but an amalgam of techniques creatively molded to suit the needs of a Western audience.

If I were to pick the single most useful teaching Western Tantra has to give us, it would be the message that good sexual loving is an art that does not come naturally but takes practice, like any other art. Raised in a sexually repressive society, most of us have to undo a lot of old conditioning before we can even begin to realize our full sexual potential. The assumption that good loving comes naturally is absurd and has done us a great deal of damage. Learning our bodies takes at least as much patience and dedication as learning an instrument—perhaps more, because the sexual body is an instrument that we are not merely *learning,* but rather *creating* as we go along. Our body's capacity for pleasure is not a given quantity, as we sometimes assume, but rather a variable that expands through use. Just as muscles develop through exercise, so the circuitry of erotic pleasure can be developed, honed, and refined to an extent most people never even suspect.

To excel in any art, including the art of sacred sexuality, one needs both talent and dedication, and Theresa had both. Her talent was evident even when she was a child; in fact, she did not so much become a Tantric practitioner as realize, in her thirties, that she had always been one. Tantra is a lot like gardening. Plants grow by

themselves, without our intervention. The gardener simply tries to enhance and support their growth by creating an optimal environment. In the same way, Tantra merely supports the natural tendency of sexual energy to evoke states of bliss and ecstasy. In Theresa's case, her mind and body were like rich, moist soil in which the flower of ecstasy took root spontaneously and flourished. "I remember having ecstatic states very young," she recalled.

> I would look up at the sun with my eyes closed and merge with the Creator. Or I would put my face down in the green grass, and I would merge with the grass and through the grass, with god. I also had visions of beings, which were sometimes formless bodies of light, but sometimes had faces. Saints would appear to me, and I often saw the Virgin Mary. I had a real infatuation with her. I remember believing that she was literally a virgin. I felt so disappointed when I decided it was just a metaphor. It was much worse than losing my belief in Santa Claus. My dreams were filled with images I now recognize as mystical. I would watch mandalas and icons. In my adolescence, I began having erotic mystical dreams, but in my childhood they were religious.

Throughout childhood, the Catholic church offered Theresa a refuge from her chaotic, abusive family life, where her alcoholic father regularly beat her as well as her mother. In comparison, going to church felt like going to heaven. "I went to church seven times a week for about eight years," Theresa told me. "If I was sick and couldn't go, I would feel awful. Church felt nurturing and comforting, and it was a place where my inner spiritual life was validated." At that time, Theresa's god was still a male; the notion of a goddess never occurred to her until much later. But even then, she said, "my god was never a figure with a robe and a beard. He was always benevolent, never punitive, I had an intimate personal connection with him, and I felt I needed him. Prayer was very real for me. It was not a mystery or a technique. It was a personal talk with god."

The safety and peace Theresa found in church would have sufficed to make her a devoted Catholic. But in addition, the church offered to give her a good education, something she desperately wanted and knew her father would never provide for her. I gasped when Theresa described her father's attitude:

> There was never a book in my family's home. My father believed that if you read books, you were a Communist. But I was starving for knowledge. Once I had a quarter and I bought myself a *Life* magazine, which I hid under my mattress. I just loved that magazine, it meant so much to me. After about a month, my father found it and he just flipped out. He went absolutely crazy and beat me up. But I wanted an education in the worst way, and I worried about how I might get one. School was a place where I could excel, and I became a very good student. I really wanted to please the nuns and priests, and they cared about my education. You can imagine what a shock it was when I announced to my parents that the Catholics were going to pay my way through college. And they did. The church gave me the best education.

Theresa is one of the few women I talked with who lost her virginity in a truly ecstatic sexual encounter. Just twelve years old, she fell madly in love with an eighteen-year-old boy. "Cecil and I had the hots for each other in a big time way," Theresa remembered with a smile. "So he invited me to his prom." Young as she was, Theresa felt ready to make love.

> After the prom, Cecil brought a blanket, and we went to a haystack. I knew what was going to happen, and I was very excited. I had no reservations about it at all. I was madly, passionately in love with Cecil, and he was a wild and crazy guy. He believed that anything two people decided to do together must be great. So we had full permission with each other's bodies. And he devoured me. He loved me all over. He was an experienced lover, and he wasn't inhibited. He was eighteen and I was twelve, not quite thirteen. I was young, but my hormones were raging. His attitude was so light and loving. He was the perfect person to be initiated with. It was glorious. I merged with god on top of that haystack in the moonlight,

making love with Cecil. It was incredible. Later I realized how rare our experience was, and I was so disappointed when I discovered it would not always be like that. Nature took us and moved us, and we surrendered. So I began a very active sex life with him.

For five happy years, Theresa told me, she made passionate, joyful love with Cecil. "Then," she announced dramatically, "I decided to join a convent." I was stunned; my mouth dropped open in amazement. For a moment I was speechless. Then I asked, "What on earth induced you to take such a drastic step?" Theresa sighed. "I had always loved the rituals and ceremonies of Catholicism, their rich sensuality and their repetitiveness. And to me, the nuns and priests were moms and dads who treated me better than my own mom and dad."

Then I understood how much Theresa must have yearned to be adopted into a loving family where she would be treated with kindness and respect, and how natural it seemed to her to idealize the institution which had offered her safety, support, and encouragement throughout her traumatic childhood. Also, her strong devotional bent was crying out for expression.

I loved my sex life with Cecil. We had fun and we were wild. Sex between us had been divine. But I started having deeper religious experiences. I started feeling a calling. It was a gut feeling, an overwhelming pull. I really felt I was the bride of Christ. When Cecil moved away, it seemed clear that this was the direction I needed to move in.

With years of ecstatic lovemaking behind her, Theresa knew the value of what she would have to sacrifice to join the convent. Yet for all her sexual experience, she was still a very innocent young girl who looked up to the church as the ultimate authority on all matters related to god. Fully aware of the joys of sex, she assumed that the church had something even better to offer her: knowledge of god. With childlike faith, she expected the nuns to guide her straight into the arms of a love far greater and more ecstatic than the love she had shared with her boyfriend.

To her dismay, Theresa found convent life intolerably dull. "I must try harder," she thought, pushing away her doubts. Her determination to be a "good" nun, a nun worthy of entering into god's presence, left her no room to acknowledge her mounting sense of discontent as the vital, healthy response it was. Instead, she repressed her anger and frustration and poured all her energy into becoming a submissive, obedient nun. Yet, ironically, even while cloistered life was failing to give Theresa the ecstatic communion she craved, she was making love with god every night, in her own personal way:

The minute I joined the order, I never thought about sex, and I didn't masturbate once during the two years I spent in the convent. I was sublimating it through prayer. I was having sex on an etheric plane, and in my dream life. I just let go of physical sex and found I was still having it in a new way. I went into ecstatic states of merging in the All. But I never related my personal experiences to the god whom the church was supposedly going to show me. In my mind, my ecstasies had nothing to do with religion.

I would lie in the tiny cot nuns have, with the nightstand, a crucifix, a rosary, and a prayer book, and curtains between the beds. I would lie there perfectly still. It was important to get so still I could barely feel my heartbeat. I would do this with total concentration. Then, I would call god, and I would make love with him. Whenever I called god, he always came. It would be a merging with the light. I would feel waves and undulations and intense palpitations in my heart. I would have heart orgasms. I never thought about genital sex, because I was perfectly satisfied.

Actually, I thought all the nuns were doing this. Little did I know. I didn't realize my experiences were unique. Now, with my knowledge of Tantra, I realize that my Kundalini was awake, and I had moved up through the chakras into higher vibrational frequencies. But I had no words for it then.

Without knowing it at the time, Theresa was already following the Tantric path. In the true manner of a priestess, she had centered herself in the intersection between the worlds, offering her heart as the gateway through which divine love came streaming in. The intensity of her devotion drew the Kundalini up into her heart chakra and released waves of orgasmic bliss, which can be experienced in any part of the body, not just the genitals.

If we think of sex in a narrow way, as a mere biological response, we have no way of relating to the type of mystical eroticism Theresa describes here. But when we understand sexual arousal as an indication that the life-force is streaming through us, then we can appreciate that sexual ecstasy does not depend on genital contact. We begin to see how some people can have sex every night and yet be sexually half dead, because the circuitry of their subtle body is clogged with resistance and tension. We can also understand how a celibate nun like Theresa might live a rich and fulfilling sexual life.

In her nightly communions with god, Theresa was following in the footsteps of Eastern as well as Western mystics throughout the ages who have described their path as a love affair with god, and who have described god as the ultimate lover, source of incomparable ecstasy and unsurpassed pleasure. Many medieval Christian nuns, who spent long hours meditating on their identity as the brides of Christ, experienced ecstatic union with god. In the thirteenth century C.E., Mechtild of Magdeburg wrote:

> Lord, you are my lover,
> My longing,
> My flowing stream
> My sun,
> And I am your reflection.[32]

When such mystics spoke of god as their lover, they were not speaking metaphorically. Suffused with love, they experienced a deep and complete satisfaction at all levels, including the sexual. Of course, Freud would have said that Mechtild was just a neurotic woman who sublimated her sexual frustration in this way. But if Mechtild had known Freud, she might have countered that he had his priorities reversed. From the mystic's viewpoint, sexual intercourse merely echoes the far more potent ecstasy of divine commu-

COSMIC LOVE PLAY

In Ireland, I swam with this dolphin, a huge old dolphin who has lived by himself for seven years. Many people have swum with him: autistic children, people in grief—he is like a holy dolphin. This dolphin literally drew me out in the water, and I was with him for forty minutes, with no wetsuit. He kept me warm. I was like a water creature. In the end, he rolled up, and rested his head so my eye was looking into his, and that did it. I just fell in total, unbelievable love. I started having body orgasms that didn't stop for the next four hours. They felt like cellular orgasms, as well as sexual orgasms. I don't know what dolphins are, but they are certainly whole, and very wise. It was a very deep sexual experience.

FRANCESCA

One night I had to make a difficult decision. I was on the freeway, and as I drove, I started praying about it. "Give me a sign, god. Tell me yes or no." Then, right out of the blue, I had a full-body orgasm. "Well," I thought, "I asked for a sign, and this sure feels like a yes." I realized, then, that sex has to do with a lot more than just physical joining with another person. It's an energetic opening to the universe. It's our body's way of saying yes, yes, yes.

DEBORAH

A couple of years ago I was walking through the forest, by myself. It was evening, and I was lying on the ground, watching the last rays of the sunlight filter through the trees. And suddenly, my whole body was flooded with sweetness, like warm honey pouring through me, so sensual. I don't know how long it lasted; I lost all sense of time. This may sound strange but it really felt as if a divine being had touched me and made love to me. Afterward, I felt a very full, complete sense of peace and a satisfaction that stayed with me for days.

INÈS

nion. According to the sixteenth-century Indian mystic Mirabai, nothing in the world can match the joy of union with the divine Beloved. When asked why she had no interest in worldly love, Mirabai laughed and mockingly replied: "I have felt the swaying of the elephant's shoulders . . . and now you want me to climb on a jackass? Try to be serious!"[33]

Theresa's ecstatic nightly communions did nothing to mitigate her frustration at the dullness of her daytime routines. Intuitively, she knew that to portray sexuality as sinful and evil was wrong. Two years after she joined the convent, just a few days before she was to take the final vows that would forever bind her to the church, she exploded with rebellious fury. When her rage finally erupted, it slashed and burned everything that stood in the way of her sexual and expressive freedom and saved her from making what would have been, for her, a disastrous commitment.

I was a really good nun, a perfect nun, an extremely obedient nun. And I really thought I was going to find god. Of course, I already had, internally. I was having all kinds of mystical experiences including making love to god every night. But I thought there was something else beyond that, something external, and I hadn't attained it. So I looked for god in every genuflection and in every rosary bead and in every nun's face, and I couldn't find anything. I was bored to death. I thought if I was only obedient enough or prayed enough and tried hard enough, I would have experiences that I assumed all the other nuns were having. Little did I know they weren't having them either.

I left the convent in a wonderfully dramatic way. When you started menstruating, you would go to the Mother Superior, and tell her you were menstruating, and could you please have a Kotex? You only got one at a time. It's part of the vow of poverty: you own nothing; you don't plan for the future. I had done this for two years, no problem. I would go to her, tell her I needed a Kotex, then we would walk up the staircase, and she would take out her keys. One key would unlock the door, another a cabinet. All in all, there were two doors and four cabinets she had to go through to get the one Kotex. I had gone through this ritual obediently for two years.

This month, for some reason, things were different. I get my period, and I go to the Mother Superior, as usual. She starts unlocking all these doors, and for some reason, I suddenly think, "Oh my god, they have locked away sex!" That thought had never occurred to me before. Then she hands me the one pad and I say to her, "Mother Superior, I would like to have *two*." And she says, very sternly, "Sister Theresa, you know that you can have as many as you want, but only one at a time." And I said, "I want *two!*" And she says, "No, Sister Theresa, you cannot have two. You can only have one."

That was it. Everything I had repressed and didn't even know was in me just gurgled its way up. I started screaming at her: "You fucking bitch!" I went bananas, absolutely crazy. My whole behavior was totally cathartic and spontaneous. I had not cussed in two years, and I called her every name in the book. I went ballistic on her. It was fabulous, and it felt wonderful. At the same time I was taken aback by myself, to say the least. She didn't know what the hell to do with me. I was unrelenting, and I was shaking with adrenaline. It was totally involuntary, like a river. I gave her a big lecture on sex and what I thought about the Catholic church. Finally, she said she thought I should go to my room and calm down. "That's exactly what I want to do, and I am going to pack, too," I announced.

It is probably no coincidence that Theresa's explosion occurred right at the onset of her period. At this time of the month, we are proverbially bitchy. We fly off the handle easily. We are as volatile as a tankful of gasoline sitting in the desert sun, and as prickly as a cactus. A priest in India once told me that menstruating women were not allowed to enter his temple, because they had too much fire and might literally set the building ablaze. Like menstrual blood, women's anger is red, hot, active, and potent, and once a month, it sees an opportunity to surface. The flames leap higher, and sometimes, especially if anger has been chronically repressed, the blaze may get so hot that the container explodes. As Theresa's story demonstrates, that is not always a bad thing. After all, her anger had something important to tell her. "This situation is bad for you," it was yelling. "Don't just ignore it. Do something! Get out!"

But Theresa did not pack, as she had threatened—at least not immediately. The Mother Superior waited for Theresa to calm down, and then came and convinced her that she had gone too far, that she should reconsider, and that, if she was willing to apologize in front of the community, all would be forgiven. "Well," Theresa told me, "I went into prayer, and then I decided to go ahead and do that. And I did. I formally acknowledged I had been disobedient and arrogant."

But I only stayed on for one more week. It was the week before I was to take my final vows, and I got to see my mother for the first time in two years. You can't see your parents while you are in training. My mother came, and I was so excited and happy to see her. Your parents are allowed to give you one gift, because you are about to take your final vows. But according to the rule, you don't get to keep it. You have to give it to the Mother Superior, and she then gives it to anyone in the community who she thinks needs it most. You are supposed to surrender control over it.

Well, my mother brought me a beautiful sterling silver pen, and I did not want to give it up. I treasured it so much. I lied to Mother Superior and told her my parents were too poor to buy me a present. Then I hid the pen. Throughout the next week, I kept getting up in the middle of the night with a flashlight and writing with my pen. It was a way of feeling close to my mother. The day before the final ceremony, I knew I couldn't go through with it. The pen was a catalyst. It symbolized the mother to me. I loved my mother very much, and she loved me very much. Whatever goodness and capacity to love I have came from her. They were trying to take my mother away, and I couldn't allow it. So that was it. I left.

How accurately our instincts can inform us, when we listen to them! Though still unsure of her right to sexual expression, Theresa knew better than to cut herself off from her beloved mother. Much later, she learned that worship of the divine Mother is an absolutely essential element of Tantric teachings. But even as a young girl, Theresa sensed that she was on the verge of a step that would have constituted a terrible act of self-betrayal. Instead, she clung to the motherline, the feminine lineage that connected her to her grandmothers, to the wisewomen among her ancestors, and to the goddess herself. To this day, Theresa told me, she treasures her silver pen.

Many sexual adventures followed in the wake of Theresa's departure from the convent, including a passionate love affair with a priest, and a ten-year-long marriage. "My relationships fall into two categories," Theresa explained, "those that were Tantric, and those that were not." Her marriage, though not unhappy, was not based on an ecstatic sexual connection, but satisfied her desire for family and children. The most important Tantric relationship of her life, she told me, began in her thirties, coinciding with her formal initiation into the practice of Tantra. Here is her account of her first meeting with the man who was to be both her lover and her Tantric teacher:

> Andrew came in the room, and we looked at each other. Instantly, everything in the whole room disappeared except for him, and I saw this gold dust. Everything was gold dust, and it was alive. It looked like golden sperm, moving all around. Later he told me he saw it, too. Our eyes met, and we took a breath together, and we knew right away we were connected. To this day, our breaths match impeccably. We have the same breath, exactly the same rhythm and spacing.

Such stories help us understand why Aphrodite is called the golden goddess. Like Theresa, some people perceive Aphrodite's presence as a fine gold dust, a gold powder, or a shimmering, golden cloud, while others describe a sensation like liquid gold streaming through their limbs.

Though not everyone has seen auras, they are real, and in Aphrodite's presence their radiance increases a hundredfold. "Aura" is actually a Greek word that means "breath," or "breeze." Translate the Greek term into Latin, and you have *spiritus,* another word that also means "wind" or "breath"—specifically, the breath of god. The lovers' shared breath and their golden aura are not two separate phenomena. Rather, breath and aura, divine light and divine breath, are one and the same. Both refer to the sacred energy that enlivens us from within and is made manifest both as our breath and as the shining, shimmering aura that envelops our body.

Every time you take a breath, you feed and nourish your aura. Therefore, Tantra places great emphasis on conscious breathing as a means of supplying the body not just with oxygen, but with life-force. This breath of life is especially sacred to Aphrodite. It is said that in the moment of her birth, as the goddess arose from the oceanic waters of Being, gentle breezes appeared to caress her body and carry her to shore. These breezes remain eternally at play around their mistress, signaling the presence of the holy spirit, the divine breath of life.

Breathing as one, enveloped in golden light, the lovers-to-be stood enchanted by Aphrodite's touch, riveted by the arrows of Eros. The life-force came charging in and instantly the inner lights turned on, fans whirred into motion, juices began to flow, and the inner serpent raised its head, suddenly wide awake and alert. As one might gather from Theresa's account of her first meeting with Andrew, their relationship revolved entirely around an ecstatic sexual connection. Further down the road, serious personal differences would undermine their love, but in the meantime, Theresa received a thorough training in Tantric sexuality and learned how to consciously cultivate her capacity for sacred union. Making love with Andrew, Theresa would see visions of gods and goddesses. Eventually, the intensity of the sexual experience triggered the full awakening of her Kundalini energy.

We were always making love, all the time. Several times a day, sometimes. So the Kundalini was constantly running. I would feel it dancing through each chakra, sometimes jumping around, opening and opening. Everything was opening and undulating. The sensations were intensely voluptuous, with full-body orgasms, accompanied by a cosmic sense of universal love. None of my experiences were of the painful kind that people sometimes describe in connection with Kundalini. I believe that through all the psychological work I had done, and in particular through seven years of Reichian bodywork, I had prepared myself. Also, I had lived such a rich sexual life since I was a small child. My body knew how to access that opening.

My longest Kundalini experience was twelve days. Again, it felt like gold liquid dust or golden lava flowing through me. During that time I didn't eat, I just drank water. The concept of eating food seemed strange. I remember seeing someone with a bowl of rice, looking at the rice, and thinking, "Doesn't he know that you don't have to eat food? That all you have to do is breathe?" When I looked at that rice, all I saw were atoms and molecules moving around. In those twelve days, my Kundalini moved all the way to the crown, and my consciousness settled there. I just sat in front of my altar. There was no place else for me to be, no place I could even conceive of going. It seemed like the most wonderful, glorious blessing.

All her life, Theresa has known sacred union. She knew it when, as a child, she lay on the earth and merged with god. She knew it when she and her first lover lay in the haystack, looking up at the moon. She knew it in her narrow nun's cot, when she called on god as her Beloved, and he came to fill her body and soul with ecstasy. Pondering the fact that Theresa has experienced sacred union both through devotional love and through sexual love, I asked her whether these two different routes took her to different states of consciousness. She stopped to think, then vigorously shook her red curls.

In essence, it's the same thing. The other person acts as a conduit for the experience, but then your lover just disappears. My lover disappeared hundreds of times, and I was just with the light. I knew he was in his own transcendental experience. I can take myself to bliss with meditation, too. It's a different way of getting there, but I go to the same place. It is a place I knew when I was just four or five years old, and it's a place I will always know.

In the West, we have put spirituality and sexuality in separate boxes. But these categories seem entirely inappropriate and irrelevant to the journey of a priestess. When a woman has a great capacity for sacred union, she will open into such union wherever it presents itself, be it in church or in the bedroom. In Theresa's opinion, the path of mystical devotion and the path of sacred sexual union cannot and should not be separated. From the onset of her life, her soul has waited with open arms for the embrace of the divine lover. Why, then, would she reject him when he appears to her in the form of a human man?

Theresa's life has been extremely rich and multifaceted. She has been married and has stepmothered four children. She has had several deeply passionate relationships. She has nursed one of her sons through death. Throughout all her ups and downs, her devotion to the path of ecstatic union has remained unswerving. Theresa laughs as she talks about the irony that she, who was once determined to become a nun, should have ended up as a Tantric adept. Clearly, this woman was not destined to give up the joys of love. "I have been to the top of the mountain," she says with pride. "I have known the highest forms of love. Whether or not I have a lover, I am going to teach Tantra until I am ninety years old. I will always teach Tantra; it's my spiritual path."

11

THE STORY OF A NUN

And God said to the soul:
I desired you before the world began.
I desire you now
As you desire me.
And where the desires of two come together
There love is perfected.
Mechtild of Magdeburg, thirteenth century C.E.

What does a woman do whose soul is hungry for nourishment? Where does she turn for sustenance? How does she respond to the call of spirit? For Isabelle, raised in a devout Catholic household, the answer was clear. On her tenth birthday, she announced to her mother she was going to be a nun. Her mother greeted the news with a smile, assuming that time would change her child's mind. But by the time Isabelle was eighteen, she had made her choice for good. One night, her mother scolded her and said, "I don't know what's going to become of you." Without a moment's hesitation, Isabelle replied, "I'll tell you what's going to become of me. I am going to be a sister."

Today, Isabelle is in her sixties and has been a nun for over thirty years. A short, stocky woman with clear gray eyes and fine black hair, she has a pale, open face that speaks of a life lived in service to others. Though she lacks many of the material luxuries most women in our society take for granted, she nonetheless enjoys a rich, fulfilling life. She has a strong spiritual community and loves her work as a spiritual counselor.

In recent years, however, Isabelle has been questioning her commitment to religious life and to the Catholic church. Like Theresa, she has come to the conclusion that it is both unhealthy and unnecessary to impose lifelong celibacy upon lovers of god. Where celibacy is idealized, spiritual pride will inevitably tempt people to pretend they have transcended sexual desire, when this is in fact far from true. Religious hypocrisy then breeds aberrations such as child-molesting priests and supposedly enlightened gurus who secretly have sex with their followers. If we would lead sexually healthy lives, we need to overcome the untrue and dangerous idea that our spiritual role models should be celibate.

On the other hand, celibacy does not always equal sexual repression. Religious history abounds with men and women who loved life passionately and appreciated sex, yet chose to be celibate for a variety of reasons. Until very recently, one important factor was the absence of reliable birth control. A woman wishing to dedicate her life to spiritual pursuits might naturally seek refuge in celibacy, not out of any aversion to sex, but because she did not want to devote her time and energy to raising children. Also, in many patriarchal societies, women were (and still are) given to their husbands like chattel, with little or no say in the matter. Down through the centuries, women trapped in loveless marriages have turned to the monastic way of life as an escape from virtual slavery. In the sixth century B.C.E., Sumangalamata, one of the earliest followers of the Buddha and the former wife of a shade-maker, rejoiced when she became a nun:

> At last free,
> at last I am a woman free!
> No more tied to the kitchen,
> stained amid the stained pots,
> no more bound to the husband
> who thought me less
> than the shade he wove with his hands.
> No more anger, no more hunger,
> I sit now in the shade of my own tree.
> Meditating thus, I am happy, I am serene.[34]

Today, most women have more freedom and control than Sumangalamata did. Still, celibacy can be a way of affirming, both to ourselves and to the world, our freedom of choice.

I first met Isabelle when she offered a workshop on the issue of celibacy. "Nowadays, celibacy is not exactly popular," she commented with a wry smile when only a handful of people showed up. But those who came were grateful for the rare opportunity to talk about celibacy. Except for Isabelle herself, they were all laypeople who wanted to step back from sexual involvement, for a limited period of time or forever. They named a wide range of reasons for their desire to be celibate. Some had found that relationships required more time and energy than they were willing to give. Others needed time to heal from losses or disappointments. One man acknowledged that he had used sex to distract himself from his inner process and to avoid confronting his real problems. Six months ago, he had committed himself to a year of celibacy as a means of breaking old, dysfunctional habits. An attractive young woman talked about her tendency to overgive, to say yes when she should have said no, and of prostituting herself for a few morsels of male affection. Sex, we all agreed, involves a give-and-take of energy, which often leads to other exchanges involving time, emotional energy, money, living space, and creativity. Closing our sexual boundaries for a period of time can reflect our commitment to becoming mindful of such exchanges. As I listened to the participants in Isabelle's workshop tell their stories, I understood that in an age where we tend to feel we "should" be sexually active, celibacy remains a valid and sometimes extremely empowering option.

Offering people the opportunity to talk about celibacy is important to Isabelle. With some bitterness, she told me that when she took her vows of celibacy, nobody discussed the implications with her. Unlike Theresa, whose story we heard in the last chapter, Isabelle was sexually unawakened and had no concept of what she was being asked to commit to. The fact that becoming a nun meant sacrificing her sexual life barely registered in her teenage mind. With childlike innocence, she believed what she had been taught—that the body was untrustworthy and spiritually unenlightened, and that it had to be firmly subjugated to Christian discipline. In hind-

THE GIFTS OF CELIBACY

I have been celibate for seven years, and celibacy has really worked for me. Ironically, all the years I screwed around I never knew myself as a sexual being, and it took being celibate to know myself. I became celibate because I wasn't willing to settle for less than total intimacy, and I knew that I always had settled for less. Though I had never experienced intimacy, I knew intuitively what it was, and I knew it was not about fondling body parts. Now, there is nothing left in me that would use sexuality to manipulate. Finally, I feel free of the addiction to the male. I am about to become sexual again, and I don't think I will fall back into the addiction.

OLGA

sight, Isabelle feels that the church misled her and stole a very precious part of her being.

I went to Catholic school, and everything having to do with sex was considered a mortal sin. That really terrorized me and affected me very deeply. In high school I dated, and some of my boyfriends wanted sex, but my terror wouldn't allow it. I never questioned the rules at that time. This was it, and it was harsh. There was a tremendous amount of repression.

Though Isabelle's decision to become a nun was taken in ignorance of the consequences, it also arose in response to a true inner calling.

I had my first very powerful religious experience around the question of joining the order. I was in my room praying, and a being of great light came to me. All the confusion and conflict left, and I was absolutely certain that I wanted to join the community. There was no question in me. The conviction didn't come out of a thought process, but out of a deep inner

SEX AND CHURCH

I went to Catholic school. Once a year, we would have a retreat with the Jesuits, and they would always tell us this story. In the story, there's this couple who make out in the car, which is a mortal sin. Then, they back out of the parking space into an on-coming truck and are instantly killed, so they don't get a chance to go to confession and confess their sins, and—boom! They're stuck in hell for the rest of eternity. I believed that story, and it scared the hell out of me. Sex became linked to the danger of hell as well as the danger of pregnancy. I don't know which I was more afraid of. At the same time, it heightened the erotic charge. I started having to confess impure thoughts and impure actions. I had to keep track of how many times I had them, and I would play games with myself because if I really counted all of them there would have been far too many. So I would discount some. It became an elaborate mind game. VALERIE

knowing. All the ego reasons for and against had not a thing to do with it.

Five years after joining the order, Isabelle took the vows that represented her ceremony of marriage to Jesus Christ. Among them, the central one was the vow to put her life in the hands of spirit, and to surrender her own will to the will of god. In the language of the temple priestess, we might say that she was promising to become god's lover and bride. Before taking these final vows, Isabelle had another mystical experience; god, she felt, was confirming his desire for her. Her voice full of wonder, she told me:

As I was reviewing the words of the vows I was to take in a few weeks, I felt god coming to me. It was as if god was saying: "I am the one to whom you are offering these vows." I experienced a clear calling for which I was deeply grateful. Later, when I was in great turmoil over the question of whether to stay a nun, the memory of these two events helped

> When I was thirteen, I had a very strong sense that what my Sunday school teacher was teaching me was false. It was one of those epiphanies of knowing. I just knew that it was wrong, that the Bible was not about what they said it was about. I went home and told my mother I never wanted to go back to Sunday school again, and I never did. EVA
>
> In first communion, at age seven, I had a mystical experience. I received god into myself. I remember how the light came down through the clouds on the way to church. As I was saying the prayers I felt such grace, such sweetness, such a funneling down of light into my being. But later, religion compounded my troubles, because it taught me a lot of fear and self-judgment. The nuns said it's a mortal sin if you touch yourself to climax, and I felt very burdened by that, and tormented by the fact that I couldn't keep from having "bad" thoughts. There was such a web of guilt. PAULINE

me stick it out until I had some kind of clarity about my path. I just couldn't ignore such powerful experiences.

Initially, Isabelle said, she thought of god as "a taskmaster." When we perceive god as a taskmaster, we assume that we are in need of correction and improvement. God is in his heaven, unobtainable in his perfection, and we are down here, flawed and imperfect. A chasm separates us from the divine that can never be crossed. But then, Isabelle said, a shift occurred in her prayer.

At first, I had seen god as a scriptural figure, a majestic power. There had always been a definite hierarchy and a distance. Now, I became aware of a very loving attraction, and I was flooded with love. It was very intimate and engrossing. I have never been the same since. My experience of god changed radically. It was a flowering of devotion, and looking back, I see its erotic nature, though I didn't at the time.

To relate to god as our lover is a different thing entirely from seeing him as a taskmaster. A lover is our equal. Though in certain ways we always remain children of the divine, in another way, we are also god's partners in the adventure of creation and the dance of love. In this dance, god needs us as much as we need him, and is waiting for us with all the eagerness and impatience of a young lover.

In another profound mystical experience, god appeared to Isabelle in the form of a red light that filled her with indescribable joy and love. Red is, of course, the color of passion, the color of vibrant life-force, the color of blood, the color of Aphrodite's roses. However, Isabelle hastened to add, she was not encouraged to dwell on the erotic aspects of her inner life. Instead, she firmly put aside all awareness of her sexuality. Decades passed in quiet service. Every now and then, some small indication of the passionate nature smoldering beneath rigid layers of repression would appear. Once, in response to a question about her inner life, Isabelle spontaneously described herself as a "seething volcano." Afterward she wondered, "Now what on earth made me say that?"

Then when Isabelle was fifty years old, the stifled volcano erupted full force. "What happened," she told me, "was that I fell passionately in love with another woman—not a nun, but a layperson. And she fell in love with me, too." Falling silent, Isabelle looked down, seemingly examining her hands, which lay quietly folded in her lap. After a long minute, she looked up at me with her clear gray eyes and said, "I decided to let love lead me." Demonstrating an amazing soul courage, Isabelle opened to sexual pleasure for the first time in her life, knowing full well that she was breaking two strong taboos at once—the taboo against nuns having sex, and the taboo against same-sex love. None of this deterred her. When I asked Isabelle what prepared the way for her sexual awakening, and what gave her the courage to act on such a doubly forbidden desire, she mentioned two factors.

First, there was a period during which I felt a great upwelling of shame over what I perceived as my sterility. A tremendous amount of self-hatred came up. I felt that I was a sterile, loveless woman. It was the opposite of sexual shame. I was ashamed for *not* being juicy and sensual. I raged about it week after week. Now I see that I was preparing for the plunge.

A second important event was a retreat at which I felt a strong call to a natural way of life. I thought about the words of Jesus when he said that not even Solomon, in all his wisdom, could equal the birds of the air. And I thought, "Yes, they live in harmony with nature." The night I made the choice to become sexual with my woman lover, the inner Nazi guards were all there in all their array and power and fury, trying to bar my way. But then I thought about what Jesus had said about the birds of the air. I kept asking myself, "Which path feels more god-like?" And the answer was clearly that it felt more divine to go with my feelings for this woman. So I did.

The simplicity of these words belies the immensity of Isabelle's step and the depth of courage required to consciously transgress the rules of her order. Behind these words, we see the power of the priestess at work, her commitment to following the spiritual path, no matter where it leads.

To Isabelle, who had never made love, the experience was a revelation, an utterly joyful discovery of her femininity. God, already something of an erotic presence in her life, now touched her through her own desire, her pleasure, and the joy of knowing her sexual potential for the first time. Contrary to what she had been taught about the supposedly "unspiritual" nature of the body, Isabelle now found deep experiences of the sacred arising spontaneously out of the depths of her own body. Like Alexandra (Chapter 2), Isabelle found that her sexual initiation was also an initiation into the feminine face of god:

I had never been sexually involved, and I loved it. It was marvelous. I was surprised at myself. Despite all this repression, I was never afraid of sexuality. I didn't feel any sense of shame at all. I felt a real fullness of life and love. It was very beautiful and very healing. My femininity blossomed greatly, and I learned to cherish and honor the feminine. I also began to think of god as mother, and of earth as mother. The maternal aspect of god which has been so missing in the Western tradition is very present to me now. It was an extraordinary gift.

In the Bible, sexual intercourse is called having "knowledge" of another. We all have a deep desire to be fully known, not just emotionally or mentally, but also physically. The body rejoices when it feels truly touched, recognized, and celebrated, and it grieves when we condemn it to remain forever unknown and unacknowledged. No wonder the experience of being known through her body opened Isabelle's eyes and heart to a whole new dimension of her spirituality. Finally, she knew that she was completely lovable in the eyes of spirit, and that no part of her needed to be excluded from this love. At the same time, Isabelle was leading a double life and was tormented by doubt and uncertainty.

My whole world cracked open, and I deeply questioned celibacy for the first time. Sex with my lover was so powerful and wonderful. Every two or three months, I would say: "I'm out of this church, I'm finished with it." But, of course, I had very deep bonds with the community. I was going through hell because I wanted to be a person of integrity, and yet I was living a lie. Everybody thought I was keeping my vows when I wasn't. There were only two people with whom I shared what was happening—my spiritual adviser and my therapist. Both were very supportive and encouraged me to find my own way.

Like most priestesses, Isabelle wanted nothing more than to live in harmony with her community. Instead, she found herself cast in the uncomfortable role of rebel. Whereas in the past she had approached the church as a parent to whose authority she submitted with childlike faith, she now had no choice but to depend upon her own spiritual authority. Thus, her sexual initiation translated into a spiritual initiation. Firmly and courageously, she claimed the right to make her own choices, sexually and otherwise.

According to the old framework, I was committing terrible sins and was not allowed to take Communion in that state.

But I continued to go to Communion and felt totally connected to god. I was consciously rejecting a lot of the old teachings. I was leaving the hierarchy and the patriarchy behind, and making my own choices. I was changing dramatically from being subservient to the rules and regulations to seeing myself as a person equal to anybody else and qualified to make my own decisions. I was claiming my knowledge, my power, and my authority.

Claiming her own authority is possibly the most important step that a contemporary priestess can take. Today, many of us are grappling with the challenge of becoming fully responsible, mature adults. For untold centuries, we lived as spiritual children who bowed to the authority of supposedly wiser authorities or institutions. Like all children, we often had to sacrifice our personal truth in order to conform to the rules of our religious communities. Now such authoritarian structures no longer serve us. More and more, we are beginning to explore our own, personal spirituality. And very often, sexual issues act as the catalyst, forcing us to take a stand against the collective and to make the sort of difficult decision that Isabelle faced at this point in her life. "What did you do?" I asked Isabelle. Quietly, she replied:

I didn't know what to do, so I waited. Month after month, I waited for clarity. I meditated, I prayed, and I worked deeply with my psychotherapist to clear my inner space of any old conditioning that might influence my decision. I realized I needed to not listen to any outside voices, but to go within. I knew I had to find out what was true for me and where my calling lay. I had to get below the surface of everything, down to the core of who I was. It took a long, long time. All I could do was sit and wait for insight.

And gradually, a knowing came that I was meant to renew my vows and live the life of a nun. I understood that I was meant to stay in religious life. This knowing came from no rational place, but from the deepest core of my soul.

Some may feel that Isabelle made the wrong choice, and that she betrayed herself. For many, the Catholic church looms large as a bastion of hypocrisy, misogyny, and sexual repression. Certainly, this was how Isabelle's lover saw the situation:

> My decision was very difficult for my lover to accept. She viewed the structure I belonged to as deeply repressive, and she saw me as just following the rules and regulations out of fear. But this was not true. She never understood that in me. She never understood that my decision was not made out of guilt or fear or repression, but that it arose from a true knowing.

It takes courage to share our sexual stories. Like Irene, who broke her marriage vows, Isabelle knows how quick people are to pass judgment in sexual matters. Some would judge her harshly for breaking her vows of celibacy, others for renewing those very same vows. Perhaps because I had the opportunity to sit with Isabelle and to see the sincerity and integrity of her spiritual quest, I felt only deep respect for her choice. My own path has taught me that the rational mind is not qualified to fathom the soul's mysterious, circuitous pathways.

We can all remember times when we had to make a difficult decision that would affect the rest of our lives. We all can think of moments when we, too, stood at the crossroads, wondering which path to take. What touched me most about Isabelle's story is the way that, throughout her difficult journey, she always listened to her soul and never hesitated to obey its wishes, though everyone else might disapprove. In this uncompromising determination to follow the lead of her own soul, she has found the core of her spiritual strength. Every choice she made on her journey—the choice to become a nun, the choice to explore her sexuality, and finally, the choice to renew her vows of celibacy—arose from a deep state of prayer in which she connected with the quiet voice of her innermost spiritual knowing. Like a pregnant woman, she waited patiently for her truth to gestate until it was ready to be birthed into the light of consciousness.

Whenever we do this, we step into what I call womb-space.

Womb-space is where divine inspiration can be received, where it can gestate and be contained throughout the delicate process of maturation. The womb symbolizes a quality of being that both men and women can tap into. In a culture obsessed with goals and achievements, womb-space reminds us of the value of process. To wait, to patiently sit in the dark without knowing what the outcome will be, to protect and respect that which has as yet no clear form—all these are aspects of the womb.

Womb-space is essential to any creative endeavor. The inspiration that will one day become a work of art, a baby, or a new phase of life must be nurtured in patience and devotion until it is ready to emerge. Like physical gestation, the inner process has its own timing which cannot be rushed. One must be willing to wait, as Isabelle waited, receptive and empty, day after week after month. This is no dull, dead waiting, but a vibrant, pulsating presence, an alert awareness of what is needed in each moment. Womb-space demands our humility. We are not in control of our creative process, and there is no guarantee that there really will be a birth, let alone that what is born will please us.

Not surprisingly, Isabelle has found it difficult to embrace her final decision. The chasm that separates her from the official church leadership is deep and irreconcilable. She has renewed her commitment not to the Catholic orthodoxy, but to the lineage of men and women who, for the last two thousand years, have followed the teachings of Jesus Christ. However, the price she has paid for her recommitment has been extraordinarily high. Having briefly lifted her sexual repression, she continues to struggle with the question of how to relate to her sexual energy. Her words reflect the hardship of attempting to reconcile two seemingly irreconcilable needs.

I have had to struggle with enormous rage. I felt so enraged that I was not taught that the body is beautiful and that sexuality is a tremendous gift. My deepest rage is about the existential situation I am in. I have chosen to be part of a religious order in which I have taken vows of chastity and celibacy for life. I don't question the decision and the deep place of knowing it came from. But my mind can't accept it. I just recently discovered my body, my sexuality, and my sensuality. Now, the decision to stay in religious life means that I have to say no to the full expression of it. For many months, I felt like god had played a very mean trick on me. Week after week I felt stuck in the rage. It has subsided somewhat, but parts of myself are still at war. Why am I in this bind?

Isabelle is in this bind, I would suggest, because of her deep love for her religious heritage and because of her desire to stay connected to the community she loves. The dilemma in which she finds herself is the dilemma of any individual whose spiritual life is bound to the life of an organization, a religion, or a culture, and who discovers that her personal understanding has outgrown that of the collective. The presence of dissident voices within the Catholic church is, of course, nothing new. Though the orthodox leaders might wish it were otherwise, the church has always included many diverse and conflicting strands of belief and has been claimed as a spiritual home by many whose views clash with official pronouncements.

During Isabelle's early years as a nun, she did not discriminate between surrender to the will of god and surrender to the church. Today she does. Her sexual awakening has taught her that she cannot depend on outer authorities to guide her wisely, since these authorities have, in many cases, lost touch with the feminine way and will actively repress those who attempt to reclaim their inner knowledge. Now, Isabelle's surrender is only to the mysterious force that speaks to her in the innermost chamber of her own soul. She has chosen to give herself fully to the work she loves, the work of spiritual counseling, but she counsels according to her own convictions, not according to church doctrine. Thoughtfully, she says:

> I feel my purpose is to be part of the healing of the sexual wound from within the church. In a deeper sense, I belong to the church community, but I have definitely not submitted to the official views of the church, and I often do not agree with the hierarchy. I listen, I sort through what makes sense to me and what doesn't, and I follow my own wisdom. I don't have all the answers, but neither do the church leaders. I am one of many Catholics who do not agree with the repressive teach-

ings, and we, too, represent the church. I work with many priests who are in agony and conflict over their sexuality. I feel sad when I think of all those priests who are caught in sexual deviancy. Many feel confused, and they are rarely encouraged to get in touch with their own inner wisdom.

I want to help religious people become free to open to the adventure of their sexuality, knowing the dangers and yet also knowing the possibility of a fuller life. It seems very important. They really want to open to god and to the fullness of life, but the restrictions are so great. I am very wary about telling my story publicly because I don't want to lose my credibility with people who are still caught in the rules. These people listen to what I say because they see me as a good nun. And in that role, I can effect a lot of change.

Today, Isabelle embodies strength, outspokenness, independence, inner authority, and courage, which, though often excluded from the patriarchal ideal of womanhood, are nonetheless essential to the feminine spirit and to the path of the priestess. Isabelle is recognized by her community as a woman of Spirit, a woman able to reflect back to others the essence of their own inner truth. Does she regret what has happened? "Oh, no," Isabelle says firmly, "not for a moment. I feel a lot of excitement about my life. I am learning about the body, and about the ways energy flows, and I am teaching whatever I learn. Opening to sexuality has brought passion and creativity back into my life. I have so much more spontaneity and joy, thank god."

12

THE SACRED MARRIAGE

This marriage be wine with halvah, honey dissolving in milk.
This marriage be the leaves and fruit of a date tree.
This marriage be women laughing together for days on end.
This marriage, a sign for us to study.
This marriage, beauty.
This marriage, a moon in a light-blue sky.
This marriage, this silence fully mixed with spirit.
                              Rumi, on the occasion of his son's wedding

If, as some say, the world is a school of love, then committed part-nership is the graduate program. So compelling is the urge to mate that we spend an incredible amount of time and energy looking for partners, courting them, maintaining our relationships, grieving over their loss, and starting all over again. Obviously, our obsession goes way beyond the simple need to procreate. Nature, it seems, has installed a little computer chip in our psyche that programs us to re-spond to the mating game with insane eagerness. Jung called such invisible chips archetypes; among them, the image of sacred mar-riage is one of the most potent. Like a vision of paradise, it glows and shimmers enticingly within the depths of our psyche, fueling our longing for a lifelong, committed partnership.

Archetypes are teachers, gateways to spiritual wisdom. One way or another, they ask to be lived and realized in the outer world, and as we attempt to translate the inner vision into an outer reality, we learn many of the most important lessons of our lives. When the ar-chetype of sacred marriage awakens, one woman may start to look for a mate. Another may join a religious order and become the bride of Christ, as did Isabelle, whose story we heard in the previous chapter. Either way, the archetype will lead her into situations that challenge her to develop strength and wisdom.

Consider the countless couples in world legend, mythology, literature, and art—Romeo and Juliet, Adam and Eve, Shiva and Shakti, Elizabeth Taylor and Richard Burton, Zeus and Hera, Isis and Osiris, and so on and on. People of all times and cultures have expressed their vision of the sacred marriage. Think of how many fairy tales end with the hero or the heroine finding a mate, getting married, and living happily ever after. Popular movies follow the same storyline. Something deep inside of us wants that marriage to happen very badly, and feels content when it does, as if the world were finally in order. Why do so many people cry at weddings? Is it not because weddings evoke and comfort a part of us that grieves for the loss of paradise? Creation, marvelous as it is, has shattered the original, unbroken wholeness into billions of shards, and fragmentation has brought us pain, loss, and separation. Marriage symbolizes the reconciliation of all opposites and the resolution of all conflicts. It points to the possibility of atonement, at-one-ment, the possibility of ending all alienation.

In mythology, this ultimate reconciliation is often celebrated as the marriage of god and goddess. With their union, creation begins, and through their union, a state of peace and harmony is periodically restored. Our collective psyche needs such images of sacred union, and when religion fails to provide them, it will simply look elsewhere. Every time the American people elect a new president (so far, never a woman), his wife attracts as much attention as he does, for the new god must have his goddess. Of course, the pendulum swings in both directions: she who has been deified can count on being demonized within short order. Still, people insist on having their sacred couples, if not as god and goddess or proud king and gracious queen, then at least as president and first lady. Intuitively, we sense how important the image of the sacred couple is to the entire community. The passion that fuses two into one might appear to be a very private affair, and yet the strength of our community as a whole depends on the strength of its families. And at the core of each family lies the mystery of sacred sexual union. From that core, everything else expands in concentric circles—the sharing of food and shelter, the raising of children, the involvement in community affairs, the passion for creating a livable future for the next generations.

The archetype of marriage radiates an otherworldly glow, a magic, an aura of numinousness. Once we step into its orbit, we are bewitched, entranced, captured. Sometimes, the inner pressure to live out the ideal acquires such urgency that it blinds us to reality. It can make us grasp at totally inappropriate partners, mistake projections for truth, confuse lust and love, and generally act like fools. The Australian film *Muriel's Wedding* tells the story of a woman who has fallen under the spell of the marriage archetype. Muriel is a homely girl who lives in the suburbs and who dreams, day in and day out, of her wedding day. Obsessed with marriage, she sneaks into bridal salons in order to try on creamy white satin bridal gowns and frothy lace veils. As she admires herself in full-length mirrors, she sees a woman whose insecurity, depression, and shame have vanished, a woman made whole and beautiful by the love of a man, an ugly duckling turned into a glorious white swan. Marriage, she trusts, is a miracle that will take care of all her woes and make her feel loved and complete. All wounds will be healed, all injuries undone, all wrongs righted.

We may smile at her naiveté. But most of us marry in part because of an entirely irrational pull that is, after all, not that different from Muriel's. We want to experience marriage, and we want it to work, against all odds. Even now that unmarried partnerships have become quite acceptable in many circles, we still love a beautiful wedding. We long to see the archetype of sacred marriage embodied in flesh and blood. A good marriage touches us deeply because it reassures us it can be done. Regardless of our religious beliefs, we sense the sacredness that underlies the cliché, the deep archetypal truth of man and woman joined in a committed union.

Once couples strip off the romantic paradise projections, they usually discover that marriage is part paradise, part purgatory. Fooled by Aphrodite's romantic glamour, newlyweds often assume they are just opting for a good life when in fact, they are consenting to the death of their old self. They are about to say yes not just to another individual, but to a process that will dissolve their old identity. Speaking of his own marriage, the famous mythologist Joseph Campbell said, "When I married Jean, I felt it was a crucifixion.

The bridegroom does go to the bride as to the cross. The bride gives herself equally. It's a reciprocal crucifixion. In marriage you are not sacrificing yourself to the other person. You are sacrificing yourself to the relationship."[35]

Aphrodite, you may recall, was married to Hephaistos, a lame and unattractive god whose main distinction was his extraordinary skill as jeweler, smith, and craftsman. From our normal vantage point, this makes no sense. Why would the most beautiful of all goddesses, who could have married any god she pleased, choose to marry the least attractive of them all?

But the language of mythology is not the language of daily human life. Aphrodite and Hephaistos are mated because they present two complementary messages about the mysteries of love. Aphrodite embodies the visceral sexual chemistry, the glamour, and the romance that entice men and women into the adventure of love. Hephaistos the goldsmith, on the other hand, demonstrates the great work of purification achieved by fire in the deep forge of the god, which transforms lovers into priests and priestesses of the golden light. From Aphrodite's vantage point, love looks like a delicious, tantalizing game. But for Hephaistos, attraction is merely the raw ore which must be melted down and refined in the fires of love, hammered this way and that. He knows that, like the precious metal, the gold of married love is not easy to come by. It does not lie around for the taking, but must be painstakingly mined by those courageous enough to descend into the hidden depths of their psyche and skillful enough to purify the raw ore in the fires of passion. And, as all those committed to marriage as a spiritual path know, this process of refinement is difficult work.

Of course, people marry for a million different reasons, many of which have nothing to do with love, but with a dense tangle of legal, social, economic, and psychological pressures. People marry out of a passing infatuation. They marry because they want the tax benefits, because they are afraid of growing old alone, because they want citizenship in a foreign country, or because they want a second parent for their child. Even today, many women marry to make sex "respectable." "I was taught that sex was inherently bad, but that marriage would make it okay," one woman told me. Another said:

MARRIAGE THROUGH THE EYES OF CHILDREN

When I was a child, one of our neighbors was a young married woman who was very kind to me. I was eleven or so at the time, and I always wanted to be with her and her husband. She would let me come for visits, and if I was ill she would come over with a pudding. I felt like she was a friend. She talked to me about love, and of there being different kinds of love. Sometimes she wouldn't let me visit because she and her husband wanted to be alone. In a very kind way she told me they had a special kind of love that I would know about some day. I always wondered what that would be like, and I always kept her words in my mind.   EVA

I idolized my aunt. She was a crack-up; she was fun. She would laugh and smoke cigarettes and enjoy her cocktails. When she smoked, my uncle Walter would say with his German accent, "Nasty habit, nasty nasty." But he would look at her and it was obvious he adored her. He also told dirty jokes all the time. I could tell there was something going on between them that I loved being around. Now, I know it was their sexuality.   VALERIE

When I was a teenager anguishing over my first heartbreak, the director of my school, who was a gay man, said to me, "You know, you are such an extraordinary person. I think you might have a really hard time finding a good relationship, because you are just so unusual. Don't give up. It might take you a while." He could see me suffering, and his encouragement meant so much to me. I have never forgotten that he said that. And I think he was right. Finding a true partner really is more difficult for extraordinary people. That's the price you pay.   IRENE

I didn't want to get married. It was my mother and my husband who decided I should get married. I was nineteen, and I wanted a very feminine organza wedding dress. But somehow my mother got me to buy this blue tailored suit that was much too big. The minute I got married, I felt trapped. I felt like a fly in a bottle with the cork just put on. "Uh-oh," I thought, "my mom has done it again." She got me to do what she wanted. In some ways, I married my mother. When I left my husband, I had been married fifteen years. I was thirty-four, and I had never loved a man.

A friend of mine said, simply, "I married because it seemed to be the thing to do at the time. Looking back, I can't even say that I married for love, though I probably thought I did at the time. But no, I didn't." And a third shared the following story:

I never lived alone until I was twenty. One night I woke up in a panic attack, and within the panic I heard this voice hissing at me, "You've got to get married. A woman is never safe alone. What if something happens? You had better get married." For the next weeks, this voice kept chattering incessantly in the back of my mind. I really felt as if I would die from being alone. Soon after, I entered into a disastrous marriage. I think it is very important that as mothers, we teach our daughters how to be alone, so they don't run into men's arms to escape. I want to take teenage girls out into the wilderness to empower them to be alone. Then they can enter into a relationship from choice, not from need.

Anaïs Nin said that "it is the liberating force of our awareness today that we would like to start anew and give each woman her own individual pattern, not a generalized one."[36] It is indeed high time that we bring back a sense of pluralism to our view of sexual relationships. Marriage is still the only sexual connection sanctioned by legal and religious institutions. But any relationship that supports our personal and spiritual unfolding deserves to be blessed and held sacred by the community.

Most of us were raised with the absurd notion that there is only one "right" way, only one worthy and sacred way, the way of heterosexual monogamy. "Do you believe in monogamy?" someone asked me at a recent workshop. I asked back, "Is monogamy a religion or a god one must believe in?" In my opinion, monogamy is one among many valid choices we can make for ourselves.

Western culture tends to view reality in terms of polarized opposites—good and evil, god and the Devil, the supremely masculine man and the supremely feminine woman. It distrusts everything that is not black or white—the "feminine" man, the "masculine" woman, the bisexual, the homosexual, the lesbian, the transsexual. Instead of celebrating the richness of diversity, it celebrates the intensity of extremes. But nature did not create us black and white. Each gender includes an entire rainbow spectrum of body types, sexual proclivities, and vibrational differences, which make us gravitate toward a whole range of sexual lifestyles. In addition, different archetypes are at work within us at different times, evoking different needs that demand to be honored in different ways. The needs of Hera, the goddess of marriage, are different from those of Aphrodite, the voluptuous lover. A lifestyle that suits one person does not suit another, and the needs of our twenties may not be the needs of our sixties. Our marriages will be stronger and more likely to succeed when we approach marriage as just one among many options. Only then can we consider our real needs with an open mind. Diane, who married and divorced three times, realized in the midst of our interview that she had never seriously questioned the need to get married:

> I have tried so hard to fit in, to make myself normal. Until just now, I never even considered the possibility that maybe marriage wasn't right for me. I just thought if I kept on trying, eventually I would get it right. But in fact, my best relationships, the most fulfilling and satisfying ones, have all been outside the confines of marriage.

Today, many marriages that once might have lasted are no longer likely to endure—not simply, as is sometimes said, because the younger generations have no sense of fidelity and commitment, but because an undeniable soul force is pushing people to break out of situations that obstruct their personal growth. People often lament the demise of the nuclear family and wish for the good old days when marriage meant forever. But from a spiritual vantage point, there is little benefit in salvaging a loveless, stagnant relationship. These days, marriages that are not rooted in real love and in a true willingness to commit to the path of partnership are not likely to succeed. And that is, perhaps, not such a bad thing.

In most traditional societies, the relationship between married people was dictated, down to the smallest details of their daily interactions, by religion, custom, and communal opinion. Throughout medieval Europe, personal feelings and individual preferences counted for so little that arranged marriages were quite common, as they still are today in parts of Asia. The primary purpose of family life was survival, not the spiritual growth of individual family members. If a woman wanted to devote her time to spiritual practice, she had to become a nun, which meant forfeiting marriage. Even the Indian priestesses, who were allowed to take lovers, were not allowed to marry. As a result, the path of partnership and the path of the priestess remained separate.

Today, our situation is different. Almost unnoticed, a great change has swept over our approach to marriage. More and more people are giving their spirituality the kind of intense attention traditionally associated with monastic life, and yet they are not monastics but lovers, husbands, wives, and professionals. Today many of us are attempting to merge two formerly separate ways of life—the path of marriage and the path of spiritual dedication. This is not just a question of making time for solitary spiritual practice, as well as time to spend with our mate. Rather, more and more people are realizing that learning to love their mate intimately and honestly *is* their spiritual practice; the two are not separate. In 1904, Rainer Maria Rilke articulated this new awareness of relationship as spiritual practice:

> For one human being to love another human being: that is perhaps the most difficult task that has been entrusted to us, the ultimate task, the final test and proof, the work for which all other work is merely preparation. . . . We are only just now beginning to consider the relation of one individual to a

second individual objectively and without prejudice, and our attempts to live such relationships have no model before them.[37]

Today, the human ego is trying to evolve into a powerful new organ of the soul. The entire realm of ego development, formerly viewed as a mere obstacle to enlightenment, demands to be recognized as a vital aspect of spiritual growth. The old spiritual teachings that commanded us to "transcend the ego" are simply no longer valid. The ego needs to be healed, purified, and integrated, not transcended. Dealing with the complexities of our psyche is no longer just a psychological imperative but above all a spiritual one, and committed relationships provide the most radical way of meeting it. As a form of spiritual practice, relationship practice engages and transforms the ego more radically than any other discipline. Therefore, sexual relationships have become the primary training ground for individuals who are seeking to develop a high degree of psychological maturity and are willing to undergo intensive personal transformation. Inevitably, our marriages are less simple and secure than those of our mothers and grandmothers. But what partners stand to gain is an immense increase in personal consciousness. A married friend recently told me:

> What people like us are trying to do has never been done. Certainly our parents were not trying to achieve that level of honesty and consciousness and intimacy. I know many people who are doing this, and none of their parents did. I don't feel alone, but I do feel we are pioneers. I feel guided by a force greater than ourselves, as if the planet were asking for this. I believe there is some kind of maturational movement to our process, and that we are evolving toward greater realization.

Today, spiritual evolution is no longer the privilege and intention of a tiny minority. Our species is poised to leap into a new level of consciousness, and unless we leap, we will perish. Millions of us live in this awareness; it is affecting us in a major way and changing the function of our marriages. Once a luxury, personal and spiritual growth has become a most urgent priority.

In the past, the spiritual needs of a community were usually attended to by "spiritual specialists"—priests, priestesses, or shamans who faced the special challenge of positioning themselves at the intersection of the invisible and the visible, the spiritual and the physical, and of living in both worlds at once. Today, because of the crisis of the planet, large numbers of people are walking the spiritual path while actively participating in worldly life.

As we attempt to merge the way of partnership and the way of the priestess, we are simultaneously challenged to unite personal and transpersonal love; our personal partner becomes our gateway to the transpersonal deity. Therefore, we look to our marriages to provide not only companionship and comfort but also the mystery and passion of an encounter with the divine. We want to meet as two compatible human beings, but we also want to meet as Shiva and Shakti, as Aphrodite and Ares, as Adam and Eve.

Friendship and passion, or personal and transpersonal love, are like two wings that enable a marriage to soar. As women's social and economic independence grows, we are increasingly unwilling to settle for marriages in which one wing is seriously injured. Diane's marriage to her Demon Lover, Stanley, for example, included plenty of sexual electricity and passion, but the trust/friendship wing was crippled. On the other end of the spectrum one finds marriages like Irene's (Chapter 5), which tried to fly without the wing of passion and crashed.

Before committing to marriage, we might ask ourselves not only whether we love and trust the person, but also questions such as "Do I see the god in him/her? Can I see beyond his/her most infuriating personality traits to the sacred depths of his/her soul? Does he/she honor and evoke the goddess in me?"

Even when our initial answer is yes, sustaining this vision over the years usually demands a tremendous amount of inner and outer transformation. Often, married couples fail to realize how much attention and nurturance the sacred, transpersonal dimensions of a relationship require to stay alive. Author Martha Heyneman remembers how the god revealed himself to her when she first met her husband. But over the years, she says, "I lost belief that the god was in any way resident in my husband."[38] When a deep passion comes our way, it appears to have such a strong life of its own that we easily forget what a fragile, tender flower it actually is. Once planted in the soil of everyday life, it will wither and die unless we nurture it with constant and careful attention. Especially when children arrive, the humdrum routines of family life can easily erode the parents' vision of the sacred presence within the other. Looking back over twenty-five years of marriage and child-rearing, one woman said:

> I understand why having an affair can be so compelling. An affair has none of the obligations of a marriage. It takes you out of time and space. When you are burdened with family life, getting up and taking the child to school, and the bills, and the phone calls, and the food, and making the household work—all that is a blessing, but it is also a burden. It's an incredible challenge. The daily routines and the inevitable compromises and the resentments that build up can wear away that passionate spark. In a long-term marriage, the trick is to keep that wild, undomesticated aspect alive. For us, it's very important to go away for weekends, and have adventures together.

To nurture the transpersonal connection, we must find ways of stepping outside our personal life, leaving behind the orbit of work and children and household. For one couple, a hot tub became the sanctuary they sought out when they needed to reconnect as man and woman:

> It's a space where all the details of our lives are gone, and we just meet in a naked, loving state, with no sense of hurry or urgency. I think people who are in long relationships can keep their sexuality alive by finding such simple, uncluttered spaces where the struggles of trying to live together fall away. To just meet in that simplicity as man and woman is so beautiful.

Of course, not everyone is interested in a sacred marriage or in a sacred relationship of any kind. Many people are quite content having mediocre sex once in a while, and many are content to live together without ever achieving true intimacy. Still, the trend is visible across the board. Most of my clients sigh when they think of their parents' relationship. "For them, it was so clear-cut and easy," one woman lamented. "Yes, they were miserable in a way, and I know my mother never had an orgasm in her entire life. I could never live like that myself, but I still envy the simplicity of their lives. Every-

SEX IN MARRIAGE

I know one can have sex without being fully present, but between me and my husband, that is no longer possible—we are too close, too intimate, too deep, and we feel what's going on right away. For me, having sex is the ultimate meditation. We don't have sex just for the sake of sex. Sometimes weeks go by when we don't feel sexual. We wait until the time is right, and we can have a real meeting of body and soul, a celebration of love. I used to have sex because I felt horny. Now, it's about merging and sacred union. Our lovemaking is not always this cataclysmic experience, but it always has a quality of sacredness and mindfulness. It's a way we explore and honor our true capacity for union. VALERIE

thing seems so much more complicated now." It *is* more complicated, because more growth is demanded of us, and growth is always a complex process. We enter into marriage expecting a much greater level of intimacy than previous generations did, and as a result, the task of relationship has become far more difficult, more demanding. We have moved from high school to graduate school, and the homework is challenging us to the limits.

The challenge we face in merging the path of partnership with the path of the priestess is unique, exciting, and revolutionary. In this process, we are pioneers, explorers of new and uncharted territory. Is what we want in the depths of our heart possible? We are not sure. Most of us find that our parents' marriages do not model the intimacy, honesty, passion, and depth we yearn for. We have all had experiences of relationships and marriages begun in high hopes that ended in bitterness and disappointment. We realize that often the very attributes that initially attract us to someone contain the seeds of separation. We see that we make choices based on unconscious projections, rather than on clear-minded awareness. We flounder; we despair of ever finding the partner with whom we can allow our whole, uncensored self to emerge, the god who will meet and affirm the goddess within us, the lover who will kindle a lifelong flame in our heart.

Wistfully, one woman said to me, "I believe the sacred marriage is something that happens inside, and if you are really, really lucky, it happens outside." And even if we are one of the lucky ones who are living the sacred marriage in the outer world, the challenges are daunting. Like tightrope walkers, we maintain a precarious balance between the demands of daily life and the demands of the soul. We are unprepared for the immensity of the healing work that awaits us as we step into the sanctified space of marriage. Yet this is work that has the potential to heal not only ourselves, but our communities and the earth herself.

In her book *The Chalice and the Blade,* Riane Eisler argues that humanity is now facing a precious opportunity to choose between two fundamentally different models of society—the dominator model, in which one sex dominates the other, and the partnership model, which is based on the principle of linking rather than ranking. Eisler says:

> Women and men all over the world are, for the first time in such large numbers, frontally challenging the male-dominator/female dominated human relations model that is the foundation of a dominator worldview. . . . There is . . . a growing awareness that the emerging higher consciousness of our global "partnership" is integrally related to a fundamental reexamination and transformation of the roles of both women and men.[39]

Eisler demonstrates persuasively that partnership societies tend to be not only less authoritarian, but also less inclined to warfare. She suggests that our survival on this planet may depend upon our ability to learn and practice the ways of partnership. This means that our struggle to create viable and satisfying partnerships is not of merely personal concern but of vitally important social and political concern as well. It means that all couples who commit themselves to the work of creating a true partnership should be honored as the heroes and heroines of our times, for there is no more difficult or more important work than theirs. Flying by the seat of their pants, they are expected to do what few of our political leaders know how to do—maintain long-term relationships that are peaceful, loving, satisfying, and trustworthy.

13

THE ROYAL PATH

Praise to Vishnu his hands
fondle in secret
the large breasts of Lakshmi
as though looking there for
his own lost heart
Venidatta, seventeenth century C.E.

At close to sixty years old, Iris is a striking woman, with sparkling clear blue eyes; porcelain skin; delicate, elfin features; and a smile that lights up the room. She and her husband, David, live in a large house surrounded by redwoods and grand old magnolia trees. When I arrived to interview her, she handed me a photograph of herself and her husband. "It's over twenty-five years old," she said with a smile. It showed a stunningly beautiful blonde turning to look tenderly at a handsome, dark-haired young man. "Isn't he gorgeous?" Iris asked proudly, tracing the outline of her husband's face with her finger.

Even as a young girl, Iris told me, she knew exactly what kind of man she wanted to marry. He would be brilliant, charming, charismatic, and good-looking, and when she found him, an immense, irresistible passion would sweep her off her feet. Until her prince showed up, she would wait. In the meantime, life was rich and fulfilling. Iris went to college and then took a media job that brought her into contact with fascinating, intellectually stimulating people—artists, writers, scientists, and social activists.

Then one day, just as Iris had always predicted, Eros took aim and shot his arrow square through the center of her heart. It happened at a dinner party:

David walked into the room, and the spotlights hit his brilliant blue eyes. And something just made me gasp. It felt like an electrical shock running through my system, and I felt vibrantly attracted to him.

There was no question about whether I was going to go with this—this was what I had been waiting for. I, who had been truly hard to get, was making love to him within a day of going out with him. It was like in the movie *Thelma and Louise,* where one of them says, "Now I know what all the fuss is about." Now I knew. I was twenty-seven years old, and David was the first person who truly activated my sexual passion. I was a flower waiting to be plucked. Making love with him felt so natural and right. I was totally at ease and uninhibited. We were both just swept away. To this day, in his arms I feel at home in the universe. Such love is precious beyond words.

I could see by the light in Iris's eyes and the softness of her voice that the old magic had not worn off. This was a woman in love, a woman still amazed at the powerful magic of male and female energies drawn toward each other like powerful magnets.

Soon after the couple fell in love, David's work took him to the Far East. Of course, the separation was painful, but eventually he was able to take some time off, and he and Iris decided to spend six weeks traveling together through Asia. Iris sighed at the memory. "It was the most romantic trip of my life, extraordinarily passionate and sexually ecstatic," she told me. "We were expecting to see beggars and lepers. Well, we did. But to our great surprise, we also found we had stepped into a bubble of exquisite beauty and magic."

The highlight of the lovers' trip was a visit to the temples of Konarak in India. In ancient times, Konarak was one of the greatest centers of Tantric spirituality, and to this day, the image of god and goddess in ecstatic sexual union blazes down from every temple wall. When Iris and David arrived in Konarak, they found that because of political upheaval, no other tourists were present; they had the whole place to themselves. Wandering among the silent temples, they were stunned and amazed by what they saw.

It seemed every being on the walls of those temples was making love—the gods, the people, the animals, even the rocks and stones—everything was alive, sacred, passionately embracing. Everything was part of the dance of love. It was such a revelation for us to see this ecstatic union of opposites, and to realize how our own sexuality connects us with the cosmic creativity and allows us to know ourselves as expressions of that universal energy. I don't know of any other religious expression that is so sensual, so passionate, so sexual, and so spiritual at once. Certainly Christianity and Judaism are not. When David and I make love, that is what it feels like. We become god and goddess, and it feels as if all creation comes out of our union. For us, making love is a worship of this ecstatic creative energy. We felt that in Konarak, we had found the perfect expression of our own sexuality and spirituality.

Then we went to Benares. One morning, in the early dawn, a boatman took us out on the Ganges. The mist was rising, and more and more people were gathering on the bathing ghats. It felt like an ancient, ancient scene. We kept our distance, out of respect. But finally our boatman urged us, "Bathe, bathe!" We said, "But this is a holy river, and we are not Hindus." "It's all right," he said, "Go ahead. Bathe." So we both got in the water, and at that moment, in the river, David proposed to me. And I said yes. There was nothing else to say. There was a lot to be cautious and concerned about, but I knew I had to take a leap. I said yes, and I gulped. It felt like destiny.

I sighed as I envisioned the exquisitely romantic scene—the handsome man kissing his beautiful young lover in the midst of the Ganges, the mother of all rivers, the river of life, while all around them the ancient, magical rituals of an Indian morning unfolded.

Opposites attract, we say, and the more extreme the opposites, the more tantalizing and exciting the potential of their union. Pulp fiction and romance novels all glorify the attraction between an extremely masculine man and an exquisitely feminine woman. David and Iris happen to fit the stereotypical cliché. He is the solar hero, handsome, strong, extroverted, and dynamic, while she is the moon goddess, her luminous beauty and grace tempered by a touch of shyness. Iris herself seems somewhat embarrassed by this fact. "Our marriage seems a cliché of masculine and feminine roles," she told me.

It is not a feminist model.[40] Even though I support feminism, the truth is that most naturally, I place myself in service of the relationship. My way is to create an energy field, a field of rapport. David's path is more extroverted and action-oriented. His way is the hero's journey, the way of service, sacrifice, and social action. For me, it feels right to be holding the soul space, the gentleness, the intuition. It is right for me *not* to be out there in the warrior world. I so admire women, like Helen Caldicott, who are, but it doesn't come naturally to me. I am finally accepting that in myself. In our marriage, I have done what is most natural for me, which is to hold our love at the center of the relationship.

I have always seen David and myself as an egg, with the egg white and the yolk that belong together. We complement each other in a very deep way. I know he adores me. Who I am speaks to his soul and nourishes him. The two of us form one organism. That has been the truth of our marriage. We each hold one end of the polarity.

During the first years of their marriage, David became passionately involved in environmental activism. Iris supported him wholeheartedly and often worked side by side with him. Already deeply bonded by their love, the couple now bonded even more deeply in the process of sharing social and political values, goals, dreams, and challenges. This they have continued to do throughout their marriage. Her voice ringing strong with gratitude, Iris said:

I feel deepened and enlarged by my partnership with David. Through his environmental work, he has made such a great contribution to the world. I am a gentle soul, and on my own, my life would not have much of an impact in the world. But the love between us has enlarged my life, so that the part of me that wants to make a social contribution has in fact been able to do so.

On the ancient walls of Tantric temples at Konarak, Iris and David felt that they had glimpsed the essence of their own passionate connection. But to maintain a Tantric relationship within the context of a twentieth-century marriage is no easy task. Tantra aims at bringing male and female energies into a state of balance. As loving and passionate as the relationship between Iris and David was, it nonetheless suffered from an imbalance of power. Though Iris only realized this many years later, she herself perceived David's life and work as more important than her own and did not take her own needs and desires as seriously as his. Like many conventional wives, she tended to defer to David. "I didn't consciously value myself and my femininity as much as I valued his contribution to the world," she told me. "I didn't give myself enough permission to demand what I needed."

As so often happens, the couple's unresolved power issues eventually showed up in the bedroom. Soon, Iris became aware of feeling sexually pressured. "It's an enormous problem—the male pushing," Iris said thoughtfully.

I always told David that I would become very passionate when I felt no pressure. The sense of pressure would close me down. But something about our interaction did not allow us to break free of the pattern. It wasn't just him, it was me, too. I would think, "Oh, he's been stroking my head for a while now, he's getting bored." And before I *really* wanted it, I would initiate lovemaking. I would undermine what I really wanted.

The old (and often true) cliché has it that men make love to feel close, whereas women want to feel close before they make love. By the same token, while a man may use sex to move into sacred space, a priestess-woman often feels no interest in making love until sacred space has been established. Iris is one of many spiritually dedicated women who told me that she would just as soon not make love at all unless she can do so in a sacred way. With a shrug, she said, "Ordinary sex without the sacred dimension has never interested me—much to my husband's frustration, who would have liked to get it on anytime, anywhere."

One wonders what might have happened had Iris and David had a competent teacher to guide them through the challenges of creating a Tantric marriage. Tantra recognizes that male and female sexuality differ in important ways and that unless these differences are consciously addressed and reckoned with, they can obstruct the state of attunement and energetic resonance that sacred union requires.

Remember when you were a child, and you got on the seesaw with a friend who weighed twenty pounds more than you, so that he or she could keep you helplessly dangling in midair? To balance things out, you had to sit at the very end of the seesaw, and your friend had to slide toward the middle. Something similar can happen in bed between men and women, especially if the man's energy is very masculine and the woman's very feminine. Men are more inclined to grasp and push for sexual release, while women gravitate naturally toward a more relaxed, meditative approach that emphasizes intimacy and sensual pleasure. Feminine energy tends to be expansive, fluid, and permeable, while masculine energy has a denser, more compact quality. If lovers are unaware of this fact, the more masculine partner (who might be a woman) usually ends up setting the tone and pace of their lovemaking, while the other adapts, often without even realizing it.

In our culture, men are conditioned to act as sexual initiators. In contrast, Tantra recommends that in general, women should preside over the ritual of lovemaking, and that men should honor women as their sexual guides and teachers. By suggesting that men follow the women's lead in bed, Tantric teachings aim at creating a context in which a true meeting of equals can occur. If lovers are to meet in a place of true equality, it helps to slow down and approach lovemaking as a meditative practice, letting go of hurry, tension, and any inclination to push the river. Otherwise, one partner's sexual drive can easily override the other's need for slow, sensual exploration.

The latent conflict between David and Iris emerged full-blown

HONORING THE FEMININE

When I look back, I realize that even as a young girl in sixth grade, I was searching for sacred union. I see that now as I tell my story. I was always looking for a certain energy field. There was a longing to touch the Beloved. But at the time, I could not have articulated that. I think most girls have that longing. They are always being pressured to have sex, and they have no way of even articulating what they really want. The girl might have something precious she could teach the boy if the context were different. But the adult world does not validate her knowledge. So she goes into a defensive mode. To communicate what she knows requires a spaciousness, a soft, open way of being together. VALERIE

when, at thirty-eight, Iris decided she wanted a child. David, though less enthusiastic, was open to becoming a father and promised to support his wife as much as possible. But neither of them had reckoned with the emotional impact the baby would have on the marriage. After the baby's birth, David felt displaced and became seriously depressed. Like many men, he tended to hide his vulnerability, his pain, and his fears by withdrawing. Instead of communicating his feelings, he pulled away from his family. "David withdrew emotionally," Iris remembers. "I could no longer reach him, and I felt just awful about it."

The well of even the greatest sexual passion will run dry, in the long run, unless lovers manage to maintain their emotional intimacy. More and more, the sexual connection between the couple broke down as anger and resentment piled up between them. Soon, neither was getting what she or he wanted. Iris felt sexually pressured, while David felt sexually deprived. David felt emotionally rejected, while Iris felt abandoned with her baby.

It was really hard. David withdrew into his work and became obsessed with it, while I was left home with the baby. We went into a long cycle during which our passion went underground.

There was so much unexpressed anger between us. I have a tendency to make the best of things, and I was not really aware of how angry and upset I felt. Years later, in couples therapy, I realized how furious I really was, and how deeply I felt that David had abandoned me with this baby. But at the time, I didn't speak up for myself. I suppressed my anger and tried to be the good wife.

Then something happened that would alter the marriage forever: Iris fell in love with a woman. Though she and David did not have an open marriage, David had always encouraged her to explore sex with a woman. Iris recalls, "He had always said, 'You should know what it is like to make love to a woman, because women are so beautiful, and you will know yourself in a new way.'" And so, when the opportunity presented itself, Iris felt permission to go ahead.

While David was going off to save the world, Paula entered my life, to my total surprise. She was part Peruvian and part Native American. I have never met anyone else with such irrepressible joy, nor anyone who so deeply held the pleasures of the senses as sacred. She knew how to enjoy every moment and she lived an amazingly erotic life—everything was erotic to her. Paula was a true woman of the earth—plants grew around her, animals grew, children grew.

Paula was lesbian, and she began coming on to me. She was very aware of my deep bond with David, and she had no intention of breaking it. She was simply the all-time sensual woman who loved to seduce women, straight women as well as lesbians. It was as if she were saying, "Look at this wonderful energy, wake up to it." There was so much joy in her. At the time, David was so self-absorbed and depressed, and I was really angry at him, though I wasn't aware of it.

Paula kept flirting with me, and I kept getting more and more nervous. Finally I said to her, "I don't know how this will feel, but I'm curious, so why don't we go to bed, and if I don't like it, I'll stop." So we lay down and kissed. To my immense surprise, it felt so natural, like falling into heaven. I had always thought of myself as totally heterosexual. I had never felt any attraction toward women, or even much curiosity. But there we were, and I felt such instantaneous bliss and familiarity, as strong as what I had felt with my husband, but different. It was like the first time you snorkel, and you discover this whole world that lies just below the surface of the ocean. I had never kissed a woman, never even thought of it, and then to have this full-blown, powerful, profound experience, was so revelatory and breathtaking. There was never a sense of anything strange or perverted about it.

I fell totally in love with Paula, and she with me. I have never again felt anything similar for another woman. There was so much sensitivity and empathy and intuition between us, and the emotional intimacy was so great. We would just rest in this exquisite erotic field for hours. It felt like plugging into the universe, with total-body orgasms that just kept going on and on. Paula was a magnificent lover, who had this total understanding of exactly what my body wanted, even more than I myself did. There was never an issue of making love when I didn't feel like it. She had an absolute intuitive awareness of when the time was right. We both did—we just knew. We never did anything just to adapt or be compliant. We were both completely authentic, and followed the movement of our passion.

Iris sat silently for a moment, her face reflecting the flood of memories that was passing through her in this moment. After a minute, I asked her gently, "Didn't you tell me that you lost your mother as a young child?" Iris nodded. "Yes, she died when I was six. So much of my life has been about trying to find that lost love. Being with Paula began to heal this very deep wound of not having had a mother."

Many women, both lesbian and not, have told me how physical intimacy with a woman has helped them heal their motherwounds, especially if they were not breast-fed, caressed, or held as infants. Tara, an African-American woman raised by an abusive mother, said that since coming out as a lesbian, she'd found her deep hunger for gentleness, nurturance, and warmth satisfied for the first time in her life:

Women have represented the mother to me. They have helped me heal my motherwounds and connect with my spiritual core. They have been the loving moms that I never had. When I came out as a lesbian, it felt like a homecoming and like the deepest honoring of my soul. Finally, I have accepted the feminine. To me, being a lesbian is the epitome of love and softness and femininity. In honoring the goddess core of myself and loving her, I have awakened to my feminine wholeness. My life has been tremendously expanded through being intimate with women.

Sometimes I get scared after we have had a sexual experience. It's too good to be true. I can't believe this is happening and I wait for somebody to come and take it away, or tell me it's not real. I feel like I had better keep this a secret because I'm not supposed to have so much pleasure. It's not easy to accept satisfaction. It still feels like something abnormal. I think in our society, it's forbidden because it's so powerful.

Cynthia and I take days to enjoy sex. That's new for me. Our love is very precious, very sweet, very honoring of each other. We spend a lot of time caring for each other, resting with each other, being in the moment, caressing each other. So much of what we look forward to when we go to bed is the closeness, the cuddling, the holding, the falling asleep in each other's arms, the knowing that we are loved. It feels like a perpetual state of connection, an ongoing foreplay which in itself is enough. With men, the climax was it, and that was very important because there wasn't much else. It was the only focus. With women, that is not the focus.

I did not discover my true capacity for pleasure until I came out as a lesbian. For me, it felt like coming out of an endless, hot, hard desert into an oasis with flowing water and plenty of green. The desert was the absence of heart space and luscious feminine warmth and sensuality. Only a cactus with long spikes could survive there. Now I have rediscovered my joy. I feel like a kid that gets to play. The pleasure is almost overwhelming. How come I get to be so satisfied? How come I get to feel so good?

Tara's words convey something of the sweetness and nurturance women have to offer each other, whether or not their connection is sexual. Together, women can create a pool of golden Aphrodite energy in which each woman can bathe and emerge healed and saturated with her own feminine essence. Unlike Tara, Iris defines herself as a predominantly heterosexual woman, but she, too, feels strongly that women should not deprive themselves of physical contact with other women:

When I think of what I would like to contribute to this book, the first thing that comes to mind is the suggestion that we have been somehow suppressed and oppressed in this area. I think there is a great wasted potential among women who are single and lonely. It's something to explore with a light heart. It doesn't have to be sexual. There can be stroking and holding and talking. I have so many women friends who are pining and grieving for relationship. They are wonderful women, in their fifties and sixties, and they can't find attractive men to match them, and they deny themselves the most rudimentary intimacy. I am not talking about mad sex, but just snuggling together, being sensual together.

Besides helping her heal her motherwounds, making love to a woman gave Iris a mirror in which, for the first time in her life, she found her sexual longing fully realized. Not surprisingly, the experience awakened her to the latent problems in her marriage. She became more aware of what she wanted sexually from her husband and, for the first time, she claimed her right to demand it. Until this point, she had not valued her feminine perspective sufficiently to insist on what she wanted. Paradoxically, stepping *out* of her marriage empowered Iris to step *into* the role of powerful sexual priestess that she had seen prefigured on the temple walls of Konarak. Suddenly, her willingness to compromise diminished radically.

When I told David about Paula, he was relieved in a way. He had thought I had lost sexual interest altogether, and I think he felt less threatened by the fact that my lover was a woman rather than a man. But then he saw how powerful the experience was, and how demanding I had become as a result. I wanted to experience the same intimacy with him. And so I began to insist on making love differently. I wanted more stroking, more quiet moving toward the erotic, more tenderness, more time for opening. It was painful for him, because he knew my demands were coming out of the contrast between making love to Paula and making love to him.

Iris sighed and hugged her knees. Sadness clouded her face as she said, "I felt I would die if I lost either David or Paula. And so I clung to Paula for the next ten years. Of course, the marriage suffered terribly." And yet the love between husband and wife was so strong that even under such immense strain, their marriage held together. "Amazingly," Iris told me, "David chose to tolerate Paula because he saw how much I still loved him and how much she meant to me. I hold this as a great tribute to the strength of his love for me. However, he also responded by seeking solace in other women. This whole period was horribly painful for all of us."

"Was David ever able to give you what you wanted?" I asked Iris. Her face brightened as she nodded. "Yes," she said with a smile, "he has. But it has been a long hard road." Today, several decades after Iris and David first saw the ecstatic lovers on the temple walls of Konarak, Iris believes they are finally embodying the Tantric vision.

We are only now realizing the sacred marriage, after being passionately in love for so many years. It is only now, twenty-five years into our marriage, that I am finally insisting on how I want us to communicate. I am finally owning the value of the awareness I hold and my authority to demand that David honor that. We were always very connected and very bound to each other. But we did not have that gentle flow of energetic communication, and its lack was very painful to me. But it is growing now. As a result, I feel that we are meeting as equals for the first time, truly as god and goddess. We have achieved that balance.

This has happened only quite recently. David has caught on to something that I could never explain to him. He has figured out how to give me what I have been asking for ever since I met Paula. In part, the shift may be the result of his aging. He has always had a strong sex drive, and now at age sixty-five, he isn't as driven by it. He is finally able to be tender and patient, without holding any sexual demands in the background. The absence of grasping is essential. I feel that finally he is completely present with me. Now, that wonderful energetic field I used to feel with Paula arises just as powerfully between David and myself. The other day, he just held and stroked me for several hours. He was making absolutely no sexual demands or overtures. In fact, I made some, and he did not respond. He did not allow me to initiate anything before I was really, truly ready. When we did become actively sexual, it was glorious.

The absence of pressure is having the effect I always knew it would. It completely turns me on. We are deeply in love, and after twenty-five years, our marriage feels new. The bliss that comes through that meeting is so great. We are older but no less passionate. David stays hard for long periods. So I worship this lingam that rests in my hand for hours. There is no place we have to go beyond that. We just dwell in that state, without much thought. The boundaries dissolve, and our bodies become one. We just spent forty-eight hours in bed, stroking and talking and being close. More and more, I am having orgasms that start in the heart and move through the body. We lie side by side with our hearts touching, and breathe together, so completely in tune that it is neither his breath nor my breath, but ours. This, too, I asked him to do previously, and he would try, but now, it happens spontaneously, without any effort. An infinite tenderness and presence has been growing between us.

Normally, we are so encapsulated in the illusion of our separateness. Sacred sex can completely strip away that illusion. It is a total miracle when you transcend that separateness so that you don't know whose hands these are, whose cock and whose vagina. It is a very profound meditation, and to me, it is the essence of spirituality, as well as an ultimate healing. Intimacy is such a beautiful path of meditation, a royal path. For me, this experience of resonance or attunement is one of the great ways of knowing god. The meditative state opens the gates to sexual intimacy, and the energetic harmony opens the doors to knowing god. This is the kind of sexuality that does not die as you get older. In fact, it deepens and grows.

Over the last year, Iris and David have spent extended periods of time apart. David was struggling with a challenging creative project and needed solitude, while Iris, too, felt that she needed time to reconnect with herself and rediscover her own rhythms. Like Iris, many women, as they grow older and move through menopause, express a growing need for solitude and quiet. Iris marvels at the positive effects the separation has had on her marriage.

I always thought living together was the "right" way. Now I see that both ways, living together and not living together, have great virtues. When the spiritual core of the marriage is strong, you don't always need to be together physically. We always felt a lot of small resentments that had to do with patterns of compromising and adapting, always for the best of reasons. No matter how much we talked about them, they still left a residue of friction. Now, that resentment is gone. We are meeting like lovers again. Our relationship has become so delicious, and so sweet.

I needed this period of time apart. The relationship was always the center of my life. Now, a shift has occurred. I am putting my relationship with god, with the greater Beloved, first. And in a different way, so is David. As a result, there is less grasping between us. I think I used to expect David to give me that experience of the Beloved, and when he didn't, I would feel bereft and enraged. As a result, the marriage was fraught with a burden of expectation. Now, I see my marriage as just one aspect of my connection to spirit. The paradox is that as a result, our marriage has become more filled with spirit than ever.

The way Iris speaks of her husband, as the physical embodiment of her greater Beloved, brings the Indian devadasis to mind. They too did not live with their lovers, but honored them as the physical embodiment of their cosmic husband. Iris feels that her life is more and more becoming a celebration of Eros, a joyful worship of the exuberant dance of energy that the ancient artists portrayed so well on the temple walls of Konarak:

What I want to do with the remaining years of my life is to know god and goddess fully, in all the ways I can. I want to explore what my own rhythms are when I am not so bound up in my marriage. My passion is about waking up to life, every moment of the day. I want to become one with the sun and the flowers, with making the bed, or with my own breathing.

The categories of hetero-, bi-, and homosexuality no longer interest me. I am interested in pansexuality, in eroticizing life itself. Ecology, for example, is about our interconnectedness with nature. We *are* nature. Everything is kith and kindred. I am opening to the living quality of it all. We are not machines, and this is not a mechanical universe, but a biological, orgasmic universe.

I think of myself as a horizontal mystic. I lie under trees and look up at the light filtering down and I go into ecstasy. Every morning in bed, I do a healing meditation in which I put my hands on my body and breathe, and allow the internal energy to move. At some point, sooner or later, a kind of force field appears, like a rheostat turning on, which gets more and more intense. It brings me a great sense of bliss and often leads to a diffused, gentle orgasm. With a minimal amount of genital stimulation I can open into waves of orgasm. When my husband is around, I often call him to bed because I get so turned on. It is wonderful to know I can turn on in this way, without a partner. I can come home to myself in the universe whenever I want to.

Recently, I was on the beach with a friend, and we were watching this gorgeous sunset. The whole sky was filled with purple and red, and the rays of the sun were coming through the clouds. And my friend, who is not normally very sexual, suddenly said with a gasp, "Everything is coming! The waves and the clouds . . . everything is coming." We laughed. When I am open to spirit, I, too, feel that everything in my body and in the universe is orgasmic. My desire, at this point in my life, is to live more and more fully in that stream of energy of which we are all expressions, to live an erotic life at all times. Sex is perhaps the ultimate form of that energy, but it's everywhere. That energy makes great art what it is. It makes a piece of music soar, and it is present in every moment of intimacy. To me, that energy is sacred and infinite in its variations and possibilities. When I am in that flow, I feel aligned with god and the sacred. It can happen just looking into the eyes of someone on the street. That is the growing edge for me, staying connected with that sacred life-force in everything I do.

14

JOANNE'S MARRIAGE

he is as salt
to her,
a strange money
precious and valuable
only to her tribe,
and she is salt
to him,
something that rubs raw
that leaves a tearful taste
but what he will
strain the ocean for and
what he needs.
                    Lucille Clifton

Joanne is a tall, attractive brunette in her late fifties, with long hair, beautiful dark eyes, and full, sensual lips. When I heard her say that her marriage of thirty years was still deepening and growing, I was intrigued. Very few couples remain married that long; fewer still manage to keep their relationship vibrant and fresh. "How did you do it?" I asked Joanne."Would you be willing to tell your story?" After a brief moment's hesitation, she agreed.

"I don't know why our marriage survived when so many others didn't," Joanne mused.

But I know we put time into our relationship, a lot of time. Some all-nighters, trying to work things out. We didn't put our careers first. We put our marriage first. We changed the form of our relationship over and over again. And our marriage is still transforming. Often I think we will be together forever. But I also know that in the next minute, anything could happen. When you are committed to your own growth, you don't know where it's going to take you.

It all started thirty years ago, Joanne told me, with a blind date—surely not a common way of meeting one's future husband. Sexually, Joanne was still fairly inexperienced. Raised in a strict, Controller-dominated family, she had been taught to be a "good" girl, to guard her sexual passion like a shameful secret. Like many women, she remembered how scared she was the first time she had an orgasm with a boyfriend. "I didn't know what the heck had happened," she recalled. "I was suddenly swept away, and when I came to, I got really scared. I had lost control, and it terrified me."

When Joanne met her future husband, she was not in a hurry to climb into bed with any man. Devin took her to a movie, then drove her home and tried to make out. "I thought he was nice, but I wasn't ready," Joanne remembers. But the second time they met, Aphrodite cast her spell. Suddenly, Joanne's body turned into a bundle of humming, overalert nerve endings, each one trembling with anticipation. "The spark caught," Joanne said, smiling at the memory.

I remember my little finger touching his hand, and all my attention went into that little finger. It didn't take long for us to get into bed. It was really different from anything I had experienced before. All my passion ignited, and everything was let loose in me. We spent all night making love, sleeping, waking up, and making love again. It was incredible. I had no inhibitions. He was very free with his body, without shame, and he so relished my body that it was easy for me to open. We danced together in bed. He followed me, and I followed him. I had never, ever been with a man like this before, and I fell completely, totally in love. Both sexually and emotionally, our opening was so complete that we bonded and merged into a single body. All of my being touched his, and none of me was left out. We were so tuned in that from the first orgasm we had, we had them together. It just bowled us over. When I told him I had almost no sexual experience, he couldn't believe it.

It soon became clear that we wanted to stay together. We were able to deeply listen and hear each other at all levels. We knew we were meant for each other. We were soul mates, and our marriage seemed predestined. We just couldn't deny or walk away from the amazing depth of our connection. I had never felt such love and understanding from anybody. As a fifteen-year-old romantic, I used to sing this song, "When I fall in love, it will be forever." That's what actually happened. Since that moment, thirty-five years ago, we have been together.

Thus began an unlikely alliance between a free-spirited, decidedly nonmonogamous man, and a woman of Spanish descent raised in a very traditional, sexually repressed family. Their marriage has been no bed of roses, no fairy tale of living happily ever after, but rather a difficult and demanding ropes course that has forced them both to grapple with their shadows and discover their true strength. "We sanded down each other's rough edges like sandpaper," Joanne said. In these words, she summed up what appears to be the essential soul purpose of this marriage.

Cynics may laugh at Joanne's sense that she and Devin were destined to be soul mates. Who can say whether certain people are really "intended for each other" by divine decree, or whether certain matches are indeed "made in heaven"? Perhaps calling someone a soul mate is merely a kind of self-fulfilling prophecy—the more you believe it, the harder you will try to make the relationship work. Still, there *is* a mystery at work here. There *is* a compelling force that guides couples to come and stay together, a force that transcends simple sexual attraction, friendship, or compatibility. Whether we talk of Eros, of destiny, of inner guidance or fate, we can never entirely deny the mysterious spirit at work here.

What is a soul mate? And how do we recognize our soul mate? To call someone our soul mate is to make a statement not only about the relationship itself, but about how we hold it, how we perceive it. "This relationship," we imply, "is my meditation, my prayer, my spiritual practice." And yet, if Joanne's story is any indi-

HEARING EACH OTHER

Women need to be heard. Not fake heard, but really heard. Men need to be heard too, and acknowledged. They need to hear that they are all right. Wherever you are in your sexuality, or in your relationship—it's all right. You are not wrong, or bad, or less than. But let's grow. Let's grow together. Let's find ways of communicating. Can we commit to not walking away from our communication, when the going gets hot? Can we stay right there and see it through? Many of us have been working from old records, and we need to realize there are new albums we can play now—even laser disks. It's time to upgrade.

MERCEDES

cator, a soul-mate relationship is not necessarily more balanced, harmonious, or peaceful than any other. Quite the opposite. Like any true spiritual path, it challenges the ego in every possible way and can be fraught with difficulty and pain. As Thomas Moore says, "Marriages may be made in heaven, but they are hatched in hell." If Devin and Joanne are soul mates, then soul mates can fight bitterly and, at times, even hate each other. To find a soul mate is divine grace, but to stick through the process of working things out requires strength, humility, and devotion.

Despite Joanne's certainty as to the rightness of the connection, two serious problems raised their ugly heads almost immediately:

It became clear that Devin's sexual appetite was larger than mine. I would get satisfied and want a period of rest to let the energy build up again. Not he. He was there, ready, any time, all the time. Being sexual was a big part of his identity. Sex was front and center in his life. Devin's sexual need became a problem for us and remained a problem for many years. Though he was never macho and aggressive in lovemaking, he pressured me a lot. I had to deal with saying no, and he had to deal with my rejection. It was simply not okay for him when I said no. Making love itself was always wonderful, except when I made love without wanting to. Later in our marriage, there was a period of several years during which I kept getting bladder infections. Finally, I realized that I would get them when I should have said no to Devin and hadn't. They stopped happening once I got that lesson. It was difficult, because I couldn't be affectionate unless I was prepared to have intercourse. He would try to grab the opportunity and get upset if I wasn't willing. It was very frustrating for both of us. Fortunately, this pattern has changed over the years.

The other thing that became a problem, and continued to be a problem, was that Devin was not monogamous. He never stopped seeing other women. Shortly before we got married, he confessed to me that while I was out of town for a few days, he had slept with another woman. I didn't know how to handle this. The truth was I didn't want to handle it at all. Here was my soul mate, so what was I going to do, walk away from him? It was a tremendous conflict for me. Devin told me it meant nothing compared to his feelings for me. This just enabled me to continue in my denial. I framed the situation in my mind: "It was just a one-shot deal and it showed him that it's so much better with me." That night, I rolled over in bed and pretended to go to sleep while the tears rolled down my face. Somehow I felt that I shouldn't share my pain with him, that this part of me was secret and I shouldn't let him see it. Maybe, somewhere deep inside, I knew that this was going to be an ongoing issue, and I didn't want to face it.

We met in January, got engaged in May, and married a year later. Before we got married, Devin said to me, "I can't imagine being monogamous." And I remember shining it on. I didn't want to hear about it. Somehow, I thought it would magically work out. But Devin knew he would not stop seeing other women. He was driven, and he couldn't stop.

In these early years, the marriage between Joanne and Devin bore a striking resemblance to the mythic union between the Greek god Zeus and his wife, Hera. While Zeus was an incorrigible philanderer, Hera was the jealous goddess of marriage. Zeus looked at marriage as an institution that tied Hera's life to his own, without limiting his sexual freedom. Though he really did love Hera, he couldn't comprehend why his wife had to pour the bitter bile of jealousy into an otherwise quite comfortable arrangement. Hera, on the other hand, as the descendant of an earlier matriarchal goddess, was not about to become a submissive wife. Sexually faithful, she expected Zeus to be likewise, and could not help but perceive his infidelity as a profound betrayal. The shrewish, nagging qualities often attributed to Hera reflect the anguish of a woman attempting to create an equal, monogamous union with a partner who does not share her values.

Like Hera, Joanne held a vision of partnership as a deeply sacred path, with monogamy being an essential ingredient of that path. Yet she agreed to marry Devin without facing the smoldering conflict between her need for monogamy and his need for sexual adventure. In her ambivalence, she followed in Hera's footsteps, for Hera, too, married Zeus knowing full well that Zeus did not share her commitment to monogamy. And just like Zeus and Hera, Devin and Joanne started fighting as soon as they married.

Our marriage was really rocky from the start. We would get mad and emotional—have wild fights and then some incredible making up. We fell into this pattern of fighting and hating each other and then falling in love again. We had met each other's match. I had wanted passion, and I got passion, on both ends of the spectrum. It was so painful that after we had been married for a year, Devin wanted to leave. He said he just couldn't take it anymore. But the thought of a failed marriage horrified me, and I begged him to try and work it out.

Over the next years, Devin and I experimented with a number of psychedelics. We spent hours sitting cross-legged, looking into each other's eyes, journeying together, or making love with an incredible sense of union. It seemed that our lovemaking couldn't possibly deepen any further, and yet it did, because as we made love we also started meeting on psychic and spiritual levels. I had orgasms that went on and on. The energy just kept moving and flowing in both of us. We would look at each other and feel our connection was eternal.

Previously, neither of us had paid much attention to spirituality. I didn't know whether there was a god—maybe yes, maybe no. How could I know? But after taking psychedelics, I said, "Yes. Definitely, yes. There is something out there as well as in here." There was no doubt about it, and when we looked at each other we saw that reality within each other. That awareness helped put our ego struggles in perspective. Our spirituality became the foundation that helped us through the hard times—the realization that we were part of something bigger, and that our relationship was part of the mystery. We were on the path together as friends, side by side, rather than constantly facing each other.

I had no interest in other men, and I never gave Devin much reason to be jealous. Devin, on the other hand, slept with other women both before and after we got married. I didn't ask him many questions, though. My denial was still at work, keeping everything fuzzy and clouded. Despite his infidelities there was no question in my mind that Devin loved me. I knew he didn't prefer anybody to me, and I knew I could satisfy him sexually. And yet I was not enough for him. It was confusing. At some point, I realized Devin's need for sex was a compulsion, and I was being the codependent.

But if he hurt me with his infidelity, I hurt him through cutting him off. I believe that the price men pay for their sexual freedom is the loss of love. Women can and do cut their love off, and they make men live loveless lives. That's the weapon women use, and I, too, used it. I never left for good, but I would go cold and shut him out. That was one of the most painful things for him to endure in our relationship.

One summer, I agreed to be part of a foursome with a woman Devin had met and her husband. God, what was I thinking? I wasn't even that attracted to the husband. We set up our two double mattresses side by side, but the very first night it was clear that all the action was between Devin and the wife, and nothing much was happening between myself and the husband. One night was as long as I lasted. I couldn't take it. They were making love before my very eyes. I don't know what made me agree to this in the first place. I told Devin, "No more. I can't take any more." "Okay," he said.

But then I walked in on Devin and the wife kissing. That was it. Finally I snapped. I moved out. I took my sleeping bag and slept in the barn. I didn't give a shit what the others did. At this point, I really did give Devin up. I couldn't cope with the pain, and I came close to being cuckoo crazy. I was losing myself.

I spent the next few months on my own with my daughter. I thought my marriage was over, and it was a shock. I still believed Devin was my soul mate, and I thought, "If I can't make it with my soul mate, who can I make it with?" It was a confusing time, but at least I had taken a stand for myself. Finally, finally, I had drawn my line and was beginning to break through my denial. I had to face that if I wanted a monogamous marriage, it was probably not going to be with this man.

Gradually, Devin and I began to explore whether there was any chance of getting back together, and after several months we did. I made the demand "No more other women." Devin agreed, though he wouldn't "sign on the dotted line." And I didn't really hold him to it, either.

Cautiously, I asked Joanne why she never really demanded fidelity from Devin. She hesitated. Then, she replied, "Part of it was that I didn't want to force Devin to become monogamous against his will. I wanted him to want me, and only me." But above all, Joanne envied the expressive freedom she observed in her husband; she saw him as a role model. "There was a barrier within myself that I wanted to break," she said with a frown.

Devin's sense of freedom seemed to hold a promise for me, that I, too, could get past my inhibitions. I saw something in Devin that I longed to find within myself. He was always true to himself. In comparison, I felt tight and constricted. With Devin, I could open up sexually. But otherwise, I was pretty prudish. With any other man, I could easily have learned to live in a clamped-down, constricted way. But after being with Devin, I couldn't deny my own sexuality anymore.

And so Joanne had ambivalent feelings about her desire for monogamy. Was she simply trying to impose her own sexual repression on Devin? Perhaps, she thought, a taste of sexual promiscuity might help her break free of the Controller's tyranny. She decided to explore this possibility. "I am tired of being the martyred wife," she told Devin one day. "I am going to explore my own sexuality."

He thought that was great. He was scared but also relieved to be off the hook in terms of feeling guilty. So I went looking deliberately. I went hunting, with intent. It actually did shift the energy between Devin and myself, and it got us out of our deadlock. But I did it out of desperation, not because I really wanted it for myself. And I did not find anyone. I tried, but it really wasn't what I wanted to do for myself. In hindsight, I see that during those years, I was imposing values and ideals on myself that didn't match who I was. I am not a promiscuous kind of person, and sleeping with a guy means nothing to me without the relationship. But I thought being a sexually liberated woman meant I had to let go of my need for monogamy and act like a guy. It never occurred to me that my jealousy might have any value. I just wanted to get rid of it. God, what a mixed-up time it was!

The "mixed-up time" Joanne refers to was the seventies. A new generation had redefined sex as an easy, fun, harmless game. Suddenly, casual sex seemed almost obligatory. People who once felt guilty for wanting sex now felt guilty if they *didn't* want it. Only too eager to win men's approval, many women did their best to conform to the new rules. After all, who wanted to be called frigid, uptight, or cowardly? Like many women during this era, Joanne felt confused. She knew she was sexually repressed, and she knew she wanted to shed her repression. All around her, people were declaring that monogamy was passé, that jealousy was merely a symptom of repression and insecurity. No wonder she found it difficult to discriminate between true sexual liberation and mere mimicry of a way innately alien to her. Eventually, however, she realized that making love to other men was not the solution to her quandary. "In the end," Joanne told me, "I saw that the freedom to be promiscuous was not what I really wanted."

> I wanted to own my own desires and impulses, my own yearning for freedom. It was not just about sexuality, no. It was about authentic expression of any kind. It was about self-expression, about feeling comfortable with myself at all levels, sexually and creatively, instead of compulsively and painfully constricting. Somewhere down the line, I had internalized a voice that prohibited me from expressing myself freely. Even today, I am still working on trying to express myself and come out of hiding.

In the meantime, twelve years into their marriage, Joanne and Devin were still fighting a lot. "I used to frustrate Devin no end," Joanne recalled with a wry smile. "When he ranted and raved, I would shut down and just sit there like a piece of wood without responding. That was my weapon, and it would make him even more angry." Slowly, ever so slowly, Joanne began to grow stronger as she focused on overcoming her tendency to compromise and conform, and learned to stand her ground in the relationship.

> One day, Devin got so angry he hit me. I was totally shocked. Then, during another fight, he hit me a second time. At that moment something snapped in me; I lunged at him and I scratched him up pretty good. Then I went into my bedroom and locked the door and didn't come out for hours. When I came out, I said to him, "If you do that again, it will be the last time." And he tested me, one more time. He started at me. But instead of shrinking, I got ready to meet him, with my claws out. And he saw that I was serious, and he backed off. That was it. That never happened again.
>
> Around this time I moved into my own bedroom and I said to Devin, "I am not going to sleep with you until I feel like sleeping with you." That felt risky. But it was clear to me at that point that I had to stay true to myself. It was a tough, dry period. I hated how easily Devin lost his temper, but I was also having to face my own rage.

For Devin, Joanne's coldness evoked painful memories of his icy, judgmental mother. So often, we unconsciously pick partners who force us to confront our unhealed childhood wounds. Of course, we hope that this time, the hostile or abusive mother will turn around and love us the way we want to be loved. Instead, our partner usually resents the parental projections and refuses to cooperate. The more Devin demanded love and attention, the more resistant Joanne would become. Many women find themselves turning to stone when they feel continuously pressured to give sexual or emotional love. Men often fail to understand that beneath this unyielding resistance which can feel so hurtful lies a deep, ancient rage. Women are sick and tired of being used as mother substitutes by men still stuck in boyhood. When a woman senses herself becoming the recipient of a man's mother projections, her resentment often manifests as a sexual or emotional shutdown. Indirectly, Joanne was telling Devin, "No, I will not be your mother. You must heal your own wounds."

But if Joanne was a strict taskmaster for Devin, he, too, forced her to confront her shadow side. While she embodied the strong goddess who refuses to cater to a man's wounded ego, he in turn embodied the ancient sexual god who will not allow himself to be boxed, confined, or regimented. If one side of the truth was that Devin was driven by a compulsive need for female validation, the other side was that his soul perceived the call of Eros as a sacred call, which no power on earth could convince him not to heed. "No," his soul insisted, "I will not surrender to the Controller." No matter how much Joanne pressured him, he knew that in his heart of hearts, he could not agree to her demands without betraying himself.

Had Joanne refused to put up with Devin's infidelity, or Devin with Joanne's coldness, the marriage would have ended in shipwreck. Instead, their love gave them the strength to honor each other as teachers. Each chose to use the very behavior that so pained and infuriated them as a key to their own awakening. Gradually, Joanne took responsibility for her rage and her repression, while Devin faced and healed his motherwound. Her face glowing with wonder, Joanne took a deep breath as she said:

We really raised each other. Somewhere in there, we got tired of fighting. We finally started taking responsibility for ourselves, and stopped blaming each other. We grew up, and things got a lot more harmonious.

In the early eighties, Devin and I had a really powerful breakthrough in a training group we attended together. For the first time, I saw how much pain my rejection had caused him. To me, that was a real turning point. Throughout our marriage, I had seen myself as a victim. "The guy plays around, the poor wife sits at home. . . ." It seemed perfectly clear who was the victim. Now I saw that if I was his victim, he was also mine. We were even. I really understood how my coldness affected him. That made a big difference. At the same time, Devin really saw my pain. I don't think he had ever fully seen it before. The guilt had created a film. He had been so busy defending against the guilt that he couldn't really see my pain. It was a remarkable event. And I believe that since then, Devin has not slept with other women.

How difficult it is to love another person deeply and honestly! And yet, our desire to experience true partnership is so great that we are willing to go through all kinds of trials and tribulations to realize our dream. In order to save their marriages, men and women change in ways they would otherwise never consent to. Thomas Moore writes,

> The courage required to open one's soul to express itself or to receive another is infinitely more demanding than the effort we put into avoidance of intimacy. The stretching of the soul is like the painful opening of the body in birth. It is so painful in the doing that we often will attempt to avoid it, even though such opening is ultimately full of pleasure and reward.[42]

Joanne's story attests to the truth of these words. Through her eyes, I began to see her marriage as an evolving partnership based on a love so profound that it was able to break down and reorganize psychic structures that would not have budged under any other circumstances. We do not release these deep layers of conditioned behavior without putting up a struggle, so Joanne's marriage necessarily included equal amounts of passionate fighting and passionate lovemaking. Clearly, Joanne and Devin have been teachers to each other. Each has held the key to unlock all the other's deepest ego issues—and to grow beyond them. Like sandpaper, they have rubbed against each other and, in the process, have polished each other to a fine sheen. Today, Joanne is deeply appreciative of Devin's and her own willingness to submit to the fires in which their love has been forged. "We have healed each other," she says gratefully.

> Once, Devin wrote me a card, "To my spiritual teacher, from your spiritual teacher." We raised each other, emotionally and spiritually. He taught me to break through my denial and my tendency to play nice, and instead, to express my authentic truth. And I would challenge him on his ego trips. I was tough on him; I didn't let him get away with much.

An important turning point in many women's lives occurs when they realize how their personal struggles relate to our collective evolution. For Joanne, this turning point occurred just a few years ago, while she was moving through menopause.

I started reading Riane Eisler and other books about equality in relationships, and I started understanding the bigger picture, how down through the centuries men have been in the role of dominators, and women in the submissive role. The whole issue of submission really emerged for me then. I felt so much anger at myself for being submissive in my marriage, as well as in other relationships. I have tried to have an equal partnership with my children, too. Because of the difference in age and size it appears that you are uneven, but really, as human beings, you are equal. When you look at children as sacred vessels, then you can have a partnership of mutual respect, and still do your job as an older person who knows more and has greater responsibility. I have two adult children, and I continually strive for a true partnership with them. That is very gratifying to me.

Even as an adolescent, I envisioned a marriage that was passionate but also equal. But only after menopause was I finally determined to be an equal partner, neither submissive or dominant. I think menopause was a factor in how deep I went in that exploration. I wasn't willing to just skim the surface any more.

Sometimes we still have fights. I still find places where Devin does his controlling and I do my submitting. Even now, we are still digging up old patterns. Sometimes I get so mad I won't talk to him, and he gets mad at me too, and we will go two or three days in this clenched state. But fortunately, it does not happen very often anymore.

Like meditation and prayer, marriage is a time-honored path of transformation, a way of transcending our narrow, ego-based identity and developing compassion. However, the difficulties of this path can be so great that even soul mates might eventually give up in despair, were it not for the aching sweetness of their sexual passion for each other. Sexuality is the glue that keeps the lovers together, the sweet carrot that keeps them going when things get rough.

All too often, we discount sexual passion as being mere "chemistry." It's a primitive, animalistic thing, we imply, that has nothing to do with love or spirituality. Thus, we discount the fact that sexual feelings are one of the soul's main ways of expressing interest, arousal, and desire. In my experience, even a fleeting sexual passion holds an encoded message from the soul. And when passion endures over a lifetime, we can be assured that the relationship answers to a deep need of the soul. Therefore, any lifelong sexual passion deserves to be honored as a precious gift from the gods.

Devin and Joanne have found, to their great surprise, that their sexual attraction has not only survived but grown and intensified over the years. When they make up after a bitter fight, their lovemaking appears like a rainbow in the midst of stormy skies—a miraculous blessing showered upon their union. Good sex has encouraged them to keep going, and good sex has assured them they have not lost their way. Several times, Joanne emphasized that "without the good sex, we wouldn't have made it through."

Our sexuality just keeps getting better. We know each other so well, we can almost read each other's minds. Devin is very comfortable with his feminine side. He was always able to show himself emotionally fully with me, to follow my lead and not be the macho director. At times, I have felt very much in the male role, while he went into the receptive, more female role. We have both experienced what it's like to be the opposite sex. We trust each other so much that sex just keeps deepening. Every once in a while, we discover something new, something we've never done before, and I think, "God, isn't this incredible, there's still new territory, even though we have explored every part of our bodies with each other. It amazes me. I think, "How much deeper can you get?" But it's endless, it's endless. When we first made love, it seemed very deep. But with the added richness of sharing so much over so many years, our lovemaking has become fuller and fuller.

Before we make love, before either of us makes an actual

move, there's an energetic readiness. We have to feel connected. There are little cues, and we both know when we are
going to make love. Neither one initiates it; it's a back-and-
forth signaling. Devin has had to work very very hard not to
push for sex like he used to. Now, we don't make love unless
it feels right to begin with, but when we do, it's so good. We
take time. We light candles and play music and shower. And
we spend hours together, giving each other massages, just being together naked, and in contact.

Our sexual life together has been the greatest, highest, and
most profound experience of my life. It has also brought me
the deepest, most agonizing pain and taken me to the brink of
insanity. But between the horrors, we would always come
back to our love and to our wonderful, passionate lovemaking.
The first sixteen or eighteen years of our marriage were very
hard, but even then, we always had wonderful periods, too,
when we would fall in love all over again. Our love was the
only thing that could carry us through, and I know that it was
really the source of our incredible sex. I think the love between us was so strong that we were willing to go through
hell, fire, and damnation for it. That's what we did, and it was
worth it.

15

HALFNESS

The wife of a great Zen master had died. Some days later, one of his students came across the master as he was sitting at the edge of a rice field, weeping bitterly. Shyly, the disciple addressed his teacher: "Master, why are you weeping? You always taught us we should not get attached to anything. You said everything changes and everything is merely an illusion." The master lifted his tearstained face and said, "Yes, you are right. Everything is an illusion. But my wife was the best illusion I ever had."

Asian story

The Greek wiseman Plato claimed that our ancient ancestors had the size and shape of two human beings rolled into one, like round balls with four arms and four legs:

> When they broke into a run they simply stuck their legs straight out and went whirling round and round like a clown turning cartwheels. And since they had eight legs, if you count their arms as well, you can imagine that they went bowling along at a pretty good speed.[43]

Some of these strange creatures, Plato says, were male; some were female; and others were hermaphrodites, half male and half female. But in time, they became so arrogant and overbearing that the gods felt moved to intervene. Zeus had them all chopped in half, a cruel move from the human vantage point, since every one of these poor creatures felt devastatingly, miserably alone without its other half. Plato informs us that

> when the work of bisection was complete, it left each half with a desperate yearning for the other, and they ran together

221

and flung their arms around each other's necks, and asked for nothing better than to be rolled into one. So much so, that they began to die of hunger and general inertia, for neither would do anything without the other."[44]

Ever since, Plato says, we have all been restlessly roaming the earth in hopes of finding our beloved lost halves, and until we find them, we are doomed to feel incomplete. But when two halves find each other after a long separation, they cling together for dear life.

Is there any truth to Plato's imagery? "Definitely, yes," young lovers would say. But talk to them a year later, and they may tell you a different story entirely. No. To find one of Plato's four-armed, four-legged creatures we must look to committed couples like Iris and David, or like Joanne and Devin, who have shared a life and have bonded deeply in the process. In them, we see the two halves rejoined as one flesh and one blood. We see a union that becomes stronger with each passing year, a melding of two organisms into one. Such couples are like trees that grow side by side until their trunks merge, so that you can no longer chop down one without mortally wounding the other.

In fact, we are *not* the separate, well-defined organisms we appear to be. Energetically, if not physically, we truly *do* merge like tree trunks. The well-known healer Barbara Brennan describes the bonding between lovers in terms of energetic cords. In the following passage, she describes what happens to these cords when partners are separated, either by divorce or by death:

The cords usually get badly damaged in these experiences. I have seen all the chakras on the front of the body torn open, with the cords floating out in space, after such trauma. The personal experience of such a trauma is described as the feeling of being torn apart, or as if their better half is missing. Many people become disoriented and don't know what to do with themselves. . . . When a lot of cord damage is done in the process of forced separation, I have seen it take at least five years, sometimes seven for people to reorient.[45]

When I read this passage to Miryam, an attractive, dark-haired woman in her early forties, she nodded. Three years after her husband's death, she can attest to the truth of Barbara Brennan's observations. Just five years ago, Miryam was dreaming of finding a husband and having a baby. Nearing the end of her childbearing years, she felt truly blessed when she met Jim. Both she and Jim believed that they had indeed found their long-lost halves. "It was a match made in heaven," Miryam told me with tears in her eyes. "I knew after our second date that I could marry him." The couple fell deeply in love, married, and spent several blissful months together, while Miryam prepared for the possibility of having the child she so yearned for.

Then, out of the blue, after only seven months of marriage, Jim was diagnosed with an unusually virulent and fast-moving form of cancer. From that moment until his death only three months later, Miryam became a full-time nurse to her husband.

Who thinks about death in the throes of a new love? Yet every marriage that does not end in divorce ends in death. To bring this awareness into our relationships is no morbid preoccupation. The awareness of death puts things in perspective, keeps us humble, reminds us not to allow unfinished business and unspoken words to pile up between us. If we live as if death could occur at any moment— as it can—then we live with greater passion and a more open heart. We set aside petty grievances and forgive more readily. We take more risks and don't put off expressing our love, knowing that now is the only moment we can be sure of. The future is uncertain.

Miryam's story is unusual in several respects. It is unusual to lose one's soul mate after sharing such a brief time together, and Jim's death was unusually painful. As Miryam herself put it, "My experience was not the common one. It was so condensed." One moment, she was a radiant bride, the next a young wife hoping to get pregnant, then a full-time nurse to a dying man, and finally, a grief-stricken widow tottering on the brink of insanity. Like a skeleton, her story reveals the bare-bones extremes of human experience: love and loss, holiness and horror.

Seven months after our marriage, my husband was diagnosed. For the next three months, I lived his dying, and he had a particularly horrible death. I was seeing death, smelling it, sleeping with it. It was not an image of death I had ever seen anywhere. Nothing prepared me for the teaspoons of brown fungus that I would take off his tongue when he was in a coma. Sores all over his body, tubes everywhere, all the while he was gasping and screaming. This was his death. It was not a gentle sliding into the last breath as it is often described. Horror films pale in comparison.

Finally, with the breath before his last, he became totally calm. When it was clear that he had taken his last breath, I started sobbing with relief and sorrow. The horrible, horrible pain of his dying was over.

Throughout his illness, there were so many moving, beautiful, holy aspects to the way people responded to us and gave us love and care. From the beginning, there were angels in the midst of the blows. It was indescribably beautiful and holy, and at the same time, indescribably horrific and painful, so loving, and so intensely awful at the same time. I felt incredibly blessed. I felt the holiness of the love that just oozed out of the walls everywhere we went.

Miryam stopped, her dark eyes shining with tears. Simultaneously, we lunged for the tissue box and then laughed through our tears. For a few minutes, we sat in silence. Then Miryam returned to her story. As a Jew and an experienced meditator, she had a strong spiritual foundation. Nonetheless, with Jim's death, her innocent faith in a loving god was brutally shattered, leaving her filled with helpless rage at the power that had snatched away her beloved husband. Like Evelyn, who nursed her lover as he died (Chapter 3), Miryam had ventured too far into the land of death and did not know how to return. Though she herself was physically alive and healthy, the horrors she had witnessed gnawed at her insides like the cancer that had killed her husband. The options were clear: either she would manage to integrate her experience, or she would go insane, drowned in her despair.

There was some way in which the horror became frozen in my psyche, like an airplane circling and circling with no place to land. Where do you put such images? Where do you land five days and nights of his groaning, his animal noises, and his screaming, "Help, help me!" Nothing I had ever heard offered a container for that experience, except perhaps Auschwitz material.

My strongest fear in the first year after Jim's death was that I would become mad and bitter. I was seeing the hatred in myself, the hallucinations, the nightmares. I was observing thoughts that I did not respect or like one bit, and they scared me. I would look at my friends' children, and suddenly, I would see them aging very quickly all the way through old age and into their death. I would look at three-year-olds and six-year-olds and see it on their faces. I found this incredibly disturbing. "This is madness," I thought. I was afraid I would never stop seeing hideous images. I was afraid I would never be able to meditate again without going into horrible images of death and without weeping. I started hating everyone who meditated, because I was jealous of their experiences of light while I remained steeped in the dark. For a long time I felt like a shipwreck. One more thing and I would collapse, kill myself, or murder someone. That's how I felt.

I used to yell at god, "You fucking brute, you murderer. I am supposed to pray to you? Why would I pray to you? You killed my husband." I would pound the floor and cry into boxes of Kleenex. I would do this for hours, week after week. I was so mad at god. At times, I went through huge amounts of grief, and other times I went through mountains of anger. Often, I just wanted to strangle people who mentioned the word "god" or "spirituality."

It was a lonely and very eerie time. I no longer recognized myself, my mind, or my impulses. I started having migraines all the time and was in a lot of physical pain. I had no desires for the future; I couldn't imagine having a future. From the grief, my body started going into premature menopause. I couldn't tell whether I was a forty-one-year-old bride or a seventy-one-year-old widow. I didn't know whether I was going to make it through, and I surely didn't need platitudes. I would get furious at people who flung platitudes at me. One of my sisters sent me a postcard saying, "Here's to your fresh start." Fresh start! What fresh start? I had one foot in death. My husband was among the dead and I wanted to be with him.

It's no wonder our trembling ego shies away from passion like a frightened horse. Aphrodite's myths underscore that despite all her gentle ambience of roses, sweet laughter, and music, she is a dangerous goddess, a goddess of treacherous waters and blazing fires. On Valentine's Day, we portray her son, Eros, as a chubby baby, sweet as sugar candy. Yet when we give each other cards with crimson red hearts pierced by arrows, we unwittingly admit the truth: Eros is armed and dangerous; love can kill as well as heal. At least we can protect ourselves, to some extent, against the physical dangers of disease or unwanted pregnancy. But what protection is there against heartbreak? Who among us does not know someone whose heart was crushed by love?

Contemplating the ocean of human misery, the Buddha taught that attachment is the source of all suffering. It does not take much reflection to conclude that he was right. We *do* suffer because we become attached to things, or to people who then leave, change, or die. Attachment is a kind of glue, and when two people who are glued together are ripped apart, it hurts. Because of this simple yet profound insight, many thousands of people have chosen the monastic path. Monks and nuns do not have to worry about their mates cheating on them, leaving, or dying.

But there is a fatal flaw in this train of thought. People don't get glued together unless they are sticky to begin with. So what is this glue that makes us so prone to bonding with certain people, yet not with others? What purpose do our attachments serve? From my own experience, I know that every person I've been attached to was a potential teacher; my attachment always signaled that some kind of lesson was asking to be learned. When we avoid forming attachments, we miss out on relationships which can teach us lessons we will never learn in any monastery. Jack Kornfield, one of the foremost Buddhist teachers in the United States, was ordained as a Buddhist monk but later renounced his vows when he realized how essential it was for his personal and spiritual evolution that he walk the path of partnership:

I could do loving-kindness meditations for a thousand beings elsewhere but had terrible trouble relating intimately to one person here and now. I had used the strength of my mind in meditation to suppress painful feelings, and all too often I didn't even recognize that I was angry, sad, grieving, or frustrated until a long time later. The roots of my unhappiness in relationships had not been examined. I had very few skills for dealing with my feelings or for engaging on an emotional level or for living wisely with my friends and loved ones.[46]

As children, we used to play a game called tunnel. We would get down on our hands and knees, side by side, forming a tunnel with our bodies. Then the last in line would detach from the tunnel and crawl through the dark passageway of whispering, breathing, laughing bodies. At other times we would play leapfrog, vaulting over each other like drunk grasshoppers. In such games, children enact a basic truth. We are all tunnels, doorways, thresholds, and stepping-stones for one another. We evolve not in isolation but in community, each person taking off with the help of many others. Partnership is an adult variation of leapfrog. In our time of exaggerated individualism, it reminds us that there are certain types of gateways and tunnels and bridges we can create alone, and others we can create only in conjunction with others.

To walk the path of partnership means to sacrifice our former wholeness in order to redefine ourselves as halves, incomplete on our own. In a society that worships the strong, the happy, and the independent, this takes great courage. We are not supposed to be needy or to feel the desperate grief of Plato's halved humans, a grief that offends the most treasured ideals of our "happy" society. The very word "half" carries connotations of lack. "He is a half-wit," we say of an idiot. A foolish plan is half-baked. A deception is a half-truth. When we do something reluctantly we call our effort halfhearted. Our language reveals how much we fear halfness, how deeply we associate it with lack. "Wholeness" has become a catchword that draws the crowds like moths to the flame.

But make no mistake: those who tell us we can have whatever we want, be whoever we want to be, and have full control of our lives are merely playing into our desire to avoid the discomfort of feeling our vulnerability. True wholeness has nothing to do with getting what we want. Paradoxically, we achieve true wholeness only by embracing our fragility and sometimes, our brokenness. Wholeness is the natural radiance of love, and love demands that we allow the destruction of our old self for the sake of the new. "If anyone needs a head, the lover leaps up to offer his," says the mystic and poet Kabir.[47] Life did not intend us to be inviolable, but to be used as fodder for its workings. We are meant to be chewed up and digested and transformed into the blood and sinews of the world.

In Miryam's story, many of us will see a reflection of our greatest fear come true: the fear of giving ourselves completely, wholeheartedly to a love—and then losing it. What happens to a person who experiences this? Miryam's loss has unearthed in her a clearsighted, unsentimental wisdom and an unshakable, rocklike strength she never knew she possessed. Her next words can help us understand our distaste for the way of pale detachment and our stubborn loyalty to passionate love.

I loved my husband more than I loved life, and losing him to cancer was the deepest experience in my life. Two and a half years later, I have to say I wouldn't undo it for the world. I wish he hadn't had to suffer so much, but other than that, I wouldn't change any part of it. It broke down every last illusion of what life can ask of one, and every shred of arrogance I had, every illusion about how spiritual a person and how strong I was. I had to face how weak and ungrounded I was in my spirituality when I was really tested in the fires. Even Jesus cried out on the cross, "Why hast thou forsaken me?" Even Jesus felt god was not there when he needed Him most. In those bleak spiritual moments, you don't feel god's presence. For my growth, it was the hardest thing and the best thing that ever happened to me. Nothing else has changed me so much for the better and the wiser and the more real.

If someone had told me in my first year of marriage: "Don't get too attached to your husband; you could lose him," it wouldn't have made any difference. I was so deeply changed for the better by loving him. It was part of my spiritual awakening to love so deeply and to serve him during his illness. I never knew I had such strength in me. I believe that attachment is valuable. To have loved that deeply, and lost what I loved, and to have discovered the steadiness and strength that followed was much more transformative than thirty years spent meditating on detachment. I was attached, I suffered the loss, and I worked through it.

Overall, the experience has not made me fearful of death, but has done more to make me fearless than any other experience in my life. I saw that Jim went through an agonizing death, but I also saw that he actually did reach peace, because that is where he was headed, and no amount of drugs or fear could ultimately sidetrack his soul. That insight strengthened my sense of security about the direction in which we are headed. Now I know now in a way I previously didn't that peace is our ultimate goal and that ultimately, we will get there. I have found a phenomenal strength in myself. And yes, I am displaying it now. I couldn't during the year following his death. But now I am. And I look for it in other people and support it in them. I expect it; I can see it in them before they see it in themselves.

As I sat with Miryam, I was touched by the depth of compassion that has arisen in the aftermath of her ordeal. Before her husband's death, her life revolved mainly around personal concerns. Today, she is deeply involved in various humanitarian projects that seek to bring relief to the suffering people of the world. Having healed her own heart, she is able to sit with the brokenhearted, offering them love and a compassionate presence. Miryam sighed. Quietly, she said:

How ignored tragedy is, and how it needs not to be ignored but to be attended to! Those who suffer tragedy need so much love and help to make it through. I know how much I needed when Jim was dying. I would like to make that loving care available to people who need it. Not to wait until they commit heinous crimes because when they needed help they didn't get it. My love for Jim has opened my heart to loving others. Compassion is the main thing. Nothing else could touch me in my grief. Nothing. When people came to me with love, if their heart really opened with compassion, I felt it and it fed me, and it helped my heart to heal. When a heart breaks open, that's what it needs. If it doesn't get that, it's in a dangerous state. I have become so much more compassionate. It has been like a homecoming. This is how we are meant to live. This is what god wants of us, nothing more and nothing less. Everything else is petty.

16

THE DESCENT OF THE GODDESS

From the Great Above she opened her ear to the Great Below.
From the Great Above the goddess opened her ear to the Great Below.
From the Great Above Inanna opened her ear to the Great Below.

My Lady abandoned heaven and earth to descend to the underworld.
Inanna abandoned heaven and earth to descend to the underworld.
She abandoned her office of holy priestess to descend to the underworld.
                    "The Descent of Inanna," 2000 B.C.E.

Ancient myths tell of a dark, shadowy, spectral realm that lies beneath our own and is often identified as the land of the dead. A dangerous place, it does not welcome casual visitors; to enter or leave, one must cross borders guarded by gatekeepers so vigilant and fierce that only very few manage to go and return safely. In shamanic traditions, it is believed that those who enter the underworld always run the risk of getting stuck there and never returning, or of leaving parts of their soul behind, which leads to physical and mental illness.

From a shamanic perspective, what we heard in the last chapter was the story of a woman whose husband's death sent her reeling into the underworld without adequate preparation, and whose soul came dangerously close to getting lost there. Miryam herself sensed the importance of understanding the archetypal underpinnings of her journey. After losing her husband to cancer, she began to desperately search for stories that might help her understand the meaning of her own journey:

> I needed to find mirrors for my experience. That seemed very
> important, because otherwise I knew I would go crazy. I felt

that if someone could articulate what they had gone through and had emerged without losing their sanity, then perhaps I, too, might survive without ending up mad and bitter. I found that certain myths and fairy tales really helped me, stories in which the hero or the heroine went through darkness and came out okay. Such stories spoke of a deeper truth that I needed to hear.

When life sends us spinning into the dark, it helps to know that we have not fallen off the map of human experience, but that this is a path others have walked and survived. It helps to know that yes, this is a journey that need not end in despair or madness, but can lead to wholeness and wisdom. Stories and myths can help us see the meaning, universality, and spiritual significance of our own suffering. Like maps, they show the archetypal terrain our ancestors traveled and communicate what they discovered about the journey.

In fact, there *is* a myth that tells the story of the heroine's descent to the underworld; her passage through darkness, loss, and death; and her resurrection into a new level of empowerment. The myth has come down to us in two versions, one Sumerian, the other Greek. As we shall see, both versions have important messages for contemporary women, especially for those whose life has been affected by sexual abuse. In the United States, a rape occurs every six minutes. One in five adult women has been raped, and one in three women has experienced childhood sexual abuse. In our society, the journey of descent is therefore not an isolated occurrence, but rather a path that millions of women are forced onto.

The earliest account of descent dates back over four thousand years and was inscribed on stone tablets by the Sumerian people in the area now known as Iraq; it is, in fact, the oldest recorded goddess myth.[48] (At the end of this book, you will find information on how to order an audiotaped journey through the ancient myth.) She who descends, according to the Sumerian story, is both goddess and priestess, immortal deity and mortal woman. She was known as Inanna; the Sumerian people worshipped her as Queen of Heaven, but also as High Priestess of the Land. Much like Aphrodite, Inanna is a sensual, flirtatious goddesss, a goddess of sex, fertility, and abundance. In the joyously erotic story of Inanna's courtship and marriage to Damuzi, the shepherd king, she calls him to her bed:

> My vulva, the horn,
> The Boat of Heaven,
> Is full of eagerness like the young moon.
> My untilled land lies fallow.
>
> As for me, Inanna,
> Who will plow my vulva?
> Who will plow my high field?
> Who will plow my wet ground?
>
> As for me, the young woman,
> Who will plow my vulva?
> Who will station the ox there?
> Who will plow my vulva?[49]

After making love with Damuzi, Innana is evidently pleased, for she says:

> He is the one my womb loves best.
> His hand is honey, his foot is honey,
> He sweetens me always.
> My eager impetuous caresser of the navel,
> My caresser of the soft thighs,
> He is the one my womb loves best,
> He is lettuce planted by the water.[50]

Later, the ancient storyteller comments:

> He put his hand in her hand.
> He put his hand to her heart.
> Sweet is the sleep of hand-to-hand.
> Sweeter still the sleep of heart-to-heart.[51]

The basics of human love have changed little over the last four thousand years, it seems. But though Inanna is blessed with a happy marriage, children, and the love of her people, she starts to feel restless. Something unnamable begins to pull her toward the dark and treacherous depths. And so, she decides to descend to the realm of her dark sister, Ereshkigal, queen of the underworld. Carefully, Inanna adorns herself with a number of objects that hum with magical power—golden armbands, deep blue lapis lazuli necklaces, and the crown that signifies her royal status. Sumptuously decked out in all her finery, Inanna leaves her sunlit world behind to enter into the womb of the earth.

When she arrives at the gates of the underworld, the gatekeeper to the land of the dead warns her and asks the obvious question:

> Why has your heart led you on the road
> From which no traveler returns?[52]

Why indeed? Cryptically, the myth tells us that Inanna descends because she has "set her mind to the Great Below." Diane Wolkstein, who translated the myth with the help of scholar Samuel Noah Kramer, describes how she discussed this mysterious line with him:

> "In the first line of 'The Descent of Inanna,' 'From the Great Above she set her mind to the Great Below,' what exactly does 'mind' mean?"
>
> "Ear," Kramer said.
>
> "Ear?"
>
> "Yes, the words for ear and wisdom in Sumerian are the same. But mind is what is meant."
>
> "But—I could say 'ear'?"
>
> "Well, you could."
>
> "Is it *opened* her ear or *set* her ear?"
>
> "Set. Set her ear, like a donkey that sets its ear at a particular sound."
>
> As Kramer spoke, a shiver ran through me. When taken literally, the text itself announces the story's direction: From the Great Above the goddess opened (set) her ear, her receptor for wisdom, to the Great Below.[53]

This is an important point because it means that, from the out-set, the journey of descent is established as a quest for wisdom. It also means that the Sumerians did not share our cultural bias to-ward the light, but saw the dark, the underground, the unknown, as a suitable place to look for wisdom. Later, in Christian times, the dark underworld would become Satan's refuge, not a place one would turn to for spiritual awakening. Perhaps this is why we often find it so difficult to believe that our own journeys of descent into the dark realms of grief, loss, depression, and confusion can truly be more than meaningless glitches or shameful mistakes, best tucked away in secret corners of our memory.

"No," Inanna cries out to us, "even the goddess herself de-scends; how, then, could you feel shame at your own descent?" Her story asks us to relate not only with compassion, but above all with reverence, to our journeys through hell. Women have always de-scended to the underworld; this descent constitutes not a failure but a fact of life best faced as a challenge to growth.

On the way to the underworld, Inanna passes through seven gates, reminiscent of the seven chakras of the body. However, in-stead of leading up and out through the crown chakra, as patriar-chal systems recommend, Inanna's path leads her down and out through the *muladhara*, or root chakra, into the realm of the black Mother. Instead of seeking god in the sky, she drops down, down, down into the bowels of the world. Each gate she passes through leads her not further away from the physical world, but more deeply into its core, into the very center of the world mandala.

At each gate, Inanna is forced to surrender one of her power ob-jects, and by the time she arrives in the underworld, she has lost every one of her treasures and stumbles, completely naked, into the awesome presence of the black goddess. Ereshkigal, the primordial, implacable mistress of death, takes no account of their sisterhood but mercilessly kills Inanna and hangs her body on a meathook to rot. The four-thousand-year-old text portrays the dark Mother's ruthless stance in perfect clarity:

> Ereshkigal fastened on Inanna the eye of death.
> She spoke against her the word of wrath.
> She uttered against her the cry of guilt.

She struck her.
Inanna was turned into a corpse,
A piece of rotting meat,
And was hung from a hook on the wall.[54]

With blunt brutality, the image of Inanna's nude body hanging on the meathook like the carcass of a butchered animal confronts us with the reality of death, shattering our secret illusions of immortality. "Wake up," it says, "even the goddess herself had to die."

But as life is bounded by death, and death is bounded by life, so neither the queen of life nor the queen of death is complete on her own. "Death, thou shalt die," wrote the English poet John Donne (1572–1631). After three days in the land of death, Inanna's decaying body is sprinkled with the water and the food of life, and she rises, much as Jesus Christ is said to have risen two thousand years later. In fact, the story of Jesus Christ and the story of Inanna have much in common. Like Jesus, the Sumerian goddess was both human and divine, both priest and god. Like him, she renounced all worldly power and experienced a form of crucifixion. And as the crucifying father and the crucified son are one, so are Inanna and Ereshkigal, the golden and the black goddess. Like Jesus, Inanna was resurrected from the dead and ascended to a fuller life.

However, Inanna's story is no myth of transcendence. The resurrected goddess does not ascend to heaven, but triumphantly returns to her people, very much physically alive, and laden with precious gifts of insight, vision, power, and compassion. Inanna has found the wisdom she sought when she turned her ear toward the Great Below. Her awareness now encompasses all dualities; she has embraced the totality of life and death. Thus, her descent reveals itself as a journey of initiation into a new level of spiritual awareness and power.

Several thousand years later, we come upon the same story in the very different context of Greek mythology. Inanna has become Kore, the maiden, also known as Persephone, daughter of the earth mother, Demeter. The bare bones of the story—the goddess's descent and return—are the same, but the differences between Inanna's and Persephone's stories are striking. Persephone, it is said, is picking flowers when Hades, the king of the underworld, reaches up, grabs her foot, and pulls the terrified girl down into the underworld to rape her. This is no spur-of-the-moment attack, but a deliberate plan hatched by Hades and endorsed by Zeus, king of the Olympians. In this context, we need not go into the complex story of how Persephone's distraught mother fights to win back her daughter. Suffice it to say that in the end, a compromise is reached: Persephone marries Hades and lives with him for a third of the year, but is allowed to return to her mother for the remaining two thirds.

We see, then, how the Greek myth takes the earlier story of an organic and sacred process and overlays it with a second story about male violence and female submission. A male king has usurped the place of the dark queen who ruled over the Sumerian underworld. And where Inanna chooses to descend willingly, as a mature wife and mother, Persephone the maiden is forcibly abducted, raped, and thereafter forced to marry her rapist. Where Inanna's story speaks of a spiritual initiation, Persephone's story describes a social outrage perpetrated upon an innocent and helpless victim. Her story raises questions of how her suffering might have been prevented, and whom to hold responsible—the very questions every victim of sexual abuse ponders.

Persephone's story reflects the fact that patriarchy has, from its very beginnings, allowed women to be dragged to the underworld unwillingly, victims of a desire they do not share. Not only is Persephone abducted and raped, but her abuse is sanctified by the powers that be, in this case represented by Zeus. In a context where Zeus can give his blessing to Persephone's rape, it is easy to understand why deep down, women often feel that they have no right to complain, but should swallow their outrage and make peace with the abuser, as Persephone does with Hades. All too often, victims of abuse believe they themselves are somehow responsible for their suffering. Persephone's story can help them shed their shame and understand that our culture has, from the beginning, condoned sexual abuse and the abuse of women. Western civilization was built on the foundations laid by the ancient Greeks. Small wonder, then, that so many of us have shared Persephone's fate. We are, after all, cells in the body of the goddess, and her journey unfolds through ours.

Women's stories of sexual wounding and healing unfold in the tension between the two truths embodied by Inanna and Persephone. While Persephone is woman as victim, Inanna is woman as initiate and priestess. When a woman first confronts her history of abuse, she usually identifies with Persephone, the maiden trapped in a catastrophic onslaught of traumatic events. She rarely has any sense of participating in a universal drama, let alone in a spiritual initiation. She knows only that something has happened to her that should not have happened, that she did not want, and that she would give anything to undo.

At a much later point in her healing, she may begin to identify with Inanna, whom the myth describes as a proud priestess, "a maid as tall as heaven, as wide as the earth, as strong as the foundations of the city wall." Clearly, Innana is no victim, but rather a woman seeking initiation into a higher stage of consciousness. Like Inanna, women have always experienced life as unfolding in rhythmic, wavelike cycles of light and darkness, fertility and barrenness, joy and pain. Our menstrual cycle itself leads us on a journey of descent and return, and so, a cyclical initiatory pattern is prefigured in the very makeup of our body.

Of course, sexual abuse is *not* an initiation—not, that is, a ritual carefully induced with the intention of expanding and maturing a person's consciousness. However, a woman may respond to her experience of descent *as if* it were an initiatory ritual, and by her willingness to interpret her descent in this way, she can make it a source of empowerment. Even if, like Persephone, she was forced unwillingly onto the journey of descent, she *does* have choices as to how she responds to her past. Inanna's story assures us that even the most traumatic experience can serve as a journey of initiation and empowerment.

If we are willing, our quest for healing and resurrection can catapult us into the most profound spiritual training of our lives. As a counselor, I have worked with many clients who became radiant and powerful priestesses by grappling with atrocious experiences of descent. Many speak of their gratitude for the path their life has taken. This does not mean that they minimize the responsibility of the abusers or trivialize the horrors of their experience. Nonetheless, they acknowledge that they have become who they are by struggling with the sacred wound life has inflicted upon them. Often, the awareness of their vulnerability awakens in them deep sensitivity, compassion, and humility. They have indeed returned from the underworld with precious gifts.

Though Inanna descended of her own choice, she, too, protested vehemently when she began to realize the scope of the sacrifice required. Like every suffering person, she could not help but demand an explanation. Seven times she asked; each time, she received the same cryptic response:

> Quiet, Inanna. The ways of the underworld are perfect. They may not be questioned.[55]

Seven repetitions of the same question, followed by the same answer, ensure that we get the point. Like Inanna, we are bound to protest as we stumble down, and are likely to blame those who betrayed our trust and abused us. Yet in the end, the question of whom to hold responsible leads us to the question of our relationship with life, spirit, god, or whatever we call the ultimate reality that is the source of both good and evil. And like the response Inanna receives in the underworld, the response life gives us is enigmatic and mysterious. It will never satisfy the rational mind, but it *will* soothe the agony of the soul.

One day I suggested to one of my clients, a survivor of severe childhood sexual abuse, that she take pen and paper and imagine what the goddess might write to her wounded self. As she did so, the following words come flowing through:

> Everything I pour forth in fullness, my beauty and my decay, my generosity and my chaos. I who am the support of everything, also shatter all your supports. In splendor and in terror I burst through the segments of your mind, for I am the mind that dreamed you. You do not understand the events you have witnessed, and would alter them if the power was yours. Yet I myself bow down and salute your passion, the goodness in you and the grief. The clenched fist that you shake at me I accept; I hear you. Those who persist to the end in their passion to know me, through love or through hate, to them I reveal

myself. And those who have seen me rage no longer, but their mind falls silent, and their words dissolve into my black light.

Her words reminded me of the Book of Job, where it is said that when Job finally sees the face of god he falls silent, awestruck. According to translator and scholar Stephen Mitchell, Job "has faced evil, has looked straight into its face and through it, into a vast wonder and love."[56] His just complaints, like Inanna's complaints, and like the complaints of every suffering being, are never answered, at least not in any way his mind can comprehend. The unspeakable cruelty of life cannot be rationalized. Abuse remains abuse, torture remains torture, suffering remains suffering. Yet the descent, if approached as a call to the healing journey, can lead to a place where, without denying darkness, we nonetheless praise the goodness of life.

17

PAMINA'S DESCENT

she is dreaming

sometimes
the whole world of women
seems a landscape of
red blood and things
that need healing,
the fears all
fears of the flesh;
will it open
or close
will it scar or
keep bleeding
will it live
will it live
will it live and
will he murder it or
marry it.

Lucille Clifton

For more than fifteen years, I have been listening to women's stories of descent. These are important stories that need to be heard and honored, yet are often held in silence and shame. They speak of suffering, loss, and pain, but also of the deep longing to heal, the incredible courage that carries women through their ordeals, and the rocklike strength of the feminine spirit. Here, one woman's story will stand for many others, as an example of the initiation of a priestess into darkness, and through darkness into her own fullness.

The following pages contain only an excerpt from Pamina's narrative, which in its entirely would fill a book of its own.

Hers is a difficult, wrenching story. As you read it, remember to hold yourself in compassion, as Pamina herself did while telling it. Remember also to keep in mind the image of the voluptuous, beautiful, sensual woman Pamina has become. This is the story of a woman who has not only survived and healed her wounds, but also emerged from her descent with extraordinary strength and creativity. Now in her mid-thirties, Pamina is an artist, mother, and wife who loves to laugh, play, and celebrate. One senses a curiosity in her, an openness to the unknown, an irrepressibly adventurous spirit. Her beautiful wild soul has come through her descent intact, and the journey has made her stronger, wiser, and more compassionate. Her words convey a sense of victory and contentment:

> I have an abundant, beautiful, full life, and I'm blessed with creativity, love, and a great family. I'm not angry anymore. I'm not angry at men, and I'm not angry at my mother, either. Some people have a hard time with that. They have their own anger, and they really want me to be mad. . . . But I have accepted my healing. I have really accepted my healing.

So many women's lives have been destroyed by abuse. So many have been murdered or hurt beyond repair, both physically and psychologically. Who can say why some manage to heal, while others do not? Against all odds, some women are able to trust that healing is possible, and that they are worthy of it. Like salmon, they fight their way upstream to return to the Source with infinite tenacity, stubbornness, and endurance. Pamina is surely one of these. Like Inanna, she has grown stronger and more powerful through her descent and has returned with precious gifts of self-love, dignity, and wisdom.

Later, we will hear of how Pamina reached this place of wholeness. But first, the descent. Like Persephone, Pamina was dragged into the abyss prematurely as a maiden, a girl just on the threshold of womanhood. In a sense, Pamina's situation was even more precarious than Persephone's. At least Persephone had a mother who grieved for her and fought to save her. Pamina, on the other hand, was utterly alone. Perhaps this had something to do with the fact that the woman she calls her mother is actually her adoptive mother. Perhaps not. In any case, Pamina's mother was too disconnected from her femininity, too repressed and defeated, to understand—let alone support—Pamina's wild, hungry sensuality. "She did her best," Pamina said.

She did the right things according to what the doctors said she was supposed to do. But I remember sitting on the steps of our house with my mom, telling her I didn't feel loved. I must have been about five. She tried to reassure me, but inside I was pretty much convinced that I wasn't loved, and it didn't matter what she said.

When she was about ten, Pamina's friends rejected her, and she became an outsider at school. At home, she felt unsupported and invisible. We enter her story when she was thirteen, the age of puberty, at the time when her descent began in earnest. The following events took place over a period of three years.

I started getting really bad stomachaches. Naturally—I'm going through holy hell, and I'm getting these stomachaches because I've been holding in, holding in, holding in. Finally, one day, I passed out in the bathroom. I think I desperately needed attention. I needed someone to help me, because I was falling apart on the inside. I was taken to the hospital. You would think someone there would have had the knowledge to recognize that something was going on emotionally, but they didn't. They just asked me questions like: "Where's the pain? Does it hurt to press here?" They decided to do exploratory surgery, and while they were in there, they took out my appendix. There was nothing wrong with my appendix, but they took it out anyway. They closed me up, but something had happened in the surgery and I was bleeding internally. My stomach got so swollen it looked like I was pregnant. So they had to open me up again. They had all the student nurses come in to watch, and they never asked me for permission or anything. They had to drain all this blood out of the wound, and I was awake, wide awake. I wasn't even medicated; no anesthesia at all. I was just hurting like hell while they stood around talking about me as if I weren't there.

My roommate in the hospital was older than I was; she was in high school. She started telling me about all this sex she'd been having and the things they did in the back of the car. It seemed like a whole strange world to me. "Do people really do that?" I thought. It seemed really weird to me. "You don't really put a penis in a vagina, do you?" I thought. I just couldn't grasp it.

She had a boyfriend who came to see her. He was eighteen and an absolute doll, a cowboy type, just as cute as ever. He would flatter me and flirt with me, and I was totally embarrassed—I was thirteen, for god's sake! I ended up giving him my phone number. "Come on, come on, please . . ." he said. So I gave it to him. He was older than me, very persuasive, and I was young and totally gullible.

Soon after I got out of the hospital I got a phone call from this guy. Eighteen seems very old when you are only thirteen. He seemed more like twenty-five or thirty to me. We talked and he started asking me questions about sex. I should have gotten off the phone right away. I felt so uncomfortable, but I stayed with it, very awkwardly, stumbling. Every warning sign went up inside me, but I didn't know what to do. I felt so powerless, and I didn't have anyone to talk to about this weird person who was calling me. I didn't trust my mom, and I didn't tell her things. I tried to sometimes, but she didn't want to hear them. This guy knew that I snuck out at night and ran around with other neighborhood kids. So he said, I'll come over some night. And he did.

The night he came over, all my friends eventually went home, and he just stayed. I wanted to go inside, but he taunted me to stay on. We were sitting on the side of my house, and he started kissing me. I really didn't like it. He was a horrible kisser, one of those who open their mouth and slobber with their teeth. I said, "I want to go inside." The dew was already coming in, because it was about four in the morning. Finally, he just grabbed me and kept kissing me. I went, "Hey, cut it out!" He was a lot bigger than me. He started pushing me down on the driveway. I knew in that moment I was in big trouble.

I kept telling him to stop, but I was afraid to yell because I wasn't supposed to be outside. "I can't yell," I thought, "because I'll get in trouble; how can I explain what I'm doing out here with this guy?" He pulled down my overalls and reached down into my pants and put his finger inside of me, even though I was fighting every inch of the way. He was really moving his finger around, and later I thought he must have been trying to figure out if he could fit himself in there. Acch . . . It felt so cold and unloving and I remember thinking: "This is what third base is." First base was kissing, second base was having your breasts touched, and this was third base. My mind was going a mile a minute. I kept trying to push his hand away, but he was too strong. He ripped off my overalls and just got on top of me. He had the biggest penis— it just seemed huge—and he just rammed away. It hurt so bad. I opened my mouth to scream, but nothing came out. There was just no sound. This was right after my operation and I was not even healed yet. Then he got up, pulled on his pants, and ran.

I'm sitting there, and I look down, and there's a whole pile of blood on the driveway. I'm in total shock. I remember my mom talking about sex and telling me that sex was love. "This is sex," I thought, "I just had sex." I also remembered her saying there might be blood the first time. So I thought, "Okay." I just put my overalls on, snuck back in the house, and went upstairs. I was feeling really strange, and I knew something horrible had happened. I felt like I had to pee and I went to the bathroom. Blood. Blood pours out, huge clots of blood. "What's happening?" I think. Then I try to go lie down, but I have to go pee again. I sit down on the toilet: again, tons of blood. It's pouring out, pouring out by the quart. "Okay, I need the Kotex pads." I use every pad, and I use all the bath towels to absorb the blood. Then I think, "I've got to get a garbage bag; I've got to do something." So I get one of those huge heavy-duty garbage bags, the kind you put in your garage, and I start putting these bloody towels in until I've filled the whole bag. But blood keeps pouring out. I was bleeding to death. I didn't understand what was happening; I kept thinking, "What's going on? I've got to get my energy back."

I had a red sleeping bag, and I thought I would lie in my sleeping bag. But then I felt like I had to pee again, and the blood kept coming. Finally, I fell asleep. My last conclusion before this was: "Tomorrow I'm going to seal the bag and I'm going to take it to the woods and burn it." That was what I had decided. I thought: "I have to get rid of this, this is something horrible, I've done something horrible."

Suddenly I saw this foggy image of our maid looking at me, going, "Honey, honey, what happened? Your mother thinks you've killed a horse. What's all the blood?" She's found this huge garbage bag filled with bloody towels. I can barely talk. My mom comes up and they take me into the toilet: blood everywhere. That's the last thing I remember. The ambulance came and took me to the hospital. I had to have stitches. They thought someone had stuck a knife inside of me. That's how badly I was rammed.

I woke up to the police looking at me, asking me questions. They took me into this little room, a pale yellow room, really dingy and cold with no windows. The police were there and my parents, and other people. I couldn't see clearly; everything was just fading in and out from all the blood loss. My dad was yelling, "Do you know what you've done?"

One day, after I had been released from the hospital, my mom came to my room and brought me a milkshake. "We have the name of a psychologist," she said, "and he can help you get rid of that black X on your forehead." My parents just assumed I had seduced this guy. It never occurred to them that maybe I hadn't. My mom has always said that the way I dressed, I was a walking time bomb and was asking for it.

I remember thinking that my life was never going to be the same. Something horrible had happened, but at the same time I didn't quite know what, I was so confused. I ended up forgetting what happened. It was just all fog. I just thought it was all my fault. In my family, nothing was ever talked about. The unspoken agreement was, "This will never be spoken about." Ten years later, when I was safe, I started remembering.

Soon after this, I was sent to military school, which was a family tradition. I had just turned fourteen. It was a preparatory school for the Ivy League, a really beautiful place with a lake and horses. I had decided to go because I wanted to make my parents proud of me. But it was disastrous. Once that rape happened, I couldn't get back into my studies. I smoked cigarettes, ran away, and got drunk. I remember one guy wanting to have sex, but a penis was the last thing I wanted to see. Ugghh.

Once, I decided to leave the school. It was wintertime, and I decided to walk across the lake in a blizzard. It was iced over, but it had hot spots where the ice was thin. I just took off across the lake, and I got to the middle of the lake. In the blizzard my footsteps were filling in, and when I got to the middle of the lake, I looked around and all I saw was white, white, white all around me. To me this became a symbol of just how far out I was, how lonely and how far away from myself. I was desperate, and on some level I was trying to kill myself. Unconsciously, I was crying for help, saying, "Wake up, people. I need help!"

But nobody was noticing. I would do anything to get someone to notice me. I would throw insane tantrums. I would start screaming and have a fit. It was me trying to get heard. People just thought I was crazy. They thought, "What is wrong with her? She's just isn't normal." I can't remember what my last offense was, but finally they expelled me, and they told my parents: "Your daughter needs psychological help immediately." My parents picked me up in the car but nothing was ever talked about. Nothing was said. Nothing, nothing, nothing.

After that, I started having sex every day. It didn't matter with whom, either. I remember deciding that that's what I was going to do. I just resigned myself. I think that somehow I was trying to get back to the beginning. Somehow, I thought if I did it enough times I would be a virgin again. I had sex at least once a day for the next few years. It was a place I felt I had control. I knew what to do to make someone feel good. I became a master at pleasuring. But I never received pleasure from it myself. It was part of a long period of what I call psychological ramming, from which I am still healing. Physically, I let myself be fucked, and psychologically, I let people take advantage of me. I overextended myself, overgave, let people step on me. I had no boundaries at all.

I ran away a lot. I hardly ever went to school. I hated school, and I hated all the people there. That summer I started doing drugs. I got turned on to this paint, Krylon, that we would spray into a plastic bag and inhale. It makes you hallucinate. I got really addicted to it and I stopped eating, because I couldn't taste food anymore.

That same summer, I tried to kill myself. It was less an attempt to really kill myself than a cry for help. I cut up my arms really badly. There was a lot of blood but nothing serious. My mom was really upset because the blood stained the tiles on the floor. All she could think about was getting the bloodstains off the tiles. Cutting myself became one of the ways in which I dealt with my problems. I would break a bottle, and take the glass, and just start cutting myself uncontrollably. I would know when it was coming on. "Uh-oh, here we go, I'm going to do it." I tried to stop myself, but I couldn't. It was just out of my control. I'd slip down to the basement, sit in a really dark corner, and cut away at myself.

The psychologist talked with my parents, and they realized that I really needed help. My dad and I took a walk one night, a very rare thing. He mentioned this school for the emotionally disturbed to me, but he didn't really explain that it was an institution. He just said it was a special school and kids like me would go there. He made me feel that freedom lay just an airplane ride away. It sounded really good to me, and I got excited. I thought, "God, I'm going to get help." That's how I saw it.

On my fifteenth birthday I went to the institution. It had a girls' campus and just over the hill a boys' campus. Even though it was an institution, we could walk out if we wanted, unless we were sent to the lockup unit. I was still on a sexual rampage. The word got around really fast. I helped the guys get off, but all I got out of it was a bit of attention.

In the institution, I was put on medication. I was on very strong drugs for the next three years. At one point, I was really doing better and I asked to be taken off my drugs. They were affecting me, and I couldn't function. But my doctor said no. Instead of taking me off medication, she started giving me more. They were trying to keep me down. So I started spitting out my medicine. I became good at it; I could put the medicine in my cheek, eat a cookie, talk to a staff member, and spit out my pills right in front of them as I pretended to take a sip of milk. That's how I stopped taking my pills. I started doing my art and coming alive again.

I escaped a bunch of times. We would run away, travel and hitchhike and party and have more sex along the way. Once, something really scary happened to me on one of those trips. Somehow my friends left me in this park, in the middle of the night. They were supposed to come back and pick me up, and they never did. It's nighttime, and I'm in this pitch black park. What am I going to do? I don't even know where I am. So I decide to hitch a ride. I get in this truck with an older guy and his stepson. I'm sitting in the middle between them. I tell them where I want to go and they say, "Oh yes, we know where that is." We are all drinking beer and driving along, and suddenly I realize we're not going into town. We're going the exact opposite direction, down a dark street going out of town. I'm in trouble now.

But I was hitting it off with the stepson. We were getting along well, striking up a camaraderie, and this ended up being my saving grace. Things started getting weird, and I finished my beer and turned the bottle over. I thought, "If anybody fucks with me I'm going to break this on the dashboard and I'm going to jab them." But I wasn't sure I really had the courage to do that. They pulled into this old raceway, and the father started yelling at his son, "Go fuck her out in the back of the truck." I was saying, "Don't do it, don't do it. Don't listen to him." Then the old guy started hitting me. "Come on," he was yelling to his stepson. "You don't have a hair on your ass if you can't go out and fuck her in the back of this truck." And he kept hitting me, broke open my lip, gave me a black eye, and bashed up the side of my face. But the stepson grabbed me, pulled me out of the truck, and started running with me. I could hear the truck screeching behind us as the old guy pulled out. He was really pissed off. But the stepson liked me. He said, "I'll take you back into town." Finally, I found my way back to the house I was staying at. I was so pissed off at my friends. They just didn't care.

This next event I have hardly ever talked about. One night, I decided to run away again. Sometimes I would want to run away, but nobody would go with me, and I would end up going with people who were really seedy and dark. That night, I ran away with this girl who was one of the worst, and we met up with a friend of hers who was a bad cat, too. We all ended up taking the train to Philadelphia.

So we were down at the main train station, three fifteen-year-old girls roaming around in the middle of the night. My friends hooked up with three really dark black guys, dark in the sense of their energy. I didn't want to go with them. But they said, "Do what you want, we're going with these guys." I had no money at all. So I went along with my friends and the black guys. One was kind of quiet and shy, and I hung out with him. We got friendly. We went to some guy's house. It was really smoky, people were playing pool and doing drugs. We took drugs too, some kind of pills. I was in a dark dream, stuck in the ghettos of Philadelphia, and I didn't know how to get out.

After a while, we get in the car and drive to another guy's house, some kind of pimp. He comes to the door, wearing glasses, completely naked, with this wet dick. That's how he answers the door. The first thing I see is this wet dick, as if it just came out of somebody. I was terrified, totally freaked out. Something was going on upstairs. Some orgy or something. And everybody wants to go up there, and my two girlfriends go upstairs. I stay downstairs with the shy guy. We're just sitting on a couch talking. Then a guy comes down and asks,

"Why aren't you up there, why aren't you fucking?" He offers us cocaine, and we take it. Then the big guy comes down and starts taunting the shy man to go upstairs, and he goes, and I'm alone with the pimp, the one with the wet dick. "Come on," he says, "don't you like to suck black cock?" "Not yours," I think, but I didn't say that. I could tell I'd be dead. So he just grabs my head and he shoves me onto his penis. Then he calls his friends down, five guys, and they all rape me, one after the other.

They had thrown the shy guy down the stairs, and he knew what had happened to me. He's sat down with me and said, "We need to get you out of here." My friends didn't give a shit. I told them I was leaving, and that was fine with them. "Fuck you, I hate you," I thought. The shy guy went in the kitchen and got me a big red apple. He wanted to make me feel better. He walked me to the station and gave me enough money for the train. I cried all the way back on the train. I didn't run away for a long time after that. Eventually I forgot the whole event. I never told this story until quite recently.

The story of Pamina's descent—and what you have just read is only a small portion of the whole disastrous epic—left us both shaken and exhausted. We both agreed we needed a break. After a long hug, Pamina went for a walk, while I lit some incense and walked around my house, trying to ground myself and come to terms with the feelings of horror and outrage that were roiling through me.

Several hours later, after having shared a good meal and some healing laughter, we were ready to continue. I had a lot of questions on my mind. "How was it," I asked Pamina, "that after such a series of horrific events, you were able to turn your life around and make something beautiful and triumphant out of it? How could you ever trust in sexuality as a source of pleasure after so much abuse? How did you contact the goodness of life when everything seemed blighted with evil?" Pamina considered; then she told me about a profound moment of awakening, which she views as a major turning point in her life.

It was at an antinuclear rally. The whole day was so magical. Everything seemed connected and perfect. Everything felt ancient, as if this had happened before. At one point in the rally, I was in between all these people who had their arms around me. Something broke through in that moment. Suddenly I realized I was lovable, and I started crying. I saw that I could be loved, that I was capable of receiving love. It seems so simple, but I never really had known that before. From that moment on, my whole life changed. It all came from that one moment of feeling my worthiness.

Almost every story of of a woman's return from the underworld hinges on such turning points—usually not just one, but several. Invariably, they appear as gifts of grace, as miraculous and unpredictable as the northern lights with their immense iridescent flares of pink, green, and yellow that illuminate the night sky for a brief moment before they vanish into the depths of space. Without such moments of grace, nobody survives the journey of descent. At the same time, no matter how hard we try, we can never control or force them. Even the goddess Inanna remained powerless until someone sprinkled the water of life upon her corpse. Persephone, too, had to wait for the gates of the underworld to swing open before she could return to the land of the living.

Self-love has the power to turn our lives around. This is a truth that shines through women's stories, again and again. But what exactly is self-love? What does the word mean? It is definitely *not* the belief that we are special in the sense of "better than"—more beautiful than others, for example, or more intelligent. It does not separate us from others, but unites us with them, as Pamina united with others at the rally. The term itself can be misleading, since it seems to imply a subject—one who loves—and an object, the recipient of love. When we love ourselves, who is loving whom? In truth, there is no subject and no object. Our greater, divine Self cannot help loving, any more than the sun can help shining, for love is its essential nature. This radiance of the Self is not a mental concept, but something preverbal and instinctive, which we are born with. A woman who loves herself in this fundamental way knows that she is part of the planetary family, that she belongs here, and that she is as valuable and worthy as anyone else. When she is sexually molested, she will not think, "Oh well, I guess I deserve no better," nor will she bow to abusive religious authorities who tell her she is innately sinful and ignorant.

Pamina's turning point was truly a moment of spiritual awakening and of enlightened perception, a moment in which the veils of self-hatred were suddenly lifted from her eyes and she realized her innate value. As inhalation turns to exhalation, the thrust of her journey at that moment turned from descent to ascent. Of course, this does not mean that her life instantly become easy and wonderful. There were moments of slipping back, of doubt and despair. The ascent from the underworld can be just as arduous as the descent. But although Pamina still had many difficult years of healing work ahead of her, the direction of her journey had changed. From that moment on, she would move, slowly but steadily, from self-destruction toward self-love.

| 18 |

A HEALING MARRIAGE

Deep in love
cheek leaning on cheek we talked
of whatever came to our minds
just as it came
slowly oh
slowly
with our arms twined tightly around us
and the hours passed and we
did not know it
still talking when
the night had gone
       Bhavabhuti, circa eighth century C.E.

It seems significant that Pamina's turning point occurred at an anti-nuclear rally. Women's myths tell us that we are of the earth, and that our cycles of light and darkness reflect the rhythms and seasons of nature. Inanna and Persephone both returned from the bowels of the earth in spring, like young green shoots after a long, harsh winter. At the rally, Pamina began to identify as a daughter of the earth. Long motherless, she greeted the earth as the greater Mother, and instantly her love was accepted and returned. Once she awakened to her worth and her right to seek happiness and love, there was no turning back. From that moment on, everything changed. The descent had ended, and the journey of return had begun.

For Pamina, being in college no longer made sense. It was what her parents had chosen for her, not what she would have chosen for herself. "That was it," she told me with a big smile. "I knew I was

DAUGHTERS OF THE EARTH

*I loved to go out and lay my body down on the earth and hug
her. I loved my trees, and I knew how to receive the land into
my body. The mothering I didn't get from my mother I got
from the plants and the trees and the flowers and the clouds
and the animals, and from the smells and seasons and the colors of the sky. Life came into me through nature. I don't think
I would have made it through had I not lived in the country.
The human conditions around me were bad, but I knew of
something nonhuman that supported me, and that was both
a spiritual and a physical source. I would feel the moss on my
cheek, and I would taste the rocks with my tongue. Nature
saved me. She was my mother, my father, my lover, my sister.
She was my home, and she received me with no shame, no
judgment.* ASTRID

*I grew up in New York, surrounded by towering skyscrapers.
When I was sixteen, somebody told me that if you tore up the
concrete from the streets, there was earth underneath. I didn't
believe them. But later, I went to a college that had wonderful land around it. I used to roll down the hills at night
in the warm spring rains. I wanted to be as close to the earth
as I could. The smell of the grass and the magnolia trees
blossoming—it was so sensual, so very sensual. I remember
how ecstatic I felt the first time I camped out in the mountains. At that time, you could still drink the water from the
streams. I lay outside with my lover, and as we kissed, I felt
the stars move. Truly, the earth turned over.* DONNA

not going back to school." The time had come to find her own path.
This she set out to do by quite literally taking to the road, accompanied only by her guitar and her dog. "That weekend I went back,
packed up everything, finished off what I needed to finish and left
in the middle of the night. 'I'm going to go traveling,' I said; 'I'm going to find myself.'"

But in the course of her travels, Pamina found not only herself, but also Richard, her future husband.

I met Richard one evening in Seattle at a bus stop. We spent the whole night walking up and down the streets, talking about life, totally connected. I had finally met my best friend, and I knew it. This guy was it. My dog knew it, too. Whenever we hugged, my dog would go totally nuts with joy.

We started hitchhiking together, and we had many great adventures, but we never got sexual. I was still in a relationship with my woman lover Margrit. Nonetheless, Richard came and lived with Margrit and me in Arizona. I remember walking into his room and finding him with a whole circle of kids, all of them doing yoga together. He loved kids and would teach them. That's when I started loving him. I knew he was a key for me, and that this relationship would open me up.

One morning, while I was cleaning the place, Richard said to me, "Pamina, I think we are soul mates." I just went on dusting, doing my thing. Again, he said, "Pamina, I *know* we are soul mates." Now I couldn't escape, I had to go sit down with him. I just knew he was right. "Yeah," I said. The dog went wild with joy. But I couldn't understand it, because it wasn't sexual. Also, I was still with Margrit. My whole world seemed insane.

Soon after this, in the middle of the night, I had to go to the bathroom. And there, in the bathroom, I felt the presence of Richard's mother, who had died when he was seventeen. I knew it was her, and she started talking to me. She told me that Richard loved me, and that a lot of hard things had happened to him. I must have stayed in the bathroom for several hours. After that, I would sense her presence at times.

I kept holding on to Margrit, though, so Richard began to feel superfluous and unwanted. Finally, he took off on his own, and I didn't see him for six months. That year, my parents suggested that I spend a semester on this boat school where you traveled to several countries while attending classes on board. It sounded like fun, so I agreed. One of the countries was China. In China, we visited a huge cave. I wandered off from the group and went down to a subcave which had little cavities one could sit in. I started hearing all this noise—vibrations and sounds.

And suddenly, there she was again—Richard's mother, trying to commune with me. "Leave me alone," I said. I had never experienced anything like this before. She wanted me to write Richard a letter. I didn't want to write him, though; I wanted him to get in touch with me. But in Greece I ended up sending him a card, just because she wouldn't leave me alone.

After the boat trip, I went back to my parents' house. I really missed Richard a lot and thought about him all the time. And sure enough, he called. It had been six months since we talked, and I had only sent that one little card, and that only because his mom's spirit had insisted. Well, we started talking, and nothing had changed—the old magic was still there. For six months, we wrote letters and talked on the phone. Then we knew it was time for a visit. On our first day together, we were sitting around looking at a map, planning our next adventure, and Richard said, "We'll go here, and then there, and in that town we'll get married." I called my mom and said to her, "I think I'm getting married, but I'm not sure." She said, "What do you mean, you're not sure?" But five days later, we were indeed married.

Richard was twenty-two at this point, and he had never had sex. We were coming from opposite extremes, me with all my sexual experience, and he with none. He had had girlfriends, but he said he had never found anyone he trusted enough to have the experience with. He had that wisdom—he didn't want to just fuck. He said he really hated those guys in school who were just going out to get laid. But once we married, we started having a lot of sex, a lot of fast sex. At this point, my sexuality started changing. For the first time, I was getting in touch with my feelings, and I was no longer willing to act out sexually. Something else was coming into play . . . like love, and self-love, too. I starting closing down sexually. When we were having intercourse it started hurting. I think my body was really tired of having sex. It was a difficult thing, because Richard was just getting into sex.

I still believed the myth that you got married and had this magical honeymoon where everything is beautiful, and then you live happily ever after. It wasn't like that at all. Within weeks, the shit hit the fan. We both had really hairy backgrounds, but neither one of us knew that the other had such a hairy background. We had no clue. Richard had come from a very abusive family. His father beat him up a lot, and his mother died when he was seventeen. She had held this demand over him never to have sex until he was married. He came from his own field of shit, and neither one of us had dealt with our past. I never talked about it. It wasn't ready to come out yet.

Richard and I fought a lot. We were always yelling at each other. When I look back, I see two very wounded children coming together, each expecting the other to fix them. We had no idea we were going to remember all these horrible things that happened to us, and that we would each want the other to mother us. But even though we had big fights, I never considered leaving him. We were beginning to reveal ourselves, including the demons and the ugly stuff you don't want to show anyone. I didn't want him to see my weaknesses, but there they were. For long periods, we wouldn't have sex at all, but we would lie together and kiss and touch. For me, this was a whole new thing, being with someone who liked me and was committed to me. I had literally married my best friend.

In their book *The Good Marriage*, Judith Wallerstein and Sandra Blakeslee discuss four different types of marriage: romantic, rescue, companionate, and traditional.[57] Most marriages, they say, include elements of each type. The marriage between Pamina and her husband Richard is primarily what the authors call a rescue marriage, by which they mean a marriage between partners who have suffered a great deal and are seeking comfort and healing together.

I know many young men and women today who have grown up fearing that because they were abused as children, they were doomed to repeat that suffering in their closest adult relationships. Here is direct evidence that people who have suffered great pain can put it behind them and have a stable, rewarding marriage.[58]

I prefer to speak of a healing marriage; to my mind, the word "rescue" carries connotations of helpless victimization. In fact, the partners in healing marriages are usually anything but helpless victims—they are strong, determined survivors who heal themselves and each other through their love and commitment. Certainly, this is the gift Pamina and Richard have given each other. With the arrival of their daughter Rose, their commitment to wholeness increased exponentially. "Rose was just beautiful," Pamina said softly.

She was beautiful from the very beginning. She has been an angel. I think we would have killed each other or broken up and hated each other had she not been there to make us have a mutual focus. She kept us working through our stuff. Being a mother was not easy for me. I was totally exhausted and would use coffee to keep myself awake, and we were always fighting. But today, I see that we have really established roots of family and commitment together. That promise and that sacred commitment has been very valuable for us.

Pamina was fully conscious of the moment of conception: "Right after we made love I burst out crying and said to Richard: 'I know I'm pregnant, and I know we are going to have a girl.'" Giving birth is priestess work; it requires a woman to pass through a painful and dangerous initiation in which she journeys to the threshold between the worlds and risks her own life to help another soul cross over. In many tribal societies, women do not undergo the difficult puberty initiations men are subjected to, because it is understood that nature initiates women automatically. About to give birth, Pamina realized what lay ahead of her and panicked briefly before she stepped into her power.

I got really anxious, and I decided to take a hot shower. I squatted in the shower, and Richard got in there with me. I just cried and cried. I had suddenly realized the baby had to come out of my tiny vagina. It suddenly hit me that this had to happen, and that it was going to happen in a few minutes. I couldn't just conveniently carry the baby around in my belly. I was scared to death. I was only twenty-one, and I didn't even know how to change a diaper. Richard was so good. He said to me, "Women have been doing this for thousands of years. You are completely safe, and this is very natural." I calmed down, and right after the shower I was fully dilated.

I had a long mirror in my room, and suddenly I looked into it and there I was, kneeling and giving birth. I remember thinking, "This is total meditation, total presence." I had a real awakening in that moment. In between contractions, there was this deep silence around me, and I was seeing purple everywhere. It was an altered state. I could see all the energy in the air, and it was purple. I had no sense of time at all. It was a very sacred experience.

For the first time in her life, Pamina now had a family, a safe container in which she could uncover long-buried truths and long-repressed memories. Slowly but surely, she began to dredge up her past and hold it up, piece by painful piece, to the healing light of consciousness and compassion.

When Rose was nine months old, she was taking a nap one afternoon and I was lying next to her. I turned over and looked at her, and suddenly I remembered being raped when I was thirteen. I sat up and thought, "Oh, my god." But I still couldn't completely own that I was raped. My parents had told me it was my fault, and on some level I had always believed them. Then I realized that I had to go back and figure out what really happened. Having a safe relationship made it possible for that to happen. A few years later, I told one of my friends that I wasn't sure whether I had really been raped or not. So she said, "Well, let's go back. Let's go back and remember it." So we got on my big couch and put all these feather comforters over us, so only our heads were sticking out. And I just went back and looked, and I remembered the story, detail by detail, and I remembered being raped. That was so liberating. I was beginning to descend into my inner basement, my psychic basement, and to look around there.

The underworld is a place of isolation, silence, and denial. As women begin to ascend from it, they often realize the power of naming their truth. Deprived of the ability to name things, we have no way of asserting—even to ourselves, let alone to others—what is true, or of putting our personal truth in perspective. What we cannot name we have no power to transform. Therefore, we cannot begin to heal our sexual history until we can talk about it. This issue of naming takes on a crucial role in the healing of sexual abuse, where often everything seems to conspire to prevent the victim from telling her truth. As women return from the underworld, they often discover an urgent need for communication. They sense that to remain silent is to risk being dragged back down into the grim depths of the underworld, whereas in telling their story they forge a ladder toward the amber light of the sun. Once Pamina had named her rape, she could get on with the business of healing.

I realized that I needed to tell my parents that I did not seduce the guy, but that he raped me. So I went down to New Mexico to visit them, carrying this truth with me along with my bags. One day, as I was ironing a dress, the opportunity presented itself. I turned off the iron and I sat down with them. As always, my mom was needlepointing and my dad was reading the paper. And I told them I was raped. As I talked, my father immediately took off his reading glasses, put down the paper, and gave me his full attention. I could see the veils falling off him. But my mother just continued to needlepoint and barely acknowledged me. Her comment was, "Well, we all make mistakes, but that's all in the past, we have to go on." Another time, when I tried talking about it, she said, "Well, you were asking for it back then. That was nobody's fault but your own." I just hated her in that moment. I hated her so much I wanted to strangle her.

But my dad told me he always had wondered about this, and that it had been on his mind. It was the first time he'd really listened to me. Afterward, he grabbed me and gave me a hug and said, "Honey, I'm so glad you got that off your chest." It felt so good. I really needed that.

Remembering the rape gave me new hope. I was already on the healing path, but now I felt this incredible urgency. My meditation practice became more important to me, and my interest in yoga, health, diet, and the cosmos grew stronger. I was asking questions: What is going on? Why am I here? What is it all about? I was starting to question everything. Richard and I both went into therapy, and we learned a whole new language. We needed a language to describe the wounded person inside. We both did a lot of going back and figuring out what happened to us.

Not only did Pamina's husband give her his love, his loyalty, and his unconditional commitment to their shared growth, but also he taught her to be honest and fully present with him during their love-making.

One of the beautiful things about being with Richard was that he had no sexual past to deal with. He had enough clarity and freedom to help me find my way back. I needed him to be devoted to me, but he also wouldn't let me get away with anything. I had a lot of manipulation tools, seductive mannerisms that were phony. They were games that were not so much fun as controlling. We might be in the middle of intercourse, and Richard would say: "What's going on?" And sure enough, I'd be in a whole other world. I wasn't even in the room. I might be in the past, or in a fantasy, or not even wanting to have sex at all. All the other guys I had been with didn't care what I felt, as long as they were inside me humping away. But Richard would just stop. Sometimes I would break down and start crying. He was my friend. He was really there for me, and he gave me the space I needed. Sometimes I felt guilty. I thought, "He needs to sow his oats." But he was going through his own healing. After the incredible abuses he suffered from his father beating him up continually and telling him he was a failure, he was trying to heal and learn about being a man.

Right now, Richard needs space. It has been about six weeks since we last made love, and my old self would have felt so rejected. But he's very assuring. He tells me I'm the most delicious, luscious, beautiful creature on earth. This is the first time that I haven't felt threatened. It's so important in a relationship that each person can say no. There will be times when I will have to say no again, too. Once, we didn't have sex for about three months. But we held hands and had long hugs, and it was really nice. Sometimes I need that. It's like reverting back to dating, getting turned on all over again.

Now, we're starting to flirt again. This is our time of foreplay, and foreplay could go on for two weeks. It's a whole new way of having sex. I used to think when we were flirting, "Okay, let's have sex now." It's not like that anymore. Now we take our time and wait, and when we do make love, it's great. There's a natural ripening. I think the long periods of not having sex only used to seem so threatening because they didn't match what I was taught. I thought we were supposed to be having sex every day, and it was supposed to be incredible all the time. But sometimes it's not. Sometimes it bottoms out, and we short-circuit, and we both feel that it wasn't that great. It was a dud. But so what? Because you know right around the corner is this extraordinary moment, just waiting.

However, there can come a point at which we need to make an effort to connect. Maybe I don't really want sex that much, but maybe it's time to push myself just a little. There is a momentum in having sex, and during our long separations, we lose that momentum. Sometimes we wait a little too long, and a lethargy sets in. It's like a taut rubber band that almost rips apart. Then we have to come together. It's really important because making love creates a cellular harmony between us that needs to be maintained.

Familiarity breeds contempt, the saying goes. Some say that sexual intimacy with a single partner inevitably becomes boring over time. Everyone has heard jokes about the deadening effects of marriage, such as Peter de Vries's wry comment: "Sex in marriage is like medicine. Three times a day for the first week. Then once a day for another week. Then once every three or four days until the condition clears up."

But there is another side to the story. While some marriages are based on the shifting sands of a passing infatuation, others are built upon the bedrock of a deep and abiding passion. In a long-term relationship, passion endures only when it is sourced in a spiritual connection, the love between two souls. But when this is the case, sexuality can ripen into a loving intimacy far deeper and more joyful than the fireworks of a short-term affair. "Every time we make love it's like new, like the first time, and it keeps getting better," Pamina told me. "We've been married fourteen years, and I feel like we are just beginning. We have so much ahead of us. After all the stuff we had to go through in the beginning of our marriage, now there is some space to enjoy. We are starting to reap the rewards." Like Pamina, every woman involved in what she considered a sacred union marveled at how sex with a familiar partner could deepen endlessly. "How much deeper can we go? How much better can it get?" Joanne asked. She answered her own question, her voice full of wonder: "It's endless, endless." Apparently, men feel no different. John Gray, author of *Men Are from Mars, Women Are from Venus,* said in an interview:

> I've known my wife for sixteen years. I'm more attracted to her than I was in the beginning. I adore her. When people hear me talk, they might say, "Oh, John Gray is married to a model." But Bonnie is not that type of body. To me, though, she has the most beautiful body—she's the most perfect woman. In my marriage with Bonnie, we're more loving and the sex is better than ever before because now we really know one another. We've seen the best and worst of one another and we still love each other. That makes sex great. That's the potential that an old married couple has that a young married couple doesn't have. A kind of ecstasy, devotion and passion can arise if you know someone over the years.[59]

We have followed Pamina's journey into the depths of the under-world and back. Today, Pamina is a strong priestess who has made the choice to turn her back on the realm of the dead and live life to the fullest. After fourteen years of marriage, Pamina finds that her capacity to give and receive pleasure is still growing.

I like beautiful, gentle, loving sex. But sometimes, I like to play loud rhythmic music and have wild, animal, grunting sex. I need to be like that too. I have discovered that I like some roughness. I'm not a daisy, I'm a human person who likes to be shaken up and to shake up. It took me a while to decipher between what was healthy and what was abuse. It's a fine line. One night, when I and Richard were playing around, he did something a little rough. And I looked right in his eyes and said, "I really like that. I like it rough like that." And with total love in his eyes, he said, "I know you do." It was pure love, so deep. He was saying to me, "I'm going to give you whatever you want, and I will love and accept you."

I went back into my room, and I just collapsed on the floor in tears. I was crying, but not out of sadness. It was not a re-leasing of pain, but a letting in, a receiving. I was allowing myself to take in pleasure. Deep, deep pleasure. Physical ec-stasy. It was so good, so beautiful. For so long, I had not known how to let myself have much pleasure.

Today, Pamina's daughter, Rose, is a beautiful teenager, the same age Pamina was when her descent began. As a mother, Pamina is naturally aware of the continuity of life. She sees her journey as part of a greater story that spans the lives of her grandparents and par-ents and will continue in the lives of future generations. She knows that her own work of sexual healing is undertaken not only for her own sake, but also so that her daughter might have a freer, more joyful experience than she did. It is encouraging to see a woman so committed to shedding the ancient legacy of shame and repression, instead of passing it on to the next generation. If sexual healing is a crucial aspect of planetary healing, then every mother who teaches her children to embrace their own sexual nature and fosters in them pride and self-respect is making a great contribution to our collective future.

When Rose started asking about sex, Pamina was frightened but fully conscious of how crucial it was that she face the challenge of responding to her daughter's questions. The love and thoughtfulness with which Pamina relates to her daughter's budding sexuality inspires hope that future generations will once again come to know sexuality as a sacred, healing energy:

My daughter and I had our first sex talk when she was nine. I was so nervous about it. Rose started asking questions and I thought, how am I going to cope with this? I was afraid I would project stuff on her. Here she was, asking questions at nine years old, right on target. "What's sex?" I looked at her and said, "I'm not quite ready to talk to you about that, but we *are* going to talk about it." "Okay," she said. Days later, she's asking again. Those were a hard couple of weeks for me. What was I going to tell her?

Then, one night, we were going to watch a movie, and we were talking about appropriate and not-appropriate movies. The word "sexy" came up. I don't know what happened, but somehow, everything opened up. We started talking about sex, and the whole conversation was beautiful. We talked for ninety minutes, and Rose asked me a lot of questions. I didn't lay any trips on her; I only responded enough to satisfy her. "Do people really have to do it?" she asked. "Do men and women really have to do that?" I remember asking my mom the same thing. I couldn't grasp it. We talked about hormones. I told her I sometimes felt afraid because she's very beautiful. Rose is going to be a very beautiful woman. And I said that when a girl is young and not yet wise, boys and men may try to get you to do something that gives you the funny feeling. We call it the funny feeling when something's not safe. I told her that made me worried sometimes, and that I really want her to feel that she can tell me when she's afraid of something. "Sometimes," I said, "it can even be someone you've been friends with or have trusted."

It was really good. She said, "Well, Mama, when the hormones come you'll just guide me through it." Since then she hasn't asked a single question, and it's been quite a while now, so that must have satisfied her appetite. At the very end we stood up and she stopped me and gave me a big hug and said, "I'm so glad I have such a good mom." It made me feel really good. I just looked up to my spirit guides in the universe and said "Thank you!" It's so important to me that she be able to talk to me, to keep those channels open that I never had as a child.

One night we were lying in bed together. Something had happened that I said had been a lesson for me, and I was talking about how we are all here to learn our lessons. This was a major revelation for her. "Gosh, Mama," she said, "I just love hearing you say that you are here for lessons. It makes me feel so good; it makes me feel that you really think about things." "Yeah," I said, "I do."

19

REMEMBERING THE CROSS

The theme of balance is particularly evident in the symbolic meanings of the cross, perhaps the most widespread and ancient of all symbols. In many cultures it represents the cosmos: the vertical line stands for the spiritual, masculine principle, and the horizontal for the earthly, feminine principle. The intersection is the point at which heaven and earth meet, and the result of their union is mankind—symbolized by the cross itself.

David Fontana

In recent Western history, the dominant myth of descent has been the story of Jesus Christ, the savior who was rejected, scorned, tortured, and crucified. Because Jesus was crucified, we usually think of the cross as a symbol of suffering and death. But originally, the cross was a joyful symbol of integration and wholeness. Long before the Christian era, people used crosses to mark an intersection between two worlds. The ancient Egyptians and Indians related to the cross in this way, and the same understanding still prevails among Australian Aboriginals and Native Americans. Religious historian Maya Deren tells us that in Haitian Voodoo, the sign of the cross is drawn in flour on the ground or traced in the air to mark "the juncture of the horizontal with the vertical, where the communication between worlds is established and the traffic of energies and forces between them is set up."[60]

This concept of two intersecting realms underlies every myth about the incarnation of a divine being within a human body, including the story of Jesus Christ, who is appropriately symbolized by the cross not just because he was crucified, but above all because he lived in the crossroads between the worlds and instructed us to do the same. The center of the cross symbolizes the point where eternity blossoms in the midst of time and where infinity bursts through into the finite world. It is a place of ecstasy and healing, a place where the unity of Being is revealed to us, and where things that appear to be opposites come together. If, as has been said, "Eros is the force that unites things that are different,"[61] then the center of the cross is the true home of Eros.

When we relate to the cross with this understanding, it becomes an immensely empowering symbol for all of us who are seeking to integrate our sexuality and our spirituality. It invites us to discover that sacred point of intersection between the worlds, and to become threshold dwellers, shamans, priests, or priestesses, who live in two worlds at once. In Haiti, the cross is considered the special symbol of the love goddess Erzulie, whom Maya Deren calls "the dream impaled eternally upon the cosmic cross-roads where the world of men and the world of divinity meet."[62] These are words that might be said of all priestess women, impaled as we are upon the crossroads between our divinity and our humanity.

It is one of the great ironies of history that Christianity, the very religion that chose the cross as its primary symbol and erected crosses in every town, has obscured the amazing promise of reconciliation between matter and spirit that is the essential message of the cross. Suffering is of course inevitable on the spiritual path, but the cross does not glorify suffering or suggest that the world is inherently sinful. On the contrary, it reminds us that a meeting ground exists between body and spirit, between sexuality and spirituality, and between the human and the divine realms. The possibility of integration is real, the cross tells us; it can be achieved.

In this chapter we shall hear the story of a woman whose sexual journey has taken the form of a double crucifixion: one that sent her spinning into the underworld, and a second that set her free to begin the journey of return.

Today, Astrid is a graceful, intelligent artist in her mid-forties, with a pale delicate face framed by blond hair; a mobile, expressive mouth; and hands that flutter and dance like birds as she speaks. We met in her beautiful, spacious house, where high windows let in the morning sun, bathing a tall vase of irises and lilies in golden light. Against the backdrop of this warm, gracious environment, the harshness of Astrid's story stood out in stark relief.

When I was an infant, two of my mother's unmarried sisters came to care for me while my mother was at work. I remember their faces bending over me. The books say children are not genitally oriented, but I sure was. I had a need to touch and be touched. At seven or eight months old, I used to put a rolled-up blanket between my legs. My aunts' reaction was severe. One of them decided to beat me with a hanger, while the other yelled and screamed. I remember the gestures and the raging faces, and I remember taking in the shame. I was shamed before I could even talk. I understood I wasn't supposed to touch myself, though I had no idea why.

When I was a little older, between one and two, I would rub myself. My mother took me to a doctor, and said, "Fix it so she'll never touch herself again." I was painted with burning iodine. The burning sensation was so terrible—it went right into the core of my being and cauterized it.

Shamed for her sexual nature, Astrid spent a sad, lonely childhood with a devouring, needy, sexually frustrated mother and an irresponsible, immature father. When she was fourteen, her philandering father abandoned his family for good. For all her father's shortcomings, Astrid had worshipped him like a god and felt devastated by his departure. Three years later, her first boyfriend abandoned her. "That abandonment was the trigger," Astrid told me sadly. "It echoed my father's abandonment. It took the last piece of trust in the world I had and dashed it. I lost hope, and my attitude toward sexuality changed. I figured I was damaged goods, and that no one would want me. I thought I was trash."

Such are the beliefs that finalize the crucifixion of a woman's soul. As Astrid tumbled down into the underworld, she forgot the magnificence of her own being and decided she must be unworthy of physical, emotional, and spiritual love. Like Inanna, she had lost her crown, symbol of her inner royalty and power.

The old myths warn us that those who remain in the underworld too long are pulled into the embrace of death. Without a clue as to how to heal herself, Astrid began to think of suicide. Death surrounded her on all sides, tempting her to escape from a harsh world into its dark embrace:

Everyone in my family was dying, dropping like flies. One of my aunts died of a brain tumor. Another committed suicide, slashing her wrists and leaving a trail of blood everywhere. My uncle had a heart attack, and then my father died. I went to one funeral after another. By the time I came into my own sexuality, I felt guilty for being alive. I felt I had no right to live while everyone else was suffering and dying. I began to use sex as a way of courting death. I was very promiscuous, and in every man, I was looking for death. My body became a vehicle for the trip to the underworld, a boat on the river Styx. Once I dreamed I was in a house that had a black pool in the middle of the living room. All the ancestors were in it, calling me, "Come to us, come to us!"

Astrid did not kill herself. However, like many crucified priestesses, she expressed her despair and her self-hatred by repeatedly involving herself with men who left, abused, or betrayed her. Every instance of abuse, every rape, added to the body of evidence that seemed to prove her unworthiness. With tears in her eyes, Astrid recalled, "Once, when this guy tried to rape me, I just thought, 'This man thinks he can do this because he knows I am trash.' So I got more and more smashed up. I kept throwing myself at men who didn't value me. The truth was I just didn't care anymore. I had given up."

During this period, Astrid became pregnant by one of her lovers. Though she longed for a child, she felt too wounded to be a good mother and opted for abortion. But a pregnant woman, no matter how brief her pregnancy, is always a priestess who stands on the threshold between the worlds. Astrid's short pregnancy gave her the precious gift of knowing herself as a spiritual being on a journey through infinite time and space:

My friend was very sad about the abortion. I remember staring at his shoes, big brown oxfords that were so out of place on him, because he always wore jeans and rumpled shirts. Neither one of us could speak. And somehow, staring at those shoes and rocking myself back and forth, I went into a trance, and I had a vision. I went back in time. First I was holding on to a piece of wood. It was a piece of the cross, and it was being dragged through the streets. I was saying, "Let me help you carry this. Let me help you." And I was weeping. I was one of the women following the crucifixion.

Then the piece of wood changed and became a plow. I was in the South during the Civil War, and all the men had gone. I was having to work the land, and I was waiting to see whether my husband would come home. Then the scene changed again and I was in New England, at a prayer rail in an old New England church, and the congregation was swaying and singing.

That baby gave me one thing I had never had in my whole life. I went through time with that child, before I had to say good-bye to it. Never until I held my dying mother in my arms have I ever felt anything so powerful. So I just said thank you to the soul of my baby. The images were very strong and very real. I *was* that woman in those three places. It could be genetic memory, it could be karmic, I don't know. But I know that it was real, and it was a much-needed gift. I was about to terminate what ended up being my only chance to have a child. I very badly needed that vision. Then the room came back into focus, and my lover went home. After he left, I washed the floors. I needed to do something very simple and ancient. No mops. I got down on my hands and knees and I washed that floor.

Slowly but surely, Astrid continued to spiral down into a pit of misery and psychic disintegration brought on by sexual self-abandonment. "I was sacrificing myself on the altar of my self-hatred," Astrid said of this dark period in her life. Such misguided self-sacrifice is a recurrent theme in women's sexual stories. We are gullible in our innocence, and will sacrifice our soul, our lifeblood, our integrity, and our wholeness, much as primitive people believed they had to feed their gods with the flesh and blood of human victims. For Astrid, her father and her first boyfriend were such false gods, and she was the worshipper at the altar of their judgments. When they abandoned her, she concluded that she had no value and proceeded to abandon herself.

Disconnected from the soul, the sweet nectar of sexual pleasure turns to bitter poison. The blessing of sexual union becomes a meaningless, hollow fake, a debasing insult to body and soul alike. Sex then becomes, as Astrid so aptly described it, "a boat on the river Styx." Wrapping her arms around herself for comfort, Astrid recalled:

> I was very promiscuous. But at the same time, I would also spend long weekends at a monastery meditating twelve hours a day. I knew I was fighting for my life. I knew that I was capable—and sometimes ready and willing—to throw my life away, and I knew that only something as powerful as spirit could hold me in it. But my spirituality was just as split off as my sexuality. I would flip from the ascetic lifestyle at this monastery to ultimate debauchery—drinking and casual sex. Both my spirituality and my sexuality were very powerful, but each was in a compartment of its own, and they did not touch. It would take me many years before I could allow spirit to touch and heal my core. It took me years and years of hard work to integrate my sexuality and my spirituality. The chasm was so deep.

Here we see the sundered cross at its most extreme—the vertical, transcendent axis confined to the monastery, the horizontal to the bedroom. If they never intersect, neither can enliven and fertilize the other. Approached as a sacrament, sexuality can place us right in the center of the cross where we know ourselves as two-in-one, body *and* spirit, human *and* divine. But without the spiritual component, sexuality becomes flat, stale, and self-destructive. Similarly, our spirituality withers and shrivels without Eros. And so, Astrid's life remained barren as she swung back and forth between spiritual asceticism and sexual debauchery. In Astrid's life, as has been the case in our collective journey, the horizontal beam of sexual pleasure was ripped from the vertical beam of spiritual communion, one beam tossed to the left, the other to the right, where both lay barren and disempowered.

"That which was dis-membered must be re-membered," says

Ken Wilber, and he continues: "This re-membering or re-collecting or re-uniting is the Path of Ascent, which . . . is driven by Eros, by Love, by the finding of greater and greater union—a higher and wider identity."[63] Paradoxically, this path of "remembering" begins with a second crucifixion, one that does not impoverish and deplete the soul, but enriches and strengthens it. The wounds of the first crucifixion must be healed by a second one, which ritually marks the end of the descent and the beginning of the ascent toward a fuller life. This is the crucifixion of the nonessential self to the essential Self, which both Inanna and Jesus demonstrated. Instead of offering ourselves up to the false idols of the ego—prestige, appearance, pride, acceptance, praise—we will have to offer up the inner demons of fear and self-hatred. We will have to give up old ways of being, old addictions, old friends, old attachments, old patterns of thought or action, so that the new can emerge.

Often, this true crucifixion coincides with the lowest, most desolate point of our entire life. So it was for Innana, so it was for Jesus. Similarly, by staging an extraordinarily visceral crucifixion, Astrid's psyche informed her that the time had come to crucify her old self, so that her resurrection as a priestess might begin.

> I was traveling between the Greek islands, and I was a mess, a total mess. I got on a small, really crowded boat. A storm was whipping up, and as soon as we got out there I knew it was a mistake. The captain was yelling to get everybody below. But I had sailed a lot and I knew that was the last place I wanted to be. Instead, I went up to the prow of the boat, and I took the lines, and I lashed myself to the deck, smack in the center. The prow would dip in and the salt water would come over me, but I was in the center point of the boat, which I knew to be the safest place.
>
> And then I realized I had crucified myself. I had tied my waist down and my arms as well, with my arms stretched out. The captain yelled and yelled at me. But I was not about to move. I shot him this look that was pure madness and let him know not to touch me. He knew I would have killed him. I would have thrown him off me. He realized that I was a crazy woman—truly, I was—and he let me be. Soon I was salt-

encrusted, my hair was wild, and my skin was leather. And as I was going through this storm, I felt the two sides of my body, the two poles. One side was light and the other dark, one was good and the other evil. One side was suffering and the other joy, one wanted to die and the other wanted to live. The polarities were coming through my two arms as I rode through the storm.

That night I had a dream. The voice of my inner guide came and told me that I needed total transformation. Until now, I had been wounded over and over, and each time I would merely heal the surface layers of the wound. That surface healing was of no use to me any longer. I had to be radically transformed.

Astrid's crucifixion occurred in the midst of the Aegean, the ocean that gave birth to the golden goddess, Aphrodite. Its heaving, angry waters mirrored the storm that raged within Astrid's own nature, where Aphrodite had been so sorely neglected and abused. By whipping her waters into a frenzy, the golden goddess was shaking her priestess awake and calling her home. For too long, Astrid had denied and debased her sacred feminine essence. Though Aphrodite herself has a reputation as a promiscuous goddess, she abhors the promiscuity that follows in the wake of self-abandonment. Aphroditic sex is never an expression of self-hatred, but always of authentic, though not necessarily abiding, passion.

In her crucifixion, Astrid enacted a ritual of commitment to the path of integration. This consecration to wholeness is one that thousands of us have made, or are on the verge of making, in these times of global crisis. Coming out of denial, we have begun to acknowledge our fragmentation. Carefully, we are taking the beams of our life's cross, placing them at right angles, one on top of the other, and hammering them together with the nails of intention, penetrating wisdom, honesty, and passion.

In pre-Christian times, the cross was sacred to the Great Mother and symbolized the tree of life, which grew in her garden of paradise, its boughs heavy with the luscious fruits of duality. By lashing herself to the mast of the ship, Astrid spontaneously enacted a ritual of rebonding to the tree of life, to the Great Mother, and to her world—the world of nature, sexuality, and engendered love. Binding herself to the tree of duality, Astrid accepted the equal value of pleasure and pain, suffering and joy. There, in the midst of the opposites, she found a point of balance she had previously never known. Centered in her inner lingam, her inner mast of truth, she began to release her compulsive pull toward death and gratefully accept the precious gift of her life and her female body.

Listening to Astrid, I was reminded of medieval images of the crucifix that show fresh saplings bursting out of the dead wood. Today, the tree of Astrid's life is indeed swelling with new buds and green shoots. Soon after her profound experience of crucifixion, she entered psychotherapy for the first time and embarked on a long, arduous healing journey. Finally, after decades of self-abasement, she was ready for radical transformation, ready to take a stand against the all too familiar voices of self-hatred. "My therapist gave me the first safe container I ever had," Astrid remembers fondly. "The power of listening is so great, and she listened to me for seven years."

Deeply wounded as Astrid was, the healing journey has not been easy. For many years, she continued to gravitate toward inappropriate lovers. "For the longest time, I still believed I was not good enough for a man." She sighed. "It was not physical shame but soul shame—deep, deep soul shame—that made me throw away my body." Finally, after several years of intense inner work, the deepest core of her wound began to surface. But this time, instead of dreaming of death, she had the strength to embrace her pain and to feel it all the way through.

> I cried and cried and cried. I had just moved across the country and was living in a town where I had no friends. But three couples I had just met saw how overwhelming my grief was and decided I shouldn't be alone. So they passed me around from house to house. Finally I was in a place where I was receiving care, instead of giving it to others, and slowly, I came through my pain. And you know what? I didn't know these people from Adam. My family and friends could never have done this for me, but these total strangers were doing it. It was

just extraordinary. It was the beginning of the true release. It came in wave after wave after wave. It had taken me forty years to get to that point.

In Africa they say, "It takes a village to raise a child." Similarly, it takes a whole community to bring a woman back from the underworld. As our wounds reflect a collective wound, so also our healing concerns the entire community and can never occur in isolation. Even Inanna, goddess though she was, would never have returned without the support of her best friend, Ninshubur, nor would Persephone have returned without Demeter's help.

Today, Astrid has reclaimed her sense of self-worth, and has remembered her powers as a priestess. "Now," she says proudly, "I have a lover who truly respects me."

Making love has become a sacred experience. There have been times in making love when I have felt a goddess over our bodies, and I would invoke her, because through her blessing, our lovemaking could become a healing. I am at a point now where I need my loving to be contained in spirit, in sacredness. Nothing less can satisfy me.

As you look around Astrid's beautiful, elegant living room, it's easy to feel a strong feminine presence. The rooms are spacious, beautifully appointed, quiet, and gracious in a way that conveys welcome and ease. Astrid has claimed for herself the ancient role of woman as keeper of sacred space, guardian of home and temple. Having a home that radiates peace, beauty, and harmony is important to her, not only as a source of solace and nurturance for herself, but also as a container into which she invites other women for regular gatherings.

My intention is to create a place that can hold a group of women and be a mother to us all. Here in my apartment, I am trying to create this. I don't feel that I have to be an expert to do this, or that I need to know any more about psychology than any of the women who gather here. It's very basic—for most of my life I so badly needed safety that I instinctively learned how to create it. Now that skill is something I can offer to others.

Having planted herself in the crossroads between the worlds, Astrid knows how to touch upon the sacred in the midst of the here and now. Her words reveal how deeply she has embraced her incarnation:

In a way, I feel my journey is just beginning. I have learned a lot about what it means to be a woman. As women, we learn so much from our bodies. Men go out on their heroic quests. They go out, up, and away. But we have no choice but to live here, in our bodies, with all our cycles. We need to suffer willingly and consciously, allowing life to burn and consume us. To be a woman means to be open to the joy and the sorrow both, to feel the births and the deaths as they pass in and through the body and the soul. It means serving the spirit that is trying to come into being, honoring what wants to incarnate through us, allowing ourselves to be vessels of new life.

20

HEALING THE MOTHERWOUND

Every mother contains her daughter in herself, and every daughter her mother, and every woman extends backwards into her mother and forwards into her daughter.

C. G. Jung

At a recent workshop, I invited a group of women to talk about mothering. Words like "protection," "unconditional love," and "nurturance" flew through the air. Women spoke of their mother as a source of comfort, security, and encouragement. One woman said:

My mom would always come help when her daughters had babies. It was the most wonderful experience. She loved her children, and she loved her grandchildren. She just adored babies. She stayed for three weeks and took care of everything. You hear horror stories about people's mothers coming, but for me, it was manna from heaven, the blessing of the universe. She cooked great food and kept the house clean and took care of everything. We got along great. For me, that transfer of roles was very important, my mother coming and helping me become a mother myself, and seeing her as the grandmother of my child. That was really special to me.

There was a moment of silence. Then an angry voice called out: "My mother wasn't like that at all. She was a bitch. She was always angry." Others nodded. They began calling out the attributes of the dark mother: the judge, the merciless critic, the ice queen, the betrayer of her children, the tyrant. "My mother really didn't want children," one woman remembered.

> She was angry, and it came out in the way she touched me. To have her brush my hair was always painful, and I would flinch when she touched me. I used to think there was something wrong with me for feeling like that. Now, I realize she was depressed, and her mind wasn't anywhere near her fingers. She really didn't want children. When I was born, she was terrified, totally unprepared, and alone. Without realizing it, I absorbed her feelings, and I have never had children myself.

If you were not well mothered, you are not alone. Very few women can honestly say that they were. Among the last several generations, positive mothering, especially in regard to sexual attitudes, has not been the norm. Only rarely do I hear a woman say that her mother loved her unconditionally, nourished her in body, mind and soul, and gave her a positive sexual role model. Millions of adults in our society lack the solid inner foundation of self-esteem and assurance that good mothering provides. Listen to a woman's story of descent, and you will invariably hear the story of a failed mother-daughter relationship. "Relationships in our culture are in crises around mothering," says Jungian analyst Marion Woodman.[64]

To understand where our mothers and grandmothers were coming from, we must consider that they belonged to the first generations of women who lived not only in a patriarchal, misogynist culture, but also in a fully industrialized society. Until quite recently, most people's lives were intimately linked to the turning of the seasons and the organic rhythms of the earth. Even if a woman suffered abuse, her journey from birth to death was graced by the ancient beauty of the land and the innocent spirits of animals who mirrored to her the essence of her own feminine nature. What four millennia of patriarchy were unable to accomplish, industrial society achieved in less than one century. As it stripped the earth of her natural resources, it also deprived us of an environment that could reflect our nature and severed our connection to the earth and to

THE LESSONS
WOMEN LEARNED

I grew up believing that the sounds and the smells of sexuality were bad. You were supposed to erase them quickly, like douching after sex. There was a lot of shame. I thought anal sex was totally kinky. So was any kind of pinching or slapping. Anything unusual was kinky. You made love in a darkened room with wineglasses and soft light, three positions only. For a long time, I wouldn't dare appear without makeup. I thought nobody would accept me without the trappings. I would even wear some makeup to bed. So I always had on this artificial face. My hair was straightened and puffed up and sprayed like an artichoke, the Jackie Kennedy look. My hair can't have been very nice to stroke at that point.

ANYA

the earth's slow, rhythmic cycles. Simultaneously, it normalized the clock-bound, frantic, heady way of life that now dominates all those who live in the belly of the industrial beast. This loss of connection with external nature has triggered a painful and dangerous disconnection from our own intrinsic nature.

In the forties and fifties, the ideal American woman was portrayed as a pert concoction of makeup and nylons, with girdles to flatten her swelling belly and brassieres to mold her breasts into geometrically perfect cones. She was anesthetized to the rage that simmered within her; her sweat had to be deodorized, her blood shamefully discarded, her births hidden behind the walls of sterile hospitals, the screams of her labor stifled with drugs. One senses a terrible rejection of the body, of the heavy clay and soil and mud we are made of. Just beneath the sterile surface, shame roils and bubbles like toxic waste. How could such a woman surrender to sexual pleasure in all its delicious, primal bestiality?

The shadow side of repression is pornography, which has become a multibillion-dollar industry, for the hidden, forbidden side of life will insist on exhibiting itself, one way or another. If one side of the coin displays a phony, superficial, plastic-coated asexuality, then the other will show human beings reduced to mere bodies, genitals, cocks, cunts, breasts, nipples, and mouths. Pornography insists on the primitive, simple, predictable elements of sexual arousal: the glistening wet cock gliding into the pink, blood-swollen vagina; the breasts with nipples erect and tender; the tongue that licks; the mouth that sucks and the hands that stroke and caress; the sounds of sex and the shamelessness of it.

We may shudder at the way pornography ruthlessly presents people as mere tools for sexual gratification. Pornography can, and often does, demean and abuse women. On the other hand, the crudeness of pornography also points to an essential aspect of the Great Mother, who is not only gentle, sublime, and ethereal, but also primal, crude, and vulgar in her lust and her creative frenzy. She is the female body that opens, gaping, to give birth, in the midst of mucus and blood and excrement. She is raw life—primordial, wild, and untrammelled by the values of polite society. She is the creative force within us that must express itself, no matter how offensive or repulsive it might look in the eyes of others. When twelve-year-old Alexandra demanded to be given the jar in which her ovary and tumor floated (Chapter 2), she did so because something within her recognized her organs as expressions of the goddess. This, however, was no chaste madonna, but a fleshy, messy goddess whom Alexandra's parents considered repulsive and ugly.

No wonder the men and women of the hippie generation were possessed by the pressing need to reclaim their earthiness, their animal nature. This need continues, and still cries for recognition. A woman in her late seventies laments the hatred of her sexual body that kept her childless:

> Oh, I would so dearly have loved to have a little baby of my own. But that instinct was absolutely squelched in me. Somewhere deep within, I was taught that giving birth was an awful thing. Even to this day, a terrible revulsion rises up in me about the process of giving birth, how it is dirty and bloody and repulsive. This is one of the most terrible things in my psyche I have struggled with. It made me revile the very thing I wanted so much.

It is probably no coincidence that this woman was herself not welcomed into life, as babies need to be. The very first message she received was that as a female, she was a disappointment and a failure.

> I was born in my grandmother's big brass bed, and my grandmother absolutely insisted that this first child was going to be a boy. Well, it wasn't a boy, it was me. My grandmother had already had these charming announcement cards printed up announcing the birth of Anthony James. They had no name for a girl. No one had even thought about a girl. So for several days I had no name.

From the moment of birth (and perhaps even in the womb), we begin absorbing our mother's teachings about sex and gender. Much of what we learn is never stated explicitly. As children, we observe her attitude toward nudity, her ways of expressing or withholding affection, her behavior around her husband and other men, her moments of embarrassment, her silences, her body language. In the beginning, a mother carries her daughter's body within her own. Later, it's the other way around—we carry the imprint of our mother's body, along with her values, her beliefs, fears, hopes, inhibitions, and memories. Pamina spoke of her need to periodically exorcise her mother's body from her own:

> My mom is really repressed and tight; her shoulders are like iron. I don't think she knew how to guide me, because she really never embraced her own sexuality. I have to keep reminding myself that I don't have to see the world through her eyes. When I get tense, I sometimes think to myself, "This is mom's body. It's not mine." Then I have to go light my candles and take off my clothes and dance and have a wild night with myself.

If we would reclaim our true feminine nature, we must do so from the inside out, unraveling the centuries of shame that are knotted into the fibers of our muscles, speaking the unspoken truths our mothers held in silence, feeling the once-forbidden feelings.

Often, women's resentment will not allow them to forgive their mothers for their shortcomings. But eventually, we must acknowledge that they, too, were victims of a collective malaise. They, too, were alienated from their mothers and from their own femininity. Most of them were shamed for their woman's body, their sexuality, and for desires that refused to conform to traditional ideals of womanhood. We are the unmothered daughters of unmothered mothers; the lineage of pain and alienation has haunted us for generations. "I don't blame my mom anymore," Pamina told me.

I used to blame her for everything that happened to me. But slowly I began to see the sadness of her life and to forgive her. She never really lived. My grandmother never took pictures of my mom as a child because she was supposedly too ugly. So she was wounded, too. And what about *her* mother? How far back can you go? At some point, you have to let your mama off the hook.

In hindsight, many daughters of emotionally or physically abusive mothers acknowledge that their mothers were not so much cruel as terribly frustrated and consumed with helpless craving for a fulfillment they could barely define, let alone obtain. Their anger reflected the anguish of feeling trapped in a cage of social expectations. Maturity brings many women the realization of how their mother's failures reflected a larger cultural failure. To recognize our wounds as personal manifestations of a collective wound helps us understand who our mothers were, and how they became that way. When one of my clients became pregnant with her first child, she began to draw closer to her mother. In the process, old blame and anger gave way to compassion and understanding.

Last week, my mother shared with me how much pain she feels. Her whole life has been filled with pain. When we were little kids, she lived through so much fighting, so much hatred, and she didn't know what to do. She envies me and my husband for having a different way, and she says, "If only I had known." When she gave birth, she was taken to the hospital and drugged out. Yesterday she said to me: "There is so much we weren't told or taught." She feels like this era is very important and she grieves that she feels too old to be part of it. I keep thinking what it's like to be her age and to feel that her life was mostly about being cut off from herself. She never had the incredible opportunities for growth that I do. She just had to hold the family together.

Another woman, herself a mother, dreamed that she was given a valuable statue of a priestess. But as she examined the figure more closely she saw, with a twinge of disappointment, that the priestess was not queenly and beautiful, but old, hunchbacked, and dressed in rags. Reflecting on her dream, my friend realized that she had not expected her inner priestess to be vulnerable or wounded. But as a guardian of threshold space, the priestess is always human as well as divine. Instead of allowing us to escape into a world where all is well, she calls us to confront and heal the wounds of our personal and collective past. She embodies the goddess, but she also shares our human journey. Can we begin to see that, like ourselves, our mothers are wounded priestesses? Can we acknowledge their beauty and their spirit beneath the layers of repression?

Today, as the feminine returns to power, a collective momentum toward healing is building. Some greater force is supporting us in doing what our mothers and grandmothers could not do, not because they lacked courage or commitment, but because the times were simply not ripe for the reversal that is now occurring. Healing is possible today that was impossible only fifty years ago. And as we heal ourselves, we also open to the possibility of our mothers' healing. Instead of seeing them as authority figures, we begin to see them as sisters. They, like ourselves, are spiritual beings who continue to evolve until the very last moment of their lives. At any time their soul may burst forth in a flowering of beauty and consciousness that catapults them beyond the limitations and the conditioning of a lifetime.

This is something Astrid, whose story we heard in the preceding chapter, has experienced. Astrid's relationship with her mother was difficult from the start. Like Pamina, Astrid could not help but blame her mother for her own descent. And yet, by the time her mother's death approached, Astrid had come far enough in her own

ACCEPTING OUR MOTHERS

My mother was never able to say, "I love you." As children, we would confront her about it and she would say, "Well, can't you see all the things I do for you?" Just before the birth of my second child, I told my mother the truth for the first time, which was that I had never felt she loved me. "You never, ever told me that you loved me," I said. In that moment, I just broke down and sobbed and sobbed as I have rarely cried in my life. Later on, my mother and I got to be quite good friends. She never was able to say, "I love you," though. The best she ever managed was to tell me, somewhat belatedly, that I had really been "a very good girl." I laugh when I think about it, because by then I was sixty years old.

SARA

My mom and I have come to a place where we accept each other, although she can't really understand my life. I am a lesbian, and there is just no box in her brain that could fit this in. She once told me that she drove a long distance to go to a parent support group for people with gay and lesbian children. She picked one in a different county so she wouldn't run into anybody she knew. She said all these parents were crying about having done something wrong to cause their children's sexual behavior. She said, "That wasn't the place for me because I didn't do a goddamn thing wrong. I think my daughter is crazy and if I can't get any support for that then what am I doing here?" And she left. I laughed. I told her, "Mom, you don't need a support group. You've got a whole support committee in your head."

TARA

healing process to feel ready to support her mother. To her amazement, she found that she was witnessing a birth as well as a death. As she lay dying, the old woman was simultaneously giving birth to her own self, the self that had previously never been allowed to emerge.

I nursed my mother to the end, and I was able to give her everything she needed during that time. When I arrived at her house, I thought: "Okay, be prepared. I'm going to walk into her room and she is going to try to devour me." But instead, she looked at me and said, "I didn't want you to come." I was astonished. "Why?" I asked. And she said, "I wanted to do this by myself." It was the first time in her life she had ever wanted to do anything without help.

Nonetheless, she accepted my support. We had four weeks before she died, and what she did was so amazing. She just kept going through layer after layer, taking responsibility for her life. Before her death, she let life pass through her for the first time. She really opened. Some people do the most incredible inner work at the very end. She talked about her fears of dying, about what she had done and not done in life, about surrendering and letting go and how hard it is. She was there, fully present, and for the first time, she was not expecting me to live life for her. It was the most healing thing for both of us. Before she died, she finally claimed herself and released me. I will be eternally grateful for that. We became so close that when I saw she was ready to die, I crawled into bed with her, and I said, "Let go, Mother. . . ." And she did. So there it was—her spirit was in the room, filling the room as it left the poor withered body.

The joy that has come out of this, the growth and creativity and love of life are just astonishing. When my mother died with that openness, and that depth of connection between us, I was able to open the door of my heart again that had been long shut, mainly out of my need to protect myself against her. I have just gotten stronger and stronger every day since then.

In this encounter, Astrid and her mother transcend their previous roles and meet as two women who are both moving toward wholeness and who both yearn for love, tenderness, and the embrace of spirit. Thus, the cycle closes. The mother's wounds were transmitted to the daughter, whose pain compelled her to undertake the journey of healing. Her healing in turn prepared her to bear witness to her mother's healing, setting in motion a vibration of love that began with mother and daughter but has since spiraled out into the world to touch many others in Astrid's life.

Through our physical mothers, we are initiated into the archetype of the divine Mother. If this initiation is botched, we develop mental and physical patterns that prevent us from receiving nurturance later in life. But unmothered sons and daughters need not remain wounded adults. Through our very wounds we are led to the medicine. The archetypal Mother lives within us, in all her complex majesty. And because this is so, we need not stay stuck in the role of wounded victim. We have the power to heal, to transform, and to go beyond past conditioning.

In India, men used to call me Mother. Unmarried and childless as I was, this seemed strange at first. But then I understood it was a mark of respect. These men were acknowledging me as an embodiment of the divine Mother. To them, I was a *Shakti*; this strange, magical Sanskrit word means "goddess," as well as "force," "power," and "primordial energy." Shakti is the sacred feminine in her totality.

We all know women who were raised by terrible mothers but nonetheless developed a solid core of self-love and healthy pride and became good mothers to themselves and others. Internally, they have connected with the good mother whom they never knew externally. Roseanne, whose story we heard in Chapter 1, is an example. Raised by a violent, extremely wounded mother, she has become a healer of the sickness that injured her.

> I believe that when I was given a body, I made a promise to god that I would speak for the children of the world. I feel that is my purpose in life. As my own children have grown up, I have moved from personal motherhood into a more universal form of motherhood. Children on this planet are suffering too much. And it isn't just babies, either. I see the suffering in people my own age. They too need the mother to put her arms around them and tell them that they are loved and that they are unique, wonderful beings. They too need someone to tell them to please love themselves. My desire to give love has expanded to a whole universe of people.

In certain Buddhist images, the Mother holds a bowl filled with healing medicine in her hands. It is our responsibility to bring forth that medicine. The awareness of our wounds, which are also the earth's wounds, calls forth our compassion, courage, and determination. Without this connection to the sacred feminine, how can we be healers to ourselves, let alone to the earth? How can we silence the wailing within our hearts? How can we comfort and nourish the wounded children within ourselves and the world? Though at times we might feel like motherless children, we have the power to call forth the Mother on our own behalf and on behalf of our families, our communities, and the earth. Rooted in the knowledge of our feminine power, we can extend a mother's love and compassion to ourselves, as well as to others and to the earth.

21

THE MAKING OF A PRIESTESS

Not all women are ready to be teachers, but we all need to start preparing for our role as teachers and as priestesses. Women once knew the realms of magic. They understood how to work magic. We still can use those powers. It may sound like hocus-pocus, but when you really get into the subtleties of what energy fields are all about—we have it all at our fingertips. We need to unlock the tremendous knowledge within us. We need to take down the walls and break out of the patterns society has stuck on us. We are so afraid to admit that we are magic. We are so afraid somebody is going to think we are witches. I want to be called a witch. A witch is a wisewoman. I am proud to be that. It is an honor to have that wisdom flowing through my veins. I am a priestess, and I create spaces and rituals in my life to embody that. I bring that with me now wherever I go. I feel it is a great honor to be thought of as a priestess.   *Shoshana*

To enter Naomi's house is to step out of the frenetic urban world into a serene, exquisitely elegant temple. The senses are gently caressed by the deep blue of a vase against a pure white wall, the luxuriously thick rose-colored carpet, a subtle whiff of incense. In the garden, a tangle of wisteria rises, heavy with purple blossoms, and the delicate tinkle of a wind chime comes wafting in. Every object in Naomi's house has been selected and placed with evident care, chosen both for its beauty and its vibrational impact. Like many priestesses, Naomi has a keen, refined awareness of how energy moves and how the energetic currents within a house, a room, or a body might be brought into harmony. She knows that beauty is a great healer, and that beauty is just as essential to the happiness of the soul as food to the body. Cradled in beauty, the body relaxes, and the mind moves into a state of balance.

Some women hide their priestess like a crazy aunt they are embarrassed to be seen with. Not Naomi. Everything about her—her love of art, poetry, ritual, and dance—expresses the awareness of one whose soul is awake and alert. Her dark eyes, her sensual mouth, and her brown curls could have belonged to an ancient Greek priestess, perhaps one of those who presided over the oracle at Delphi, or over the Eleusinian mysteries, where the initiates relived Persephone's descent to the underworld.

But Naomi's sensual radiance is a hard-won gift. She is now in her early fifties. For the first forty years of her life, her soul was trapped in the underworld, where her body hung on the meathook like Inanna's, swaying in the wind. Only in the last years has she begun to trust that she has truly been reborn, her feminine wholeness restored.

Naomi's descent began in infancy, when her father began to sexually abuse her. She remembers how he used her infant body to masturbate, and once almost killed her when he ejaculated in her mouth and left her choking on his sperm. The abuse continued for many years. All the while, her entire family participated in the pretense that nothing was amiss. Today, Naomi remembers these events. But until she was almost forty years old, she completely repressed all memories of the abuse. "The story I thought I was living was not the real story," she said.

All the things I believed about my life and my sexuality were false. I believed that I belonged to a decent middle-class family of wonderful, warm, affectionate people. I was popular and well-adjusted, and got good grades in school. My father was supposedly one of the pillars of the community. He taught Sunday school, and all my friends thought he was the greatest. If I describe him as I saw him for most of my life, he sounds like an intelligent, creative, caring man.

Like many victims of abuse, Naomi survived only by shattering into pieces. Unable to stay present in the face of such incomprehensible torture, her inner being splintered as the agonized psyche tore herself away from the tortured body. "I recently remembered the moment my personality shattered," she recounted. It happened one nightmarish day when her father took his daughter—just seven years old—to the house of one of his friends to be gang-raped. While this was going on,

> a kind of guardian presence appeared and said: "Come on, we're leaving. We're not staying in this body." I was already fragmented into "we" by then. This guardian took my hand and started pulling me away from my body. I was flooded with incredible grief that I had to leave my body forever and I could never go back, because it was too awful to stay. First I cried, "No, no, I don't want to leave." But then I looked at the scene around me and was convinced. "Oh, I see. Yes, I guess I'll come with you. I really can't stay here." From then on, I just lived somewhere else, dissociated from my body.

As so often in listening to women's stories of descent, my heart ached and my mind reeled with disbelief and anger. How can such things happen? How can a father do such a thing to his child? "And yet," Naomi continued, "even in the midst of such horror there were moments when a great feminine presence seemed to reach out and comfort me."

> I can't believe I'm not totally insane. But as much as those horrible realities were there, I was also living with a constant protective energy that was so much a part of my consciousness that I took it for granted. I didn't think, "Oh, I have a guardian angel." But now, I see that I did. I remember going into closets and sitting there. I would feel this incredible presence which later I completely forgot about. It was a huge, healing, female presence, like a guardian angel or like the divine Mother.

Had I not worked with dozens of survivors of sexual abuse, I might well have doubted the horrendous stories Naomi told me, as she herself doubted when the memories first began to surface. However, she had always remembered certain telltale incidents. For instance, there was the time she was ten years old and turned to her father for comfort after her mother's early death. Instead of comforting her, her father ended up lying on top of her, body to body. And there was the time he kissed her on the lips and stuck his tongue in her fifteen-year-old mouth. Like many abuse survivors, Naomi had no standard of what was normal and what was not, so for many years she discounted such events as insignificant. Having constructed an illusionary reality that kept her from going insane, she was not eager to face the truth.

Her body, on the other hand, never forgot. Affectionately, St. Francis called the body "Brother Donkey" for the way it patiently carries the overload of our psychic baggage, our unprocessed pain, and our unfelt emotions. Incorruptibly truthful and innocent, the body is a great spiritual teacher and a powerful catalyst for transformation. As an agent of the soul, it may insist that we heal our wounded psyche, even when the conscious mind resists with all its might. When she reached her thirties, Naomi's body began to protest. "Look here," it said, "this baggage is too heavy for me. You're breaking my back." Naomi heard her body's complaints, but still felt too terrified to face the ugly truth.

For years, I would wake up in the middle of the night shaking and sweating. My teeth would be rattling, and my whole body would shake for about an hour. I think it was releasing some of the terror triggered by a certain time of night when my father used to abuse me. Sometimes I became afraid I was having some sort of attack and would die. It happened two or three times a week for years. But when I woke up in the morning, I would push it aside like a dream. I never talked to anyone about it. I just pretended it didn't exist in the daytime.

Until Naomi was forty, her sexual life followed the predictable pattern of a woman compelled to recreate the abusive scenario over and over, hoping beyond hope that this time, the story would have a happy ending. Sadly she said, "In my twenties, none of my sexual experiences were based on real relationships. They were just chance encounters with men." Somewhere, she hoped to find that knight in shining armor whose love would fill the dark hole in her center and replace the loving father she never had. With every new lover, her hopes would soar. "This one is it," she would think; "my savior has arrived." Instead, every relationship ended with yet another rejection, another abandonment, another experience of abuse. Her face darkened by pain, Naomi says,

> I was unable to protect myself or to take care of myself in the simplest ways in relation to men. If I met someone who was nice to me, I would go to bed with them. Everything I did in the hope of leaving the abuse behind just carried me deeper into it. Sometimes, I feel so ashamed about this. At other moments I feel enraged. But in the last few years, I have mostly felt compassion for the person who suffered so much for so long.

Eventually, Naomi's quest for acceptance and belonging led to her involvement with a religious cult. Happily, she joined what initially looked like a wonderful new family, headed by the wise, gentle father of her dreams. As a thirsty wanderer lost in the desert greedily gulps down murky, polluted water, so a starving priestess often gratefully accepts whatever spiritual community she can find. Her vision blurred by need, she bows down to corrupt authorities while silencing the legitimate voice of doubt. And if, like Naomi, she has been habituated to abuse, she will rush into the baited trap as eagerly as a starving mouse who chances upon a fat, juicy piece of cheese. "I hadn't yet faced my sexual abuse," Naomi told me, "and I thought this spiritual practice would be my salvation. At the time, I felt that I had found my spiritual home. In retrospect, I see that I was looking for a daddy who would love me unconditionally, as well as a spiritual family."

Her new substitute parents taught Naomi a series of powerful spiritual techniques, all designed to lead her out of the body into a state of transcendent bliss. Given the excruciating trauma Naomi's body held, we can see why she, like many victims of sexual abuse, eagerly embraced the ideal of transcendence and readily took to a path that supported her dissociation from the body. After all, if there was one skill her abuse had taught her, it was how to leave her body in the blink of an eye. In hindsight, Naomi says that although these practices did indeed evoke states of disembodied ecstasy, they also deepened her fragmentation.

Through the cult, Naomi met and eventually married a man who seemed the epitome of everything she wanted. He was deeply sensitive, intelligent, a wonderful lover—and he shared her spiritual path. Finally, things seemed to be going well for her.

But deep down, Naomi knew that things were not what they appeared to be. Her dreams were telling her. Her body was telling her. Within the cult, there was blatant evidence of manipulation and abuse, which she tried hard to ignore, preferring a dysfunctional family to no family at all. In truth, Naomi's life was like one of those houses that Californians, who have perfected the art of denial, like to build right on top of faults in the earth. Everything looks fine, but you know that one day the earth will rumble and roar and the walls will be left standing at odd angles, like teeth in need of braces. Naomi sensed the hidden fault lines but was too terrified to acknowledge them consciously. Over the next years, she and her husband became important functionaries in the cult and moved to the Midwest to take jobs at its international headquarters. "I felt that this was my spiritual destiny," Naomi said.

> And so I gave up the life I had built for myself to go with my husband to work for our spiritual master. I left everything— the school I had founded and the whole community of people who really cared for me. Once we got there, I found it was like being in the military. There was all this secrecy and demand for obedience and punishment if you had thoughts of your own. I kept thinking that if I just meditated and chanted enough, I would be able to adjust. But I became more and more depressed. All I thought about was dying.

Then, after forty years of denial, adaptation, compromise, and repression, life finally took Naomi in its powerful jaws and shook her wide awake. Probably, Naomi's marriage acted as a trigger that caused the memories to surface. Living with a man and having regular sex was bound to open certain long-locked chambers in Naomi's consciousness.[65] Piece by horrifying piece, a series of images from hell began welling up, forcing Naomi to remember her past and to face the overwhelming truth of who her father had been and what he had done to her. Month after month, she found herself engulfed in unbearable hopelessness and despair.

For a priestess, her body is the ground of truth. But if she has been abused, staying present in the body may be almost unbearably painful. To her, staying in the body feels like imprisoning herself in a small cell haunted by all the demons of her past. Nonetheless, Naomi knew this was exactly what she needed to do. Intuitively, she sensed that, as her body held her deepest wounds, so it also held the key to her healing. And not surprisingly, her first major breakthrough occurred in a bodywork session. After months of hard inner work, a roar of rebellion finally arose from the guts of her tortured body, signaling the resurgence of the life-force:

> I did a lot of work with a bodywork therapist. I would go into states of terror and relive the abuse and scream. Then I would feel totally helpless and cry and cry. I went through the same cycle over and over and over, month after month.
>
> One day, the turning point came. I started into the same old cycle of terror and grief and helplessness. Then all of a sudden, a wave of rage rose up from my pelvis. I found myself up on my knees on the massage table with my arms raised and my fists clenched, screaming: "No! No! No!" I kept screaming it over and over and I could feel the life-force shooting through my body. It was like a reversal of centuries of abuse happening within my body, propelled by rage.

After this first eruption of her healing rage, Naomi felt a new sense of strength and a new determination to speak her truth. Aware of certain problems at work, she decided to write a memo cautiously suggesting that some changes might be in order. To her utter shock, the cult authorities, with their paranoid sensitivity to criticism, reacted with immediate and ruthless brutality. Between one moment and the next, Naomi found herself "spat out like scum," as she described it, by the organization she had devotedly served for many years.

> The day after I gave them the memo, my boss called me in and said: "As of this moment, you don't have a job. Don't go back

to your desk, just leave the building immediately." I was in shock. I couldn't believe this was really happening.

At first, my husband was equally shocked and very supportive. He said, "I don't know what kind of dream I've been living in. I realize that the only thing that really matters is love, and I've been abusing it." He had a powerful position in the organization and he'd been turning the screws on a lot of people. He called up these people and apologized. The love came flowing back into our relationship, and I thought, "What a miracle!" Our sweet, healing love was back.

But on Monday, he went back to work and they brainwashed him. He became totally cold. "Get off my back," he told me, "I can't keep my heart open in this place, so stop nagging me about it." That was it. I went into a spin as I watched everything in my life collapse. I lost the spiritual teaching that had held me together through all the adversity. I lost everything—my marriage, my home, my work, my money, my community, and my friends.

Sometimes, liberation from a life of falsehood comes disguised as disaster. As the false father idols fell, Naomi's entire life, based as it was on submission to abusive male authorities, came tumbling down. Stunned, she realized that the big earthquake she had always feared had finally struck, devastating everything she prized and exposing the hidden underpinnings of her world. No longer could she deny the fault lines that her previous life had straddled. Like Astrid, Naomi had invited an experience of crucifixion, which signaled the death of her old identity. Finally, she had reached the turning point at which her descent was to end and her ascent would begin.

For the first time ever, Naomi now committed herself totally to her own healing journey. Her most daunting task was to clear up a mountain of toxic waste and fallout material accumulated over a lifetime of abuse and self-betrayal. Recognizing the all-important need to reenter her body, Naomi continued to see a trusted bodyworker. Slowly, ever so slowly, tender green shoots of new life started pushing through the cracks. The hard work began to pay off when, at the very bottom of the rubble, Naomi discovered the sexual priestess, the messenger of the goddess from whom wave upon wave of healing ecstasy emanates. Here is Naomi's account of what happened in another bodywork session:

> As I was lying on the massage table, I started feeling a powerful surge of energy. At first, I thought it was fear, but as I stayed with it, it opened into an intense, expansive sexual feeling. For a moment, I worried about what my male bodyworker might think if I really got into my sexuality lying there on the table. But I'd been working with him for over a year, and I trusted him enough to let go.
>
> This incredibly powerful, sexual energy kept building and expanding, and I allowed it to run through my body. Then, I found my body wanted to move in certain ways in order to let the energy flow. If I didn't move, the energy would get stuck. I started arching into positions and moving my hands into mudras [sacred gestures] that looked just like pictures I have seen from ancient temples. I could feel how turning my wrist in a certain way, or moving my finger even a fraction, would alter the flow of energy and open it up in a different part of my body. I became more and more ecstatic. I could also sense that what I was doing was deeply affecting the bodyworker. I had moved out of my personal self into the sacred ground of the priestess, a priestess of the sexual rites.
>
> Afterward, I got dressed. The bodyworker was sitting there, overwhelmed and stunned. "I feel that I am in the presence of a goddess," he told me. I said, "Yes, but it isn't personal." He was married, and I certainly was not going to have sex with him. I could see he was in the thrall of this primal female energy that had been moving through me and had filled the whole room. It had connected him with something he was longing for, and he was teetering on the edge between personalizing it—thinking he was in love with me—and understanding that this was an impersonal archetypal energy. I was so filled with this energy that it was easy for me to be absolutely impersonal without denying the spiritual power I was embodying.
>
> He said, "I love working with you because the way you deal with energy is so inspiring and so powerful. My wife isn't

like that." And I said: "She is." In that moment, I really knew that I was speaking for all women, and that all women are like this. This is our heritage; we *are* this primal force. It can be covered over, but it's there. Speaking from an altered state, I said, "I understand that you may not see this in her, that maybe she doesn't even see it in herself, but she's a woman and it's there. There are ways you can uncover it together so you can both be fed by it."

In this moment, Naomi had become the archetypal priestess, a woman so fully surrendered to the goddess within that her normal ego identity melted away, leaving her in a state of total union with the goddess herself, who evokes the deepest adoration in all who behold her. As priestesses throughout the ages have done, she offered her body as conduit to this vast, primordial power that streamed through her and sent her bodyworker into an ecstatic state of shock. "I am She," Naomi might well have said in her state of sacred union. Christian authorities have sentenced many mystics to death for such supposed blasphemy. In Hinduism, on the other hand, our identity with the divine is accepted as a matter of course. To say "I am She" is merely to state the obvious. The real question is to what degree we *realize* our identity with the divine—not just intellectually, but in an immediate, visceral way, as Naomi did in this instance.

Having worked with women for many years, I know that such experiences of sacred ecstasy are more common than we generally assume. However, women often hesitate to talk about them, especially if they occur during states of sexual arousal. If a man could be crucified for owning his divine identity, what kind of welcome can a naked woman aglow with sexual fire expect? No wonder we often decide to lock such experiences in a steel box, upon which we write in big letters: PRIVATE. KEEP OUT! No wonder we veil our true beauty, our power, and our magnificence; we're afraid of being called arrogant, presumptuous, inflated, or just plain crazy.

Naomi's story highlights the difficulty of embodying the priestess outside of temple space. Priestesses have always invoked and embodied divine energies. They have always served as channels through which the goddess herself might appear to bless the community. But in cultures that understand the nature of sacred power, the worship of the divine presence within us always occurs in a ceremonial and ritualized context and does not encourage ego inflation. Homage is paid not to the personality of the channel, but to the deity.

Naomi, on the other hand, had no sacred container in which to receive the presence of the goddess. There she was, lying naked on a massage table, moving into states that would formerly have been surrounded by ritual, prayer, and ceremony. Very few modern Western people have any understanding of how to initiate contact between human and divine energies, or how to respond when such contact occurs spontaneously. Because our religious traditions discourage identification with the divine, we have no experience in relating to a person through whom a deity speaks and acts. Stunned by the power of what transpired, Naomi's bodyworker confused the woman with the goddess—or, as a Jungian would say, he fell prey to a full-blown anima projection. Fortunately, Naomi was conscious enough to not be seduced into the role of seductress. She recognized that her bodyworker needed to offer his love not to her, but to the vast transpersonal power that was moving through her. Her clear awareness of the nonpersonal nature of the experience protected her from accepting his projections and falling into the trap of ego inflation.

Listening to Naomi's story, you may think, "Well, nothing like this has ever happened to me. I guess I'm not a priestess." But having extraordinary experiences is not the point. The basis for Naomi's union with the goddess was her willingness to honor her body as the ground of her being, to enter fully into her experience, and to express whatever she might find within herself, no matter how dark or ugly it might appear. The horror of her old identity strengthened her commitment to radical honesty; she had nothing left to lose. When rage appeared, Naomi became one with her rage. Similarly, she became one with her terror, grief, doubt, hope, resentment, and disbelief. Thus, when the goddess appeared, Naomi became one with her, embodying her not in the spirit of arrogance but in deep humility. By following the shimmering thread of the truest truth she could perceive, she was led toward the nameless yet profoundly sacred and luminous core of her being.

Slowly but surely, Naomi became more and more attuned to herself as priestess, shapeshifter, and shamaness. Accordingly, she began to value her own sexual energy in a new way. No longer was she willing to sacrifice her body for mere crumbs of male attention. Rather, in an outflowering of clear minded self-knowledge, she claimed for herself the sexual powers of the ancient priestesses:

Still in this altered state, I thought, "I want to do a sexual ritual." So I called my husband, from whom I had recently separated. I said to him, "I want to give you something. If you want it, be at my apartment at six o'clock. Bring some flowers or fruit. Don't ask any questions. It will take around three hours. If you want to come, those are the conditions. If you don't, that's fine."

My husband had been very drawn to the notion of woman as sexual priestess, and he saw me as a woman who held that energy. But in our marriage, he became really frightened of my power. He was attracted, but when we got close, it terrified him and he felt that he had to dismantle my power and take control of it. I guess that is the story of patriarchy as a whole. I think the shroud of our shame makes it hard for us to see that we really are priestesses of the goddess, and that we live in a world where people still come to us because of our function as her representatives. But there is no sacred context for this anymore unless we create it ourselves.

I bathed and put on a gown and put flowers in my hair. When my husband arrived, I gave him a beautiful robe to wear. I lit candles, and I wrote out these statements with blanks to be filled in, one set for me and one set for him. They said, "I dedicate this lovemaking to . . ." "I bring to this lovemaking . . ." "In this lovemaking I ask to be healed of . . ." After writing this down, we did a Sufi dance where you put one hand on the other person's heart while your other hand is raised. In this way, we danced together to a very beautiful piece of music. Then we entered into an embrace. All the while I was filled with this goddess energy. And our lovemaking was completely sacred. There are no words for it. My husband was absolutely ready to receive this. He totally opened to it. I feel thankful that our relationship ended in this sacred way.

Then we made a mistake. We were lying together talking about our life in a very sweet, loving way. Then he started touching me again and we got aroused and tried to make love again. It didn't work. We were back in our personal selves, and all the elements of conflict and dysfunction returned immediately. It was like cheating. In a way, I'm really glad we did that, because it was so graphic. I saw how sacredness could exist within a certain space, and as soon as we moved outside that space and were trying to use our sexuality in a different way, nothing worked. It was just not happening. We tried to make love a couple of times, and then we realized it was not the thing to do. Then he got dressed and left.

The "mistake" Naomi speaks of is particularly interesting, because it clearly demonstrates the difference between personal and transpersonal love. At this point in her life, Naomi could embody the goddess to her former husband, and he could embody the god to her. They could step out of their personal lives in order to meet as vessels of the transpersonal sacred masculine and feminine. However, the doors to their personal relationship had closed and could no longer be opened.

To embody the sacred, as Naomi did in her bodywork session and again in this sexual ritual, is one of the greatest blessings a priestess can receive. For those of us who were raised with the notion of a distant, inaccessible God, there is tremendous relief in discovering that we can feel the holy presence with the same immediacy as a lover's touch. This sacred knowledge gives a woman a healthy pride, a pride rooted in knowledge of her true Self. In her book on women in Tantric Buddhism, *Passionate Enlightenment*, Miranda Shaw says:

To know oneself as an embodiment of the divine is to gain access to the ultimate source of spiritual authority within. The man or woman who knows God within is no longer dependent on outer intermediaries. Women must discover the divine female essence within themselves. This should inspire self-respect, confidence, and the "divine pride" that is necessary to traverse the Tantric path. Divine pride, or remembering one's ultimate identity as a deity, is qualitatively different from arrogance, for it is not motivated by a sense of deficiency or compensatory self-aggrandizement. This pride is an antidote to self-doubt and discouragement and an expression of the pure Tantric view. When a woman reclaims her divine identity, she does not need to seek outer sources of approval, for a firm, unshakable basis for self-esteem emanates from the depths of her own being.[66]

A woman's healing journey always relates to the healing of the collective. In Naomi's story, this interlocking of the personal and the collective is very evident. Naomi was abused, as women in general have been abused. And as women collectively are doing, she has reclaimed the sacredness of her feminine essence. Naomi herself is very aware of the way her personal journey mirrors the collective.

I see my life in the context of a planetary process. All my conflicting stories exist as simultaneous truths. I am an abused child. I am a middle-class girl. And I am also a primal, powerful feminine force. My story is a story of reversals, where everything I had believed about myself was shattered and an entirely different truth emerged. The reversal that has happened in my life is like the reversal that's happening now around patriarchy. Over the last five thousand years, women have been abused. In my own life, I wonder why I didn't just stop accepting abuse and say no. But the truth is, I couldn't. In the same way, it has not been possible for women to reclaim their power until now. I feel that I am one among millions of molecules working to heal abuse on a planetary level. The primal feminine is turning over; it's inevitable now. It is happening, and we are part of it.

The contrast between the contracted misery of Naomi's abused victim self and the glorious, expansive majesty of her awakened awareness could hardly be greater. Out of the complete collapse of

Naomi's former life, a new beginning has arisen. Having broken her allegiance to repression and abuse, she has been initiated into an awareness of her connection with Aphrodite's wild joy and her deep, oceanic sexuality.

One night, as Naomi gazed at the moon, she received a deep healing of her feminine essence. Even after leaving the cult, she had feared the power of its male leaders who had deemed her a spiritual failure. But in this moment she knew with utter certainty her oneness with that eternal, vast, primal feminine spirit who waxes and wanes, who descends and returns, who dies and is reborn.

That night, I lay on a cliff above the ocean in the bluish-silver light of the full moon. My body felt so alive in that light. As I communed with the moon, I had the feeling that she loved me, and that her love and endurance were becoming part of my own flesh and my mind. Watching her face, I was having a silent conversation with her. I had been so afraid of the authorities in my spiritual organization and so devastated by their judgment. That night, I felt the eternal love and power of the feminine and her primal vastness. I saw how that vastness went before everything and would continue after everything else was gone. From that vantage point I looked down at the temple I had served for so many years, and at all those great spiritual authorities, and they looked like little boys playing in the dust—frightened, cruel boys. They were just nothing. I thought of all these great spiritual hierarchies that men have created, and they all were nothing. Waves of validation of the feminine within myself flowed through my body, which had been so denigrated before. It was a deep healing. Once you have seen the truth, you know it and you don't forget.

22

SEXUALITY AND EVIL

Everything is good and perfect in relation to God but not in relation to us.
Rumi, thirteenth century, C.E.

Women's stories of descent make one wonder about evil. How does one relate to a man like Naomi's father, who orchestrated his own daughter's gang rape? And what about Theresa's father, who, after his twenty-one-year-old daughter returned from the convent, came to her apartment one night, forced his way in, and raped her? How does one come to terms with such events, and how does one explain the strange fascination evil seems to have with sexuality?

Biblical mythology describes evil as an angel, Lucifer, who once was god's most devoted servant but then began to resent his limited role and wanted to be all-powerful in his own right. Etymologically, the word "evil" is related to "over"—Lucifer is the angel who overstepped his limits. The name "Lucifer" itself means "Bearer of Light." Lucifer is in many ways an exact portrait of our own ego. Like Lucifer, the ego bears the light of consciousness, and like Lucifer, it has a tendency to overstep its limits. As Lucifer's purpose was to serve god, so the ego's purpose is to act as a devoted ally of the soul.

The Bible claims that Lucifer's rebellion was caused by his arrogant desire for godlike powers. Instead of being a part, he wanted to be the whole. This is a desire we all share. Why? Because everything that is partial is destined to change and die. Our ego does not like to acknowledge its vulnerability, its mortality, or its limitations, any more than Lucifer did. Frightened as we are, we too grasp for little morsels of power to mask our ultimate powerlessness. The more our ego contracts in fear, the more it pulls away from the soul, just as Lucifer separated from god. The devastation of our planet provides a shocking demonstration of what happens when the terrified, power-obsessed ego is allowed to run amok. Alienated from spirit, it wrecks havoc as it desperately tries to outrun its own inevitable death. There is only one medicine that can heal this ego sickness, and that is sacred communion. Only the immediate embrace of spirit can melt the core of terror that gives rise to evil. Only direct experience of what the Buddhist teacher Chögyam Trungpa called "the basic goodness of the universe"[67] can convince the petrified ego to soften, open, and relax.

A person whose soul has been taken hostage by the rebel ego is in a difficult position. He or she longs desperately for the ecstasy of sacred union, for a fallen angel is still an angel. But the condition for sacred union is ego surrender. To experience sacred union, the ego must offer itself as fodder to the cycle of creation, birth, and destruction. This the rebel ego refuses to do. Even in the midst of sexual union, it would remain untouched, undissolved, unaffected. "Let me see," it says, "whether I can possess that sweet fruit of paradise without surrendering, without consenting to my own death or acknowledging my fear."

We see, then, why evil might have a special obsession with sexuality. Evil recognizes the divine nature of sexual energy and senses that the genitals are instruments of a sacred power. Every act of sexual violence is also an assault upon the embodied Creator, whose power evil resents and would like to destroy. In a strange, horribly twisted way, the rapist acknowledges the creative spirit as it shines through the sexual body, just as Lucifer acknowledged god through his rebellion. Intuitively, he or she recognizes what our culture denies—that sex is an oyster which hides the priceless pearl of sacred union. The rapist wants that pearl, wants it desperately, yet cannot accept that nothing less than love will convince the oyster to open. The more he (or she) fails to satisfy his hunger, the more his anger swells. Many sexual crimes reflect the rage of men who, in a perverse way, punish women for failing to give them the sacred experience they crave. They will not or cannot surrender to love, the great dissolver of ego, but neither can they escape their need. So they slink around the edges of the sanctuary, seeking opportunities to snatch away the holiest of holies, eager to possess that which cannot be possessed.

Evil is not a problem unique to certain individuals but a collective problem, a problem of the species, a disease of the human ego. As with the common cold, nobody is exempt. Even if we never have done and never will do an evil deed, we would be fools to ignore the potential for evil that lies within us all. As the Buddhist teacher and peace activist Thich Nhat Hanh points out, all things are interconnected, and all beings on this planet *interare*. Because we interare, nobody is only a victim of abuse or only a perpetrator. The potential for violence lies in every one of us, as does the responsibility for healing the sickness it reflects. Thich Nhat Hanh, himself a survivor of the Vietnam War, wrote a poem after hearing about a tragic incident that occurred on a refugee boat:

> I am the 12-year-old girl, refugee
> on a small boat,
> who throws herself into the ocean after
> being raped by a sea pirate,
> and I am the pirate, my heart not yet capable
> of seeing and loving.[68]

To those who assume that evil must be approached with an attitude of moral condemnation, the complete lack of judgment in Thich Nhat Hanh's words may seem strange, even disconcerting. Moral outrage seems like a natural response to acts of evil. But our judgments are self-serving. We feel the need to set ourselves apart from the evildoer and to assure ourselves and our community that we have nothing in common with the criminal, that we are altogether different and better. Our condemnation distances us from the condemned, and such distance reassures and comforts us.

"I am the 12-year-old girl," says Thich Nhat Hanh. What happens in the rape of a twelve-year-old girl? The psyche of a child is extraordinarily soft, porous, and permeable. Children are like dry sponges, rapidly soaking up the information and energies that come their way. When a child is sexually violated, he or she cannot help but absorb the abuser's energy, for energy is like water—it flows from the eyes to the genitals, from the fingers to the heart, and from one being to another. The nature of sexual contact is such that inevitably a mingling not only of bodily fluids but also of psychic energies occurs. The most devastating effects of sexual abuse at any age, but especially in childhood, relate to the fact that the abuser invades the victim's psyche as well as her body. A portion of the abuser's energy then remains lodged like a deep, festering splinter within the psyche of the victim. Virtually all victims of childhood sexual abuse I have worked with anguished over the recognition that the abuser's energy had entered and penetrated them.

Survivors of childhood sexual abuse often grow up to be highly psychic individuals (Pamina and Naomi are fairly typical in this respect). Their psyches are like pieces of pottery handled much too roughly before they were fully hardened. As a result, they developed rips and tears through which outside energies, both human and other-dimensional, could easily enter. Naomi believes that over the years of abuse, a demonic entity or "ghoul" was transmitted to her from her father:

> I read a book by a psychologist who believed that the problems of many of her clients were caused by psychic entities. While reading, I started having really bizarre physical reactions. So I wondered whether such an entity might have attached itself to me. A friend offered to lead me through a process of talking to the entities and telling them to leave. While we were doing this, I suddenly saw a fat, gross, Japanese man from around the seventeenth century. He was a troublemaker, a short-tempered, perverse bully who was living in my body. I saw very clearly that he had previously lived on my father, and that he had attached himself to me when my father abused me. I realized there is a whole category of abuse entities which live off the combination of sexual stimulation and fear that is so characteristic of abuse. Abuse is great ghoul food. The abuse fragments you, and in that fragmentation

there is space for these entities to enter. I saw how parents can pass such entities down to their children.

Energy itself has no constant form. Necessarily, each one of us will perceive it in our own way. Whereas Naomi speaks of ghouls, Pamina describes deep gashes in her energy body:

About three years ago, while I was lying in my bed, I saw my body as a blueprint. It looked like a three-dimensional architectural design. I think we all have a blueprint of our body. In this blueprint, I noticed these black gashes, like long jagged triangles. When I saw them, I knew they were there because I had allowed people to abuse me and step on me. I knew right away they were injuries, and that they really needed to be tended to. They were leaks from which I was losing energy like one loses blood from a wound. "Yes," I thought to myself, "they are real, and they are deep."

When Persephone is abducted by Hades, she is warned not to eat the food of the underworld. Despite the warning, she *does* eat, and so takes the dark essence of the underworld into herself. Persephone, the maiden, still has the psychic porousness of the child-priestess who all too easily absorbs the truths and untruths of her environment. Sometimes a woman internalizes the falsehoods of the underworld gradually, over years. Other times, they pierce her like an arrow in a moment of shattering trauma, as when Naomi's father took her, at age seven, to be gang-raped by his friends:

One of the guys said to me, "Your daddy says you really like this." His remark went right into my nervous system. At that moment, shame entered my body at the deepest level, and that shame has never entirely left me. I took in the belief that this horrible, terrifying, painful torture was happening to me because in some way I had asked for it. Part of me thought, "Oh, I guess it must be my fault that they are doing this to me."

No matter how we describe it, the fact is that the abuser's energy penetrates the victim and takes up residence within her. When a woman connects with the darkness that has penetrated her flesh, she often experiences nausea and vomiting, along with the desperate desire to expel the toxicity that has been ingested. Darkness threatens to engulf her not only from without, but even more insidiously from within her own psyche. Deep despair arises as she faces the fact that all her attempts to repress the abuse or leave it behind have failed. The revolting, slimy creature still sits in her belly and has no intention of leaving.

When a woman returns from the underworld, she must face the fact that she has brought the darkness back with her and that she will never be the same. Her former self has died, as Inanna died in the underworld. Before her descent, she was an innocent child, like Persephone, the maiden. Now darkness has entered her and lives within her. As yet undigested, it sits heavily within her stomach. And since she rejects the evil yet feels it moving within her, she feels stuck and hopeless. At this stage, it is likely that she will grieve for her lost innocence and rage against her abusers.

But beyond the grief and beyond the rage, she may find that though the road she had intended to walk—the wide, comfortable road—has been blocked by a mudslide, there is another path, though a stony and difficult one. This path begins with a woman's recognition that since all her attempts at spitting and sweating and cursing out the evil have failed, she will have to digest it. She will have to stop treating it as a foreign object and claim it as hers to transform. Instead of insisting, "They did it to me. They are guilty and I am innocent," she must take the next step of saying: "I and they are one. Their darkness now lives within me. This is my wound, which only I can transform and heal."

This path of ingesting the darkness and claiming it as ours to work and struggle with, ours to transform, is the path of the shaman. Shamanic healers do not merely observe and diagnose at a distance. Often a shaman is initiated through serious physical or mental illness. This confrontation with sickness, suffering, and death familiarizes the shaman with the terrain he or she is destined to explore on behalf of others. "The shaman," says Joan Halifax, "is a healer who has healed himself or herself; and as a healed healer, only he or she can truly know the territory of disease and death."[69]

In a sense, we are all being forced onto the shamanic path today. Why do so many teenagers wear black these days? I remember how in my teenage years, I, too, chose black as my daily uniform—black clothing, black hair, black nail polish. I remember how comforting my black coverings felt. Black felt strong and clear. Behind the decisive clarity of black, I could hide my pink vulnerability, my multi-hued confusion, my many shades of passion. Black was a way of signaling to the world that I saw the threat of annihilation, that I was a child of the nuclear age who walked and lived with death at my door. Wearing black was my way of broadcasting that I had swallowed the evil of the world and was struggling with it day and night. Black was my despair, as well as my defiance. And black was also a question: Is there anything else? Is there anything beyond death? This was not a question that could be asked of the god of light. Intuitively, I, like many of my generation, was searching for a spirit whose darkness was greater than the darkness of our times and deeper than the darkest evil. Today, millions of children and teenagers are crying out for the wisdom teachings of the dark Mother. Naturally, their well-meaning parents would prefer them to follow the path of light, the golden path, the path of innocence and goodness. But the presence of darkness and evil in our world is too overwhelming to ignore, and children are desparately trying to establish their own relationship with it.

Many shamanic healers become healers only after spirit forces them to. Similarly, nobody asks to become a victim of sexual abuse. However, we *can* choose to relate to our descent as an initiation. Though this is not a form of initiation one would wish upon anyone, in hindsight many women have made peace with the path their life has taken. In Pamina's reflections on the meaning of her descent, the blossoming of a deep spiritual awareness is evident. When a woman calls her journey a descent, as Pamina does, she implies that her suffering has meaning and that her journey reflects certain universal patterns. The choice to see her life in this way is one which only she herself can make. Having passed through Ereshkigal's dark realm, she now carries her knowledge of the dark as a source of strength and wisdom. To her, black is no longer the color of evil but the color of strength and wisdom. Having healed herself, she has become a healer to others. She knows, through hard-won experience, what Thich Nhat Hanh means when he speaks of interbeing.

In a women's circle, I was able to let out my scream. I had been trying to find that scream for a while, the scream that came from the very bottom of that black pit. When I let out that scream, I felt like a vessel. It came through me, and I heard it move way out over the sea. I felt so connected to the dark goddess, like an open black vessel with the sound pouring through. Now, when I sing, I make sounds that come from the depths of my being. Not just beautiful sounds, but sounds that come from the harsh, dark places. When I sing about violation, I know what I am singing about. I was cracked open, and as a result, I know the inner places that people go to, and I can do good work with them. I can relate to people who suffer. I have not only experienced healing for myself, but I am able to give to others, too.

I've learned something from the rapes. I don't think anything happens without our participation. Even though I was attacked and raped, on some level I feel I invited it. In my healing, there was a point where I really needed to establish that I was raped, I was violated, they were the perpetrators and I was the victim, and it was a really bad, wrong thing. And that is still a truth. I had to be mad. I had to be angry and grieve. But there's also the truth that I have my own divine plan, and I do have a higher Self. My soul has lessons to learn, and I have to embrace those experiences. Those intense rammings were wake-up calls, even though I would never want to have them again. If I deny that, then I'm not embracing my life and my truth.

Naomi comes to very similar conclusions. Usually, victims of abuse need to firmly "take their own side" for a long time before they can even consider taking any responsibility for the violence that wrecked their lives. All too willing to blame themselves, they need to identify as victims, until every cell of their body knows that

THE BEAUTY OF BLACK

What draws me to lovemaking, as well as to meditation, is the possibility of expansion. The expansion is not always into light. It can also be into the Void or into darkness. In moments of total surrender, I have entered a profound darkness, yet a darkness that shines, that sparkles, that has a light to it.

Once, I did a twenty-four-hour meditation that involved looking at myself in a mirror. During this time I experienced all kinds of phenomena—beings and past lives and so on. At one point, a light came out of the mirror that was so strong it knocked me off my chair. But in the end, I was sitting there, fully aware that it was midafternoon and I was looking into the mirror, and there was nothing there—nothing. Total blackness. My mind had stopped projecting. That blackness had a quality I had never seen before and never saw again.

ANYA

they were innocent and that what happened to them was not their fault. The process that gradually transforms rage and pain into acceptance can never be willed or forced, but must occur naturally, like the blossoming of a flower. And yet, at a surprisingly early stage in Naomi's healing process, her dreams began pointing toward another dimension of truth, the truth of our interbeing, which Thich Nhat Hanh expressed in his poem.

For about five years I had been working up to remembering the abuse. At one point, I felt stuck in my spiritual practice, and I asked for a dream about the obstacles I was facing. That night, I had a very important dream.

In the first scene, I saw all these babies, all dressed in white, incredibly pure and innocent and beautiful. They were on a beach. Then a group of big men came and started throwing them around and ripping them apart, and an overlay of my father appeared on these men. In the next scene, I was standing on a road. Farther down the road, some men were raping a woman. But I didn't do anything about it; I just stood there. In the final scene, a young woman showed up who was a friend of mine and whose own abuse memories were just starting to surface during this period. She and my sister came to me and said, "We don't know how to tell you this . . . It may be hard for you to accept this . . ." They kept beating around the bush without coming out with any information. Then, I realized they were trying to tell me that in a former life, I had abused them.

I believe that the three scenes of this dream showed me three roles I had played, as victim of abuse, as a passive witness who fails to intervene, and as an active perpetrator. And this entire dream came in response to my question about what was obstructing my spiritual progress at that time. I do believe that my family was together before, and that I have enacted the three roles of victim, witness, and perpetrator.

I hesitate to talk about it, though, because it's so awful when people who were sexually abused are told, "It must be karmic; you must have been a perpetrator in a previous life." This is like saying, "It serves you right." I feel very sensitive about this. I cannot accept any view that condones or minimizes the horror. Some people try to find the redeeming aspects of being horribly violated. They want to know what gifts this experience brought me. There is a time and a place to ask those questions, but it's so important to realize that sexual abuse involves unredeemable devastation, terror, and suffering. That's it, period. It's the underworld. At a later point, you can say, "Well, my trip to the underworld was so useful, and I learned so much from it." But sidestepping the horror misses the whole point. The suffering of such abuse as I experienced is irredeemable and inexplicable, and there's no reason for it, except that the world is full of pointless cruelty.

Still, there *is* another level of truth where I feel I made a choice to experience these kind of horrors, and to be articulate about them, so that now I am able to speak for a whole cluster of people who have had similar experiences.

Naomi's struggle to transcend the roles of abuser and abused, victim and perpetrator, led to a powerful visionary experience in which she glimpsed the unfolding of her soul's evolution in a drama that spanned many millennia and culminated in a battle between herself and the forces of evil. As she describes the events of this mythic battle, we see her establishing herself firmly as a priestess of the Light, who reclaims her powers and uses them to envelop, devour, and transform the darkness that she herself helped unleash.

I remember a lifetime, a very ancient lifetime, in which I was an apprentice to a priestess of the dark forces. A ritual took place in which the priestess collected dark energy in order to then unleash it. She was offering this energy to the dark forces in order to gain some kind of personal power in return. A young boy who was to be sacrificed was wheeled into the temple courtyard on a huge carving of a black bull. He was crouching by the bull's leg, and I recognized him as my former husband in this lifetime. I was helping the priestess amidst sounds of chanting and strange metallic noises. There was a swirling of black energy and then, as the boy was killed, an explosion of destructive energy was released. I remembered participating in this ceremony, and then seeing the destructiveness of the outcome. At that point, I made a vow that I would never again abuse power, and that I would always choose to be abused rather than be abusive.

The day that I saw this particular life, I also saw that the dark energy I had helped unleash many, many centuries ago was still at large, and that until now, I had lacked the spiritual power to confront it. That very night, all this dark energy started collecting around me. Then it descended and attacked me. I was engulfed in darkness and evil. Although it terrified me, I also saw that now, five thousand or so years later, I possessed the skills to transform the darkness, and that I needed to do this. But it challenged me to the limit.

I understand now why there are so many stories about the war between good and evil. That's what this was. It was a battle of sorcery between the dark, destructive forces, which I myself had helped create, and the creative life force. I tried to radiate love from my heart into this energy, but the beam from my heart was puny compared to the vastness of this evil, and it just swallowed me up and spun me around. My personal love was much too tiny to confront this immense force. "Okay," I thought, "that didn't work. What else can I do?" I had to change my consciousness in every way I knew to find some way of containing this energy. It was a long, long process. First, I had to overcome the terror of feeling the evil and relating to it. I knew that the terror itself could easily kill me. So first, there was a battle with my own fear. When you're paralyzed by fear, you can't use your creativity, so I knew I had to master my terror in order to win this battle.

That was the first stage. Then I tried all these different techniques. I tried calling on every positive energy I knew of. That didn't really work, either. I must have used hundreds of techniques, and the adjustment of the dark force to what I was doing became more and more refined. In the last stages it was as if I were holding my consciousness in my hands, and I would make a tiny adjustment and see how that affected the energy.

Finally, I expanded my boundaries and identified with the part of myself that is timeless. I had to keep expanding my sense of who I was. I had to go way back to the beginning of time, which doesn't really exist, because there is no boundary there, and way forward to the end of time. I had to go to the ends of space, and I had to expand until I was a vast, infinitely huge presence of love. Then it seemed as if I were blowing white smoke into black smoke, so that the particles mixed and the color became gray. I kept pouring in more and more light until the dark energy was diffused and finally dissolved. At this point, it seemed as if the darkness lost its strength and the magnetic power that held it together as an entity dissipated.

It was important for me to acknowledge the power of the dark in order to battle it. I could not say, "This doesn't exist." I had to accept that it *did* exist, that it was real, and I had to face how powerful and vast it was, and then I had to create a state of consciousness that could contain and dissolve it.

When the infusion of love became great enough, the magnetic power of the darkness was broken, and I fell back into myself.

This process lasted through most of the night. For the rest of the night, I had visions that predicted my life for the next three years. Until this moment, I had experienced abuse over and over again, and everything I did in the hope of leaving it behind would carry me deeper into it. This night was a key and a turning point that marked the end of the abusive cycle. However, it took another three years for the inner changes to be integrated and manifested in my outer life.

I don't believe in the devil, but I have experienced the reality of evil. I choose to believe that the divine is in control, and that evil is not. There is no proof of this, but it is my choice to see things that way because it works; it would be hard to live and not believe this.

23

THE TIGER MOTHER:
GUARDIAN OF BOUNDARIES

i found god in myself
& i loved her/i loved her fiercely
Ntozake Shange

At one point while Pamina was institutionalized, she spontaneously began painting tigers—huge, vibrant animals with bold green eyes, twitching tails, and muscular bodies that seemed poised to leap off their six-foot-long canvases. For hours, days, and weeks on end, Pamina was completely engrossed in bringing forth the archetypal images that her unconscious sent her during this time of need. "I think I was calling on them for strength and protection," she remembered. "Each time I painted tigers, I was in absolute chaos and despair, and I just holed up in my room and painted."

"Your fascination with tigers is as ancient as humankind," I told Pamina. Since the dawn of history, tigers have been portrayed as symbols of vibrant strength and as fierce allies of the goddess. Sculptures dating back to the sixth millennium B.C.E. show female figures accompanied by lions, panthers, or tigers. Sometimes the great cats stand by the goddess's side. Sometimes they guard her while she gives birth, and sometimes she rides them or holds one of their cubs in her hands. A bond of mutual protection is evident—as the cats protect the goddess, so she protects their young. In India, the Tiger Mother is to this day one of the most beloved Hindu goddesses. The tiger's golden-black stripes reflect the knowledge she embodies—how to live in the light without avoiding the dark, how to honor death within life and life within death, how to reconcile the soft, voluptuous sensuality of the golden goddess with the ruthless, uncompromising fierceness of the black Mother who can kill with one swipe of her paw.

Western religion has abolished all images of the goddess, with the one exception of the Virgin Mary, and even she has been defanged and declawed, domesticated, stripped of her sexuality and her instinctual wildness. With her delicate beauty and her otherwordly radiance, Mary does not embody the fierce, fiery, juicy energy certain women need to access in order to become whole. With her sharp fangs, ripping claws, and sinewy strength, the Tiger Mother reflects an essential but often underdeveloped side of our own feminine nature. She is, first and foremost, a protectress of the earth and of all earth's creatures, for whom she feels the same fierce mother love that a tigress feels for her cubs. Only a fool would risk getting too close to a tigress with her cubs: cross her boundaries, and you are dead meat. And so the Tiger Mother is also worshipped as the guardian of sacred boundaries and as the ultimate warrior queen. Though our religions ignore her, our collective unconscious remembers her well. Just as she showed up in Pamina's paintings, so I also see her showing up in women's dreams, always at times when they are dealing with boundary issues.

As has often been noted, the rape of the earth and the rape of women go hand in hand. If we would become protectors of the earth, we must first learn to protect our own boundaries. Sexual self-protection in particular is an important issue for every woman. When we let loose our sexual magic, we become alluring and magnetic, like Aphrodite herself, who attracted suitors the way a honey jar attracts ants. So how do we fend off unwanted attention? How do we avoid abuse without denying our soft, yielding sensuality?

The traditional patriarchal solution is to have every woman attach herself to a man who, in return for his protection, treats her as his sexual property. This arrangement is not only degrading to everyone involved, but also leaves millions of single women unprotected. Hopefully, future generations will know a less violent, abusive world. In the meantime, we had best befriend the Tiger

Mother within our own psyche. When a woman embodies the Tiger Mother, she manifests a calm dignity and strength, which people perceive and intuitively respect. Her confidence flowers out of a deep, cellular knowledge of her sacred nature, and this knowledge affects all who come into her presence. She feels strong and she knows her own worth. If threatened, she will fight unto death, yet at the same time, no creature is more tender, more voluptuous, or more sensual than a tigress.

Our first step in reconnecting with the Tiger Mother is learning how to say yes and no and mean it. For many women, this is a daunting task, trained as we are to be compliant and please others. You may recall how both Iris and Joanne (Chapters 13 and 14) lamented their tendency to give in to their husbands and have sex when they really didn't want to. But more often than not, the body refuses to lie and will broadcast the truthful no that lies hidden behind the false yes. Like many women, Joanne suffered from recurrent bladder infections. The healing that no amount of antibiotics were able to bring about occurred naturally once she learned to say no. Unfortunately, few urologists or gynecologists ever talk with their female patients about the fact that many vaginal and bladder infections are caused by sex that is either unwanted, too fast, or not sensitive enough. One woman told me:

> My husband used to want sex in the crack of time between a meeting and a party. "Let's have a quickie," he would say. To me, that meant, "Let's have a meaningless, one-minute genital contact." But I thought I was supposed to be able to do that. I had no sex education at all and no one to talk to. I thought that I should be able to enjoy that. While I was married, I was constantly sick with bladder infections and many other symptoms. I didn't realize that my body was asking me to pay attention to myself. The minute I got out of the marriage, my health was terrific.

One of the nation's most successful programs for preventing teenage pregnancy is based on teaching teenage girls how to say no to sex. Shockingly, many girls who participate in the program say they never realized they had a right to say no.[70] Whenever you feel guilty about saying no, just try to remember the queenly assurance with which a cat communicates her likes and dislikes. Pleasing herself is her main purpose in life, and she is determined to do the very best job she can. But don't expect everyone to be pleased when you say no. You may recall how Roseanne's husband claimed he had a right to be sexually serviced (Chapter 1). You, too, may find yourself accused of selfishness or disloyalty, as cats often are. But this is selfishness at its best, selfishness born out of self-love. Without such selfishness, we lose sight of what we want and need for ourselves. One woman told me, "My whole life I have had to discipline myself to get up in the morning and ask myself the question, 'What do I want for me? What does my soul need from this day?'" We need to cultivate this good selfishness, so that if and when we make love, we do so to please ourselves, with the playful sensuality of creatures completely at one with their own instinctual nature. Then, our yes will mean yes, and our no will mean no.

In a culture that values female compliance, many women learn early in life to stifle the Tiger Mother's exuberant vitality. She is too wild and independent, too sensual and threatening for polite society. Though she reflects essential qualities of the feminine spirit, we are often told, when we embody her, that our behavior is "unfeminine" or "selfish." So we learn not to growl, not to bare our teeth, but instead to smile and be "nice" while others violate our boundaries. Gentle and conciliatory, we learn to submit to casual humiliations. Why make a fuss over what nobody else seems to think is a big deal?

The Tiger Mother's message is that it *is* a big deal, that we *do* have the right to demand respect, and that our self-protective instincts are valid. How can we heal our wounded and abused planet, as long as we fail to speak up on our own behalf? To protect our boundaries is to honor the sacred presence that resides within us. In the following passage, Naomi speaks eloquently and passionately about the ecological and spiritual implications of honoring her sexual boundaries and demanding that others honor them as well:

> If it is really true that healing our sexuality relates to the healing of the planet, then our task is to refuse to participate in any kind of abuse. That awareness would empower me to do

everything possible to honor myself and my body and to heal myself of the willingness to accept or excuse abuse—or be silent about it. As a spiritual practice, this is very demanding. Various kinds of abuse enter my environment countless times every day. But I am beginning to understand that to honor myself and to prevent anyone from dishonoring me *is* my spiritual practice, as well as my pleasure and fulfillment and my commitment to the continuation of life and the healing of the planet.

Once I made love to someone who had been very respectful to me until that point. And although I am sure he meant it in a playful way, we were in the kitchen, and he came in and slapped my bottom and then pinched my cheek. "What the fuck are you doing?" I thought. But I didn't say anything. I thought, "Oh, well, don't make a big deal out of nothing." But if I really honored my body, and if I was really willing in every detail to say, "No, this isn't acceptable to me," I think I would teach myself to respect my physical form more, and I would teach everyone around me that they had the right to respect themselves in the same way. I think that would transfer to how we related to the earth, and to plants and other species. It isn't just a petty personal thing when you defend your boundaries or demand respect. It may be personal or political, but more than that it's a spiritual practice.

All too often, women sabotage their own safety and welfare because they feel they have no right to a fierceness that offends traditional Western ideals of femininity. And when their rage becomes too great to contain, they turn its sharp blade against themselves, opting for self-abuse rather than self-expression. Pamina, for example, used to literally cut up her own body with glass shards. Drugs, alcohol, depression, eating disorders, and sexual self-abuse are ways in which we typically turn our rage against ourselves.

Gently, the Tiger Mother takes the dagger of self-destruction out of our clenched fists. Planting her feet like oaks, she demonstrates its proper use. Then she hands it back. We feel our fingers curling around the hilt. The gleaming silver blade flashes in the sun, sharp

WORTHY OF ANGER

Once my best woman friend called me up weeping hysterically because she had just been raped at gunpoint. I had never been able to feel angry about my own rapes; I didn't love myself enough. But when this happened, I went into the kitchen, pulled the big meat cleaver out, stuck it in the pocket of my coat, and ran out the door. "Call the police if I'm not back in ten minutes," I yelled to my husband. I ran down the street and into her apartment building with the full intention of hacking that man to pieces if he was still there. No fear, total rage. I had that rage for her. But I still hadn't given myself permission to feel it, just for me. ASTRID

as a shark's tooth. Instead of turning it against ourselves, can we learn to let it protect us? Can we own such power, such potential to injure and maim? Can we trust ourselves to use it wisely?

Naomi says that now, in her fifties, she is finally claiming her tigerish fierceness. She openly presents herself as a sexual, sensual woman, but also as a woman who holds a dagger in her hand, a woman not to be trifled with. Her history of abuse has made her sensitive, wary, and apt to bolt at the least sign of danger. "I realize that you are dangerous," a man recently said to her. And she answered, "You're right. I *am* dangerous." As she told me about this conversation, she added proudly, "I've never been able to say that before. I always tried to pretend that I was this sweet person who wouldn't hurt a fly, just like my mother had been."

When Pamina was nineteen years old, she took a giant step in this direction. At this point, she had not yet learned to avoid unsafe situations. Women whose self-love has been injured often have a hard time discriminating between safe and unsafe situations, or making wise decisions on their own behalf. Therefore, victims of abuse run a high risk of being abused again. If you have not been damaged in this way, you may well wonder why Pamina kept exposing herself to danger, or why Naomi and Astrid kept getting involved with abusive men. Like a damaged immune system, their self-protective capacity did not function well.

When Pamina's lack of caution led her into an encounter with a would-be rapist, the stage was set for yet another repetition of the old cycle. But, she said, "this time, something was different." This time, the Tiger Mother burst forth from her in an explosion that signaled the end of her submissiveness, the end of any tolerance for abuse, the end of her willingness to be victimized.

One day I was hitchhiking, alone, in Hawaii. I was wearing an old antique slip that I had sewn patches on and loved very much. I didn't have the sense to cover myself well in those days. I was very free and open and never wore a bra, and I had no sense of self-protection. At the same time, I really felt protected that day. I was waking up to the presence of my spirit protectors. It was a beautiful day, with a pure blue sky and a sparkling ocean.

So here I am hitchhiking, and I want to get to a certain beach. I get picked up by this guy, and he tells me about a place where you can hike up some cliffs and walk to the beach. So I say, "Great, take me there." We pull up and walk out to what is supposed to be a trail, and the guy attacks me. And I am thinking to myself: "This is not going to happen. I am *not* going to get raped again."

And suddenly, something was different in me. "No fucking way," I thought. He was taking off his pants and I could feel his penis against me, this yucky thing. But I really felt that I was being watched spiritually, and I just knew this was not going to happen. I was thinking "No, no, no." Then he ripped my beautiful slip apart. That was it. My rage just exploded, and I screamed at him, "What the fuck do you think you're doing? Do you know this is an antique? Do you know how much time I've spent mending and caring for this slip? Do you know how many generations it has come through? Who the fuck do you think you are, tearing at my clothes like this? You just cut this out right now."

I don't even know what came over me. Immediately, he

jumped up and said, "I don't know what's happening, but I can't do this to you. Can I take you out for dinner, can I drive you back to town? What can I do for you?" I just couldn't believe it. This was a big breakthrough, the way this power had just come through. There was something about ripping my skirt that brought my fury out. It was great. That was a big victory day for me.

A petticoat may seem a trivial thing, yet women have always poured their soul into their handiwork and have always known that a piece of fabric, a quilt, a hand-knitted or hand-sewn garment can contain the spiritual power and the blessings of those who made it. Pamina's slip put her in touch with the spirits of her foremothers, and with a collective field of feminine power and feminine rage. As she reconnected with the archetypal Tiger Mother, a powerful energy radiated from her and instantly, almost miraculously, transformed her attacker's behavior.

Like many victims of abuse, Pamina hid her beauty for several years. "I didn't want to be noticed, so I became really plain," she recalls. "I didn't wear makeup and I just gave up on my body." Like Pamina, many women surround themselves with a kind of mantle of invisibility. Instead of flaunting their bold stripes, they hide behind excess weight or dress in drab, unattractive clothes, or in ultra-masculine, angular business attire. Others suppress the sensuality of their body language or keep their voices childlike and weak. "If I am invisible," they hope, "maybe I will be safe. Maybe the thugs will pass me by." To the world, they broadcast, "Don't hurt me. I'm harmless. I'm not really female at all. I'm not a tigress, just a little gray mouse."

But eventually, Pamina's tigerish exuberance demanded space to romp and play. She remembers the day she decided to emerge from hiding and let her beauty shine:

One day I stood naked in front of the mirror and practically passed out. I had become so fat, and I did not like it one bit. Now, I lost those twenty pounds. I started thinking about my beauty, my womanhood. I began to value myself for the first

COMING OUT OF HIDING

For many years I tried to neutralize and hide my sexuality as much as possible, both in my behavior and my appearance. In old pictures, I look bright and intelligent and clean, sort of like a born-again Christian. NAOMI

I always tried to hide my sexuality. I didn't want my clothes to be too suggestive, and I would try to cover up, keep parts of myself under wraps. Somehow I didn't want people to know I was a sexual being. JOANNE

I used to put up this wall of sexual aloofness that would cover my insecurity. I was afraid that if I wore anything too revealing, I would be considered a slut. But I had a gay friend with whom I could let out my flamboyance, and he just loved it, and I felt safe with him. Once he bought me this pair of pinkish-red suede shoes, with high heels, ankle straps, and rhinestones down the back. They were kind of slutty but beautiful. Just recently, with my husband, I have been starting to let that side of me come out again. My sexual energy is opening up, and I am feeling the desire to fully embody this Aphrodite energy and let it be visible. VALERIE

Finally, I am able to allow myself to be female, to be beautiful, and get all decked out. I let myself buy frilly underwear instead of the practical stuff I used to buy. I started looking at underwear as this wonderful female decoration with no functional value. It's divine, sexual play. Finally, I feel my body is beautiful enough to wear it. I put it on and look at myself, and think, "I look good. This is beautiful. I'm not too fat or too short here and too long here. I am beautiful." IRENE

time. One day I looked in my drawer. All my panties were so old and baggy I had to pin them up. All those old socks with holes . . . I threw everything away. I went out and bought all new socks, all new underwear, all new bras. I went on a rampage. It was a real breakthrough for me: I was learning to mother myself.

Today, Pamina boldly flaunts her outrageous, gold-black striped beauty. She allows herself to express her authentic feelings and to be exactly who she is, without worrying whether others will approve. Erotic and fierce, sensual and untamed, she is a gorgeous, flamboyant woman who pursues her own sexual pleasure and satisfaction without apologies.

I have finally embraced my beauty. Now I no longer feel I have to hide in the presence of men. I wear whatever I want to wear. If I want to wear something exotic and beautiful, there's nothing wrong with that. I can embody desire. I don't have to shut down in the presence of men. I can say no.

Many women fear their own rage because they equate rage with violence, especially if they were raised in abusive families. Pamina's story of a violent man stopped in his tracks by an enraged woman proves just how different violence and rage can be. Rage is a red-hot jolt of voltage which demands that we take forceful action. Like a red flag, it alerts us to the fact that something is seriously wrong. As you may recall, Naomi's first major breakthrough occurred when her despair turned to rage and she began screaming out that forbidden word of protest and rebellion: *No!* Used properly, rage can give us the energy and courage we need to set right what is wrong. In contrast, a violent person makes no attempt to set right what is wrong, but merely discharges his or her rage energy by inflicting harm on others.

Wherever we find myths about the goddess, we also find stories about her rage, which assure us that rage can have a healing and even sacred dimension. Invariably such stories also reflect an understanding that female rage has far greater destructive power than male rage. In a culture where the destructive effects of male rage are so obvious, this may be hard to believe. A raging man often acts like an angry elephant who stampedes around trumpeting loudly and leaving a trail of devastation behind him. His rage has a blindness

WOMEN'S ANGER

Women's anger has inspired them to cut ties with abusers, never again to have to endure pinches, inappropriate jokes, and drunken advances while they try to chew their Thanksgiving turkey. Women's anger has catalyzed them to quit jobs with domineering bosses, to divorce battering husbands, and to break addictions to drugs and alcohol. Focusing anger precisely—onto the abuser and away from yourself—clears the way for self-acceptance, self-nurturance, and positive action in the world.   ELLEN BASS AND LAURA DAVIS[71]

about it, an unconsciousness. One can't reason with him, so one had best get out of his way until he calms down.

Female rage is very different. The rage of the goddess is highly conscious, like a blinding flash of light that shoots from her third eye and unfailingly finds its target. Where male anger seeks to penetrate its target physically, through hitting, stabbing, or shooting, female rage penetrates energetically and psychically. With one word, an enraged woman can cut her victim to the quick. If a woman uses this power in ego-based ways, she becomes a true witch who can totally undermine people's self-esteem and destroy their lives. But when she channels her rage energy toward protecting justice, beauty, and innocence, she becomes a formidable guardian of the Light. No wonder patriarchy has tried to repress women's rage by declaring it "unwomanly." In fact, our rage is very womanly indeed, and it is one of our most important and misunderstood allies. •

A Hindu myth says that once, long ago, demonic forces were devastating the earth, forces so powerful that none of the male deities could halt their destructive frenzy. Finally, in their desperation, all the gods came together and concentrated their prayers in one point. Out of the immense blaze of that fusion, a brilliant figure arose—the Tiger Mother, dressed in red, bearing a thousand weapons in her thousand arms. Instantly, filled with sacred rage, she launched into battle against the demons, and before the eyes of the awestruck gods, she cut them down as playfully as if she were picking flowers for a garland.

Like all archetypal myths, this story appears to speak of the distant past, yet in fact it addresses our current situation. It points out that the patriarchal authorities to whom we have been looking for solutions simply do not have what it takes to halt the destruction of the earth. Instead, it suggests that we should concentrate our efforts on evoking the sacred feminine, who can help us access an energy that is courageous, clear, powerful, intelligent, and large-hearted enough to save our endangered planet.

24

CUNT HEALING

In the Amazonian jungle, the first woman and the first man looked at each other with curiosity. It was odd what they had between their legs.

"Did they cut yours off?" asked the man.

"No," she said, "I've always been like that."

He examined her close up. He scratched his head. There was an open wound there. He said: "Better not eat any cassava or bananas or fruit that splits when it ripens. I'll cure you. Get in the hammock and rest."

She obeyed. Patiently she swallowed herb teas and let him rub on pomades and unguents. She had to grit her teeth to keep from laughing when he said to her, "Don't worry."

She enjoyed the game, although she was beginning to tire of fasting in a hammock. The memory of fruit made her mouth water.

One evening the man came running through the glade. He jumped with excitement and cried, "I found it!"

He had just seen the male monkey curing the female monkey in the arm of a tree.

"That's how it's done," said the man, approaching the woman.

When the long embrace ended, a dense aroma of flowers and fruit filled the air. From the bodies lying together came unheard of vapors and glowings, and it was all so beautiful that the suns and the gods died of embarrassment.

Eduardo Galeano

Body parts are powerful symbols. As the heart symbolizes love, so a woman's genitals represent the core of her feminine self. In ancient India, as in many cultures less misogynist than ours, a woman's genitals were considered her most sacred body part, the part that most clearly expressed her goddess essence. In certain Indian temples, you will see an image of the Mother's yoni, or vulva, set above the temple door, often at a height that allows people to touch it for blessing. "You are entering the body of the goddess," the image of the yoni tells us. "You are entering sacred space."

In Eastern symbolism, flowers, especially lotuses, are symbols of the vulva. At the same time, the lotus is also the symbol of perfect purity and innocence. Rooted in slime and mud, the lotus floats up to the surface of the water, where it opens its delicate, luminous petals to the light of the sun. In the same way, our sexual bodies blossom out of the earth, and in turn the lotus of enlightened consciousness blossoms out of our bodies. Lakshmi, the Hindu Aphrodite, stands on a lotus, is praised as the lotus-eyed goddess, and holds a lotus in her hand—all this to remind us that such purity and exquisite beauty are the innate nature of all physical matter. What a healing concept for us, who were raised to think of our genitals as dirty!

Women in many other cultures freely and proudly displayed their genitals. In the story of Inanna, the ancient Sumerian queen, we read:

Inanna placed the shugurra, the crown of the steppe, on her head.
She went to the sheepfold, to the shepherd.
She leaned back against the apple tree.
When she leaned against the apple tree, her vulva was wondrous to behold.
Rejoicing at her wondrous vulva, the young woman Inanna applauded herself.[72]

When I read this passage to Donna, an African-American midwife, she sighed and told me that the worst insult to a man is to call him a woman, and specifically to call him by the name of a woman's genitals. "I know this," she said, "because in the seventies, I went to a black power conference at which one man called the other a cunt and was shot seven times by the other. That was the level of insult involved." As a midwife, Donna also sees the impact of genital shame in the women she works with:

Women feel their genitals are ugly, smelly, dirty. Among hundreds of women I have examined, the number who have gotten on the table and could lie there openly, without shame, I can count on half the fingers of one hand. An older Chinese woman told me she used to be a midwife but stopped because it was too "nasty." "Nasty" is a term many women use. Black women say it a lot. They own it openly, but white women feel it, too.

"It saddens me," Donna says, "how few of the women I know really love themselves as sexual beings. Many women talk about sex, but very few are really sex-positive. They know the sacred feminine in terms of emotional connection, but not through their sexual body." After talking to Donna, I looked up the word "cunt" in Barbara Walker's *Women's Encyclopedia of Myths and Secrets*, and read:

Derivative of the Oriental Great Goddess as Cunti, or Kunda, the Yoni of the Universe. From the same root came county, kin, and kind (Old English *cyn*, Gothic *kuni*). . . . also cunning, kenning and ken: knowledge, learning, insight, remembrance, wisdom.[73]

Well, if this is what "cunt" means, one could be called worse things. One could, for example, be called a whore. But then again, Walker explains that whores were originally

Aphrodite's celestial nymphs, who performed the Dances of the Hours, acted as midwives to the gods, and inspired earthly *horae* (harlot-priestesses) to train men in the sexual Mysteries. The dance still called *hora* was based on the priestesses' imitation of the zodiacal circling of "hours."[74]

Patriarchy has caused a strange reversal of values, whereby women's bodies, once revered as the source of life, have become the epitome of everything degrading. Venus is no longer venerated, but instead blamed for venereal disease. A rift runs through our lives, severing what we do in bed with our lover (or our vibrator) from what we do and think in church, in temple, in meditation. What was once held most sacred has become the devil's domain.

Naturally, our language reflects this reversal. Celia grimaced as she talked of her vagina and clitoris. "I hate those words," she said. "They remind me of an anatomy class. They are so cold and sterile." Most of our sexual words are indeed either clinical and cool in their Latin precision ("penis," "scrotum," "clitoris") or vulgar, tainted with disdain ("cunt," "hole," "fuck") or ludicrously exotic (as when Tantric teachers talk about the man's "jade stalk" instead of his penis). Some women feel more embarassment at naming sexual organs and acts than they do about actually having sex. Yet we should not let the awkwardness of our language keep us silent. For too long, the taboo on using sexual language has reinforced our disempowerment. It is high time that we learn to speak about the physical aspects of sex openly, to name the body parts, the sexual acts, and to ask for what we want from our lovers. Language grows through use. The Eskimos would not have developed twenty words for snow unless they talked about snow a lot. By talking about sex, using whatever words we feel most comfortable with, we help birth a new language as well as a new consciousness.

Today, as the era of patriarchy nears its end, we are beginning to shake off centuries of falsehood, like wet wolves climbing out of a cold river. Slowly but surely, we are remembering the sacredness of our sexual nature and the inherent innocence and goodness of our bodies. We stand on the cusp between our patriarchal past and what we hope will be a more sex-positive future. No wonder, then, that we are creatures of paradox, bound to the past yet birthing the future. Sometimes we feel poisoned by self-hatred; at other times we blaze with light like the sun. Old lies whisper in our ears, while our heart sings to us of even more ancient truths. Our psyche is many-layered, like the earth at sites where many cultures have lived, each one building upon the ruins of the last. A client of mine lamented the fact that her entire life had been marred by sexual repression; yet, even while trapped in the coils of shame, she dreamed that she was lying naked in a lovely meadow, and that an exquisitely beautiful flower was growing out of her vagina.

Real transformation is always linked to the body and to the nitty-gritty of our individual lives. This is why how we feel about

SEXUAL WORDS

When I was seven or eight, I saw this word written on some windows: F-U-C-K. So, one day I asked my mom, "Mom, what does F-U-C-K mean?" She just smacked me across the face and told me to never say that word again. So I still didn't know what it was, but I soon got the idea that sex was bad.

MERCEDES

I remember standing in the schoolyard, talking with my friends about boys. Sometimes we talked about what we called "tantrums." I would look at a boy I liked and I would get this incredible feeling in my belly, probably down into my genitals, but I didn't even know they existed at the time. Still, I knew something was happening. We would say, "Oh! Oh! I'm having a tantrum!" I think we were having these mini orgasms, but at the time, we had no words for that. So "tantrum" became our word for this visceral feeling that was so unmistakable and pleasurable.

VALERIE

our genitals is important. Sexual healing is not just a question of abstract ideas and concepts. Ideas are valuable insofar as they contain the seeds of transformation. But to bear fruit, they must take hold in the soil—that is, in the flesh and blood of each individual, in the way we speak or do not speak, the way we eat our food, the way we meet our lovers' eyes, the way we inhabit our bodies. I emphasize this because too many women call themselves feminists yet remain in severely abusive relationships. Too many women worship the goddess yet hate their own bodies, and do not walk their talk. So many women appear confident and self-assured, yet secretly hate their bodies, their breasts, their genitals.

How do we begin to feel that our genitals are pure and sacred? Sexual healing begins with great and small acts of courage that rumble like earthquakes through our lives. Such an act of courage

One summer, I went to a women's camp. We were supposed to pick a word we wanted to reclaim for ourselves and then paint it on a banner. Most women picked words like power, wisdom, healing, and so on. Well, my word was "vagina." Nobody else picked anything having to do with sex at all, so I hesitated. But then I wrote it on my banner. Because if you can't own your word at camp with your sisters, where will you ever own it? Then I spent the next months figuring out why I had picked that word. And I understood that it related to all the shame women carry in their bodies. I knew that shame was not our natural heritage.   DONNA

In my family, there was no talk about sexuality. There were no words for sexual parts or sexual acts. My mom would call my genitals my "teedlee," and that was the only word I knew. When I was eight or nine, I got out a mirror and looked at my vagina, and wondered if there was something wrong with me. "Is this okay?" I thought. "Is this how it's supposed to be? Is there a word for this?" It's amazing how few words we have for female genitalia. Some are insulting, and others are clinical. There are no comfortable terms.   IRENE

is evident in the following story of Pamina's determination to move beyond rape and torture to reclaim the sacred core of her feminine body. The horror she feels as she looks at her scarred vagina is the horror we all feel when we contemplate our collective history. From such horror, and from the courage to face and move through it, compassion and healing arise.

After my first rape, my vagina was stitched up. Then, during the home birth of my daughter, the whole base of my vaginal wall ripped and had to be stitched up again. If I had gone to the doctor, I would have had an episiotomy, where they go in and actually cut your vagina, so that you have a perfect scar. Well, my vagina is a very wild place. It's not smooth and perfect. It's scarred and very intense. I go through a lot of feelings when I touch it. After that birth I didn't masturbate for two years. I just couldn't bear to touch it.

One day, I grabbed a mirror, and I said, "I am going in the bathroom and I'm going to see what it looks like down there." That was so powerful for me. It took a few sessions like that for me to even start digesting the incredible transformation that had occurred. I was horrified at first. My vagina just didn't look the same. It looked like something pretty hellacious had happened down there. Back then, I was just starting to own my vulva again. "That's not my vagina," I thought. "That's not my vagina at all." For a long time, I didn't want to have sex, and I didn't want anyone to touch me there. I didn't want to have anything to do with that part of my body.

I am still in the process of healing, and I think it will be a lifetime process for me. I have a lot of feelings locked up in there. But in the last year I have had a lot of breakthroughs. I have broken through a big door, and now I am traveling in a new field.

We are in tremendous need of sexual healing, and certain courageous men and women are now providing opportunities for us to heal. Unfortunately, in our culture, many people despise those who earn a living through any activity related to sex—not just prostitutes, but also men and women who give erotic massage, sex surrogates, and sex educators. Since patriarchy has turned everything upside down, it is no wonder those who are trying to set things right are afforded little respect. After returning from a Tantric sex workshop, one woman shared:

I feel that the sexual explorations I have experienced are among the bravest and freshest work I know of that is being done today. This work is reviled by the outside world, and yet it seems to me truly holy work, so worthy of honor and gratitude. It turns everything upside down and allows you to see that many things are exactly the opposite of what you thought. This work is utterly radical and revolutionary in reversing the prejudice of centuries, even more radical than spir-

EROTIC MASSAGE

I do erotic massage, and it is important to me that I take pride in my work. We need to break the equation of sexual work with sleaziness. For women, the traumas we have had are held in the yoni. As priestesses, we have three thousand years of abuse stuck in our bodies. Where do we go with that? If we are very lucky, we get a lover with whom we can really work it through. But that is very unusual. I myself had nowhere to go with it. It wasn't the kind of thing a normal therapist could deal with. So I know how valuable it can be to have a safe place to explore the memories that are held in the sexual body and feel them. NINA

ituality, which is acceptable now. So much suffering in our culture could be reversed and stopped if only people could experience this kind of sexual healing. If all these women whose bodies don't look like *Playboy* models' could shed their shame and experience the utter sacredness of their being . . . I believe that this is the work that needs to be done now.

One of those courageous women who helps others in their sexual healing is Betty Dodson, author of *Sex for One*. In her book, she describes how, early in life, she came to the conviction that she was deformed:

Around the age of ten, I wanted to see what I looked like "down there." One afternoon when the house was empty, I got Mother's hand mirror and went into my bedroom. Sitting by the window, the sunlight pouring in, I looked at my sweet little child's genitals and was instantly horrified. There hanging down were the same funny-looking things that dangled from a chicken's neck. Right on the spot, I swore off masturbation and made a deal with God. If He got rid of those things that hung down, I promised to stop playing with myself, keep my room clean, and love my little brothers.[75]

Of course, neither she nor god kept the bargain. Instead, Betty Dodson not only learned to love her vagina, but now teaches other women to do the same and helps them let go of the common fear of being "deformed." Teaching women to love their vaginas and give themselves sexual pleasure is not a common profession, and certainly not one most people would consider spiritually significant. Yet what could be more spiritual than teaching self-love? And what kind of self-love are we talking about, if it does not include our creative organs? Betty Dodson concludes, "We will be more civilized and humane when beautiful genital imagery along with a positive attitude about masturbation is part of the sex education of every American boy and girl. Now and then there are signs of progress, though. Just the other day I saw a friend's teenage daughter wearing a shocking-pink button that said, VIVA LA VULVA."[76]

25

SPITTING NICKELS AND
BREAKING FREE

*After college, I went back to my parents' home and started hanging out at the local
bar. I was twenty, a virgin, and really miserable. There was one guy, Tommy, who
had been my best buddy for many, many years. We used to talk about everything.
One night Tommy said to me, "You know what you need?" "No, what?" I said.
And he said, "You need to be able to stand on your head stark naked and spit nickels if that's what you want to do." "Yes!" I said. "That's exactly what I need to do."*

*Tommy said he wanted to take me to the seashore for the weekend, and I thought
that was a fabulous idea. I went home and told my mom, "Tommy and I are going to the seashore this weekend." And my mom said to me, "You are not. Not with
Tommy." You would think, me being twenty years old, graduated from college, I
would have said, "Yes, I am, see you later." But I didn't. I called Tommy and said
"I can't go, my mom won't let me." And I just fell back into my despair.*

*But Tommy said, "Let's get a hotel room at the Holiday Inn and hang out there.
You can still stand on your head stark naked and spit nickels." He was wonderful,
so dear. So I said, okay. I didn't think of him romantically at all, he was just my
best friend. But here we were in this room with a bed. And we were just laughing
and having a blast. So we started making out, all in the spirit of "Whatever you
want to do, you just do it." That's when I had intercourse for the first time, and it
was perfect. We were such good friends. I needed to break free. I realize just now
that it was in fact a deliberate act of breaking free, from my mother, from the church,
from all the repression. Doing the very thing I wasn't supposed to do.* Valerie

How do we heal the wounds of shame? How do we regain a sense
of pride in our sexual nature? How do we break free of repression?
These were questions the women I spoke with kept returning to.

Concepts are not enough; awareness is not enough; and the theoretical belief in our own purity is not enough, either. Awareness is important, but to anchor it in the body one must take action. What action? That depends. You may recall how Alexandra (Chapter 2) arrived at the sexuality workshop that was to transform her life trembling with fear, with bowed head, so as to avoid looking at the erotic images on the walls.

Whatever steps we take to break free, our actions must help us remember that we can be bigger and wilder and freer than we thought. When women talk of the things they have done to overcome their sexual inhibitions, many tell stories they would never tell their mothers. For Roseanne, raised in a Mormon environment, liberation began with a visit to a sex shop.

When sex shops first came to my area, I wanted to go see one. But I was scared. Decent people just didn't do that kind of thing. Then I thought, "Okay. It's time for you to admit to the world that you are fucking. Just go in there and admit you are interested in sex." I was dying of shame, but I went. Someone came up and asked me if they could help me, and they took me on a tour and showed me all the different things. "What a difference to the attitude I was raised with!" I thought. "Here are all these things people use to pleasure themselves, and they are actually talking about it, and clerks who have never seen me before are perfectly relaxed showing me what a dildo is, and explaining why one would want a large versus a small dildo versus a vibrator." It was a wonderful acceptance of the sexual part of me.

Eva, close to eighty years old, had her own story to tell about breaking old taboos. She was raised in a terribly repressed family; her religious community only reinforced her sexual inhibitions. "At the age of forty, I was still a virgin," Eva said. "But I had a wonderful therapist who recognized my dilemma and helped me with my sexuality. One time, he ordered me to go to a little chapel that was open all night. He told me to go there totally naked under my coat and masturbate." I stared at Eva, wide-eyed. "And you . . . ?" Eva nodded solemnly. "I sure did. I danced, and I lay down on the altar and masturbated. I tell you, it really did cause a breakthrough. It helped me tremendously. Shortly after that I was able to enter into the first sexual relationship of my life."

Self-pleasuring (a more positive term than "masturbation") is an immensely powerful tool, which has helped many women befriend their bodies and their sexuality. Self-pleasuring allows us to focus entirely on our own experience, without the distraction of a lover's presence, and so to discover what truly pleases us, as well as to explore the subtle ways in which we habitually hold tension or block the flow of energy. Pamina, in particular, talked about what a powerful healing tool self-pleasuring has been for her. Many readers will recognize, in her account, their own habitual patterns of tensing against pleasure instead of letting go into it, and of abusing their bodies rather than truly making love to themselves. By practicing consciously, with a meditative intention, Pamina learned to open to more and more profound levels of pleasure.

I read several books on masturbation, which was good for me, because it made me feel that I was not the only one doing it. I started taking advice, and practicing, and I would make it a special time for myself.

I prefer to speak of self-pleasuring instead of masturbation. But at first, it really was masturbation, in the sense that it was definitely not pleasurable. After sex, as well as after masturbating, I would feel physically sick, with sharp pains that shot through my pelvis and ovaries after I orgasmed. My whole yoni would get really sore and I would have horrible stomach cramps. Emotionally, I would withdraw into shame and would not want to be touched. This kind of tension never was pleasure, but I had had so much of it that it was a habit. Then I realized this was a form of self-destruction. My fantasies were really violent, and my actual masturbation was violent, too.

So I started self-pleasuring at home, when I had privacy and wasn't going to be disturbed. My main practice is relaxing. I'm allowed to touch myself, but I'm not allowed to be tense. Sometimes I practice in yoga postures, which are designed to relax you. I notice that when I relax, I don't go out into fantasies so much. I keep coming back to the present. I wasn't used to being excited and relaxed at the same time. But I found that as I relaxed, my pleasure would be ten times greater than before. I wasn't used to having that much pleasure, not just in my vulva but all over. Then, I started trying to bring the pleasure up through my body. Whenever I started having an orgasm, I would raise the energy up. At first, it would just come up a little bit. But now, I can really open my whole body. My vulva has become a container within which I build the pleasurable feelings. Then, I feel them rising through me, spreading through my limbs and up into my head. And I don't feel the pains anymore.

I believe that if we want to totally embrace our sexuality, we need to practice. It's like dance, like playing music, or like any other discipline. It takes practice and repetition. So I practice with myself. I feel I am becoming my own woman lover. I think of myself as my woman lover and of Richard as my male lover.

A few years ago I dreamed of a man. He was so beautiful, divinely beautiful—godlike, almost—but very human. I knew right away in the dream that this was me, my male side. But he was much older and wiser than I am. He was my friend and had come to help me deal with some of my sexual problems. That dream was one of the most important gifts I ever received. After this dream he was very much alive for me. He started coming into my fantasies, even when I wasn't thinking about bringing him in.

Now, when I go into my self-pleasuring sessions, I'm really in my dream world. The experience is physical, but I am allowing another dimension to be present. In this other dimension I heal myself psychically. My inner friend will not permit any violence. But he loves having adventures, and he participates in all my fun fantasies. In my fantasy world, there is me, and my dream lover, and often there is a third party, a part of myself that needs healing. A repressed part that I am inviting into having some fun. I repeat fantasies until I figure them out, and then they go away until a new level appears.

This year I decided, "I want to be sexual." That was a big decision. Before, I wanted to be sexual in theory, but actually I was shut down. I think we need to feel sexual for ourselves, first of all. No matter what happens, I will always be able to have wonderful sex with myself. I like that feeling. I have consciously decided to be a fully sexual women. I have made a crossover to being whole.

It is rare to meet a woman who owns her fantasies without judging herself for having them. So many of us feel ashamed of our sexual fantasies, especially when they involve incest, rape, or other scenarios we would never want to play out in real life. "I have a lot of guilt around my fantasies," Tara confessed. "They feel forbidden, and I don't talk about them. Often, they are degrading. What is wrong with me?"

There is nothing wrong with her. Like dreams, fantasies are not to be taken literally. Rather, they belong to a different realm than real life. Above all, they are not enemies, but friends in disguise who come to help us bypass energy blockages. For example, if a woman has learned that sexual surrender is shameful, she may fantasize about being forced to surrender, and so bypass the guilt at accepting pleasure—for in our fantasies, unlike in reality, rape is always pleasurable. The imaginary aggressor is actually a part of the woman's own psyche—the part that wants to break her resistance to receiving pleasure. In other instances, she may fantasize about being a slut, a woman who has no shame and is therefore free to enjoy herself. If she has internalized a lot of physical shame, she may fantasize about being exposed and examined by probing fingers and eyes. Again, her fantasy is helping her bypass the blockage.

All forms of sexual dominance and submission, whether in fantasy or in actual sex play, derive their arousing, titillating power from the fact that they aim at ritually controlling the all too righteous, repressed Controller and forcing him to surrender to pleasure. Since the Controller blocks our access to pleasure, his enforced submission can open the way to sexual ecstasy. Unfortunately, while sex games such as S & M can help circumvent energetic blockages, they can also reinforce them, especially when people become hooked on one particular sexual scenario. The real problem is not what certain individuals like to do in the privacy of their homes, but the fact that such games are just the tip of an iceberg. In a sense, we should be grateful to S & M aficionados for making visible the collective sickness and perversion that our Controller-dominated, power-obsessed, pleasure-fearing culture engenders. Consider, for instance, what the sexual fantasies, say, of an Australian aboriginal man or woman might be. It seems highly unlikely that in less control-oriented societies, many people would be interested in sexual games or fantasies involving dominance and submission.

However, as Pamina's story shows, we need not stay stuck in sexual ruts born out of shame or abuse. Changing our sexual minds is no easy task, but with consistent and patient practice, it *is* possible to actually undo old conditioning entirely. The first challenge is to decipher the encoded message our fantasies deliver—to "figure them out," as Pamina says. The second (and far more difficult) task is to consciously release the tensions and inhibitions we discover in the process, and reeducate the body. If you have ever practiced Buddhist Vipassana meditation, you will notice how very similar the challenges are. Can we allow our fantasies to arise without drowning in them? Can we anchor ourselves in the present moment by remaining aware of our breath and of our physical body? Can we greet with compassion whatever arises?

In essence, all sexual power games are either imitations or perversions of the dance between the small self and the greater Self, or between the soul and god. In the divine presence, the soul surrenders naturally and spontaneously, and in such surrender, it finds its ultimate satisfaction. In dominance-submission games, one ego play-acts the all-powerful Controller-god, while the other takes the role of submissive creature. Usually, however, this drama is enacted without any spiritual awareness, and is contaminated by strong overlays of dysfunctional human family dynamics.

What happens when lovers consciously hold the dominance-submission issue in a spiritual light? One woman, Valerie, said that recently, she has been aware of a growing desire to enact her desire for spiritual surrender in a sexual way. Valerie has been happily married for several years, and knows that in the context of this deeply loving and trusting relationship, she can enact the dance of dominance and submission without feeling humiliated or diminished, as she inevitably would if ego were submitting to ego.

Recently, I started having fantasies of my husband taking me, dominating me. "Do whatever you want with me" were the words that came up, but I was too embarrassed to say them. Still, we have been talking about it. In the past, I could not have allowed this kind of ravishment, which is not like rape. All my old ideas about men and needing to be equal and be in control got in the way. There used to be a way I kept my body hard so I could be sure of having some dominance and never being completely submissive. It was a posture I used that kept the humiliation at bay. Now, I am allowing my softness. I can surrender and feel it as humbling, not as humiliating.

It's so akin to spiritual self-surrender. "Do whatever you want with me" is my prayer to god as well. "May my will and your will be one." But in sex, the vulnerability is so apparent, with this man who is much bigger than me. If I really surrender, I am not in control anymore. It is very much the same edge that I am riding in my spiritual development. How much am I willing to give myself over to this divine force, versus holding on to the illusion that I am running the show? When I surrender, I open to the fact that I don't know what is going to happen. How much am I willing to be present with not knowing what is going to happen next? Can I trust that it will be okay? Talking about it now, I see that the same process is being mirrored in my spirituality and in my sexuality at the same time. How much am I willing to drop my defenses around my husband?

Since few people have a relationship as trusting and open as Valerie's, it is a good thing that surrender to god—which means surrender to our own innermost nature—does not require a partner. For Naomi, who had experienced so much abuse at the hands of men, it was immensely empowering to discover that she could ex-

I CLAIM THIS FOR MYSELF

Once, while I was making love with my husband, he touched my breast. I felt my breast open like a vagina and a wave of orgasm washed through me. When this happened, I immediately thought, "I claim this for myself." I didn't want it to be connected only to him. I knew that this deep pleasure was the potential of my own body. DONNA

perience total sexual surrender without a lover. Somehow she found the courage to participate in a ritual in which women undressed and danced naked for each other as a means of healing their shame and blessing their sexuality. Given her history of sexual abuse, nothing could have been more terrifying than the thought of revealing her sexual essence to a group of total strangers. Still, she chose to do so, because she sensed how closely her sexuality was entwined with her spiritual path. Something within her—call it the soul, the inner teacher, the priestess—insisted that she challenge the voice of shame and reclaim the innate innocence of her primal nature. In opening to the streaming of her sexual energy, she opened to her soul, to her feminine essence, and to her true identity.

"In part, the experience was so wonderful," Naomi recalls, "because it did not involve any partner at all. It opened into something that does not have to be contained in a relationship. It was just my life energy, and all women's life energy." But for Naomi, it took immense courage to open to this experience.

I was fat and out of shape, and my body didn't look that great. To be naked in front of women was a big issue for me, and for many other women as well. But we all realized that it was totally irrelevant what kind of body you had. It was your vehicle for healing, whether you were old or heavy or skinny. Each woman had a radiance and an unspeakable beauty that was very physical, no matter what she looked like.

I was totally terrified, because in my experience, sex meant humiliation. My whole body was shaking. But as I danced, my terror subsided quickly, and a wave of connection to these women flowed through me. Everything I felt in my body seemed to be cycling back to them. All these nuances of my energy and my sexuality were being mirrored in their faces. It just escalated. Finally, this joy started coursing through my body until I was rolling around on the floor like a little animal and kicking my legs and laughing. It wasn't dignified or beautiful. It was a joyful, ecstatic exuberance exploding through my body. That radiated out to the other women, and they were all coming unglued with laughter too. Oh, it was just incredible!

Afterward, I was stunned, just stunned. "This must be the way I was born," I thought. I could see that my sexuality had a steamy depth, as well as a playful, profound joy, and I saw how it was different from the other women's sexuality. I saw how my sexual energy could evoke the same kind of energy in their bodies and faces and touch something in them. I saw how each woman's sexuality was unique and healing for all of us. This was my real essence that had been locked up and buried until now.

Some months later, I repeated this workshop. Again, I danced, and I could feel how much more deeply I had connected with my body in the meantime. I felt less fear, and I could feel my cells pulsing. I was more mature, present, and conscious, and my energy was much more sexual. The first time, I had connected to a physical joy that was almost child-like. This time, I experienced my sexuality as an intense, penetrating, transforming power that is not afraid of darkness. I could feel my sexual energy riding on an ecstasy about life. I knew that the women in front of me were feeling what I felt. Their mouths were hanging open with amazement, and they were totally mesmerized. By their reactions, I saw the immense power of this fearless, healing sexuality. I felt like a masterful surfer riding a huge wave of energy. I could negotiate it with joy and pleasure to the benefit of everyone, and to the great physical pleasure of my own body. I had an orgasm that time, though I was not touching myself. The energy moving through my body was being augmented by all these women until it exploded.

Then I became hysterically happy, and I was rolling on the floor laughing again. Oh, this joy is possible! It had been covered with layers of dust and with this encrustation of suffering and abuse. I finally knew that my identity as victim was not my final story. My real nature had always been this kind of ecstatic, joyous explosion of life.

26

INITIATIONS OF THE
FEMALE BODY

Birth in other cultures is Initiation. This is not only because it marks what anthropologists have called a rite of passage in the life phases but because it naturally stimulates and awakens the sleeping snake power. Birthing is a woman's organic opportunity to become empowered through a challenging, physical encounter with the forces of life and death. A birthing woman actually stands on the edge of life and death, at the doorway between them, and (in service to the race) brings a new soul from there to here. What could be more shamanic than this? No wonder Native people say that warriors who dance the Sun Dance do so in order to match the experience, and call up the courage, of a woman in labor.

Vicki Noble

Donna is an African-American woman in her late fifties. She is also a professional midwife who has delivered hundreds of babies and has guided their mothers safely through childbirth. Quiet and soft-spoken, she seems to rest peacefully in her body, like a bird at home in its nest. Her very presence is so soothing that you begin to relax just by being around her. Everything about her, from her gentle, singsong voice to her rust-colored clothing, feels earthy, full, ripe, and nourishing. One of the first things she tells me is that in her eyes, the female body is a great spiritual teacher that leads us through a series of powerful initiations—menstruation, pregnancy, birth, and menopause—which transform us in dramatic ways and have no male equivalent.

Donna works in a hospital that serves primarily poor women and women of color, and racial healing is as much a part of her

FIRST MENSTRUATION STORIES

My mother told me nothing about menstruation. I got it early, at eleven. I thought I must be dying. My mother told me it was the curse, but then she also called it "the friend." I couldn't figure out why she called it both the friend and the curse. Was it good or bad?
ASTRID

My mother took me to see a movie about menstruation. It was in a town hall, and there was a large auditorium full of women with their daughters. But she never talked to me.
DONNA

I was the fifth child in a family of eight, and yet I knew nothing about menstruation. I remember how terrified I was when I started bleeding. Something about it made me feel guilty, as if I had done something wrong and should be ashamed. But I also felt very powerful and grounded in my body. I knew men didn't

work as sexual healing. Like most midwives, she is underpaid and overworked, and yet she derives a deep sense of satisfaction from what she does. Midwifery is one of the most ancient priestess arts. A midwife holds a field of sacred energy that encompasses, holds, and nurtures. She may patiently wait with a woman, but when she sees that the time has come, she will help the baby move into the light of the world. As we talked, we realized how similar the work of a midwife is to the work of a counselor or therapist. A counselor, too, must be alert to the clues that signal readiness for movement and birth, whether birth means the expression of an emotion, a new insight, a decision, a breakthrough, a shift in consciousness, or a healing.

"What drew you to this work?" I asked Donna. In response, she told me that as an African-American woman, she began her journey with the need to grapple with the complexities of her cultural and political heritage. "Race is always there," she emphasized. As a

*do this, and I knew it was associated with babies. There was a
drenched feeling. I felt the blood coming from the top of my
head down, painting me in red. I felt like I was channeling down
this power.*   TARA

*When I got my period, my mom gave me some Kotex and she
showed me how to put it on a little harness. So I went and put it
on. I remember so clearly walking around and pulling and picking at the thing. "This has got to be some kind of joke," I
thought. I felt like I had a tire between my legs. "You can't be serious. I am supposed to walk around like this?" It seemed so
dumb. It would either stick out in front or in the back. It was a
totally uncomfortable nuisance. Then came the bras. My mom
said to me: "It's time for you to start wearing a bra." "Oh no, I
don't think so," I said. But she insisted. They were called training bras, as if I was a horse that needed to be broken in. So I had
this thing on, and it felt so stupid and uncomfortable. All my
sexual parts had to be harnessed into these awful contraptions.*
                                                               IRENE

young child, Donna remembers being taken to hear Malcolm X. "I
received a strand of race consciousness from my environment," she
said, "that led directly to my involvement in the civil rights movement and the peace movement." Later, Donna left her predominantly white college because, as she put it, "I wanted to be building
the black nation. That was what mattered to me." However, she
continued,

What that meant in practice was attaching myself to a man
and being his auxiliary. It was 1967, and I didn't see the sexism
in this at the time. Early feminism was a white movement, and
it did not reach black women until much later. We had not yet
named sexism. There was a strong Muslim influence, too. I remember leaving a conference in disgust where it had been
proposed that on the street, black women should walk three
paces behind their men. This proposal was seriously discussed.

In her twenties, Donna's quest for cultural identity led her to join a traditional Yoruba household in New York; soon after, she went to Africa. "On that trip," she tells me, "I fully realized how much I was an African American. After living in a Yoruba family and going to Africa, nobody could romanticize Africa to me. I had a deep understanding of sexual politics in Africa and how difficult they are. I returned knowing my home was in America." But Donna also returned carrying a child in her womb, a baby conceived in the land of her ancestors.

In medieval pictures of Jesus's conception, a beam of light slants down from the heavens, piercing the clouds to touch the womb of the young Mary, who stands, completely open yet amazed at what is happening to her. At the conception, she is touched by the finger of God, powdered with an otherwordly dust, bathed in a light that comes from beyond the sun and the stars. The medieval mystic Hildegard of Bingen celebrated Mary's motherhood in her luminous poetry:

> Alleluia! light
> burst from your untouched
> womb like a flower
> on the farther side
> of death. The world-tree
> is blossoming. Two
> realms become one.[77]

For most women, conception is not quite such a mystical experience. Still, many women do know when they have conceived and feel that they have witnessed a sacred and miraculous event. "In my mind's eye, I could see the sun and the moon coming together," one woman marveled. "I felt my whole body change. I knew instantly I was pregnant. Nothing had ever felt like that. Everything became exquisite and numinous—colors glowed, and cereal tasted incredible."

Sperm and egg merge, and the arch of a great shimmering bridge reaches across the vastness between the worlds. When Donna conceived, she, too, felt the spirit worlds reaching out to touch her. "I had a mystical experience," she recalls. "A voice told me that I was

THE STORY OF AN ADOPTION

I never wanted a child until I was thirty-nine, and then, all of a sudden, something took over. It was the proverbial biological clock. Suddenly, all I wanted was a child. But I tried to get pregnant and couldn't. We tried everything, including different infertility drugs. For a while, I was really angry with god for not giving me a child. "Why, why is this happening to me?" I would scream.

Then, after eight or nine months, I was able to just put it out as a question while I sat in meditation: "Why?" Just the question, with no anger. And immediately, I heard a voice. You know how it is when you hear something which is definitely not your ego. Wherever it comes from, it's not your ordinary mind. This voice said, "If you had gotten pregnant, you would not adopt. There is a child out there who needs to come to you." The answer came instantly and with total clarity. And in my mind, I saw the image of a gate being closed down. It was very powerful. After that, we elected to do an independent adoption. We sent out about 150 letters describing ourselves and our desire for a child. Six weeks later, we had a son. Today, he is fourteen years old. ALEXANDRA

pregnant. And then it said, 'You can say yes or no to your pregnancy.' Later, I had a period and so I assumed I could not be pregnant. I thought I must have been mistaken. But I was indeed pregnant." Suddenly, all Donna's attention shifted to her womb.

"You can say yes or no to your pregnancy." Donna has had ample opportunity, both in her personal and professional life, to contemplate the complex issues of birth control and abortion. She believes that in ancient times, women knew they could choose or reject a pregnancy by willpower alone.

I believe that part of men's fear of women has to do with our power to say yes or no to conception. Most of us have lost the power to choose with our consciousness, but originally, we could internally choose yes or no. We could end life in the womb. I think women can still kill with a thought. We carry a life-and-death energy that is very powerful and very different from the power of the male. I think this is one of the main reasons why men fear women.

Is it indeed possible that women once knew how to accept or reject a pregnancy through sheer force of intention? Perhaps I looked a little skeptical, for Donna went on to tell me a story about her firsthand experience of this power.

I have very consciously dealt with conception on a psychic level. Once, I went on a trip, and spent the night with a man who smoked cigarettes. All night, we made love, and laughed a lot, and he smoked his cigarettes. After I returned home, I realized I was pregnant.

Then, I had an incredible dream. I dreamed I was in the country of my womb, and my womb was a landscape. I was standing on a green hillside—lush, radiant green. I saw a young girl, and I knew that she was the child I was pregnant with. She was running down the hillside toward a lake at the bottom of the hill. I knew that once she entered that lake, she would be born. In the dream, I smote the lake with my hand and turned it to ice, so that she could not enter. As soon as I did that, she fell down unconscious and inanimate. I took her in my arms and carried her back up the hillside. At the top of the hill, I dissolved her back into her component elements of smoke and laughter.

When I woke up I felt great sorrow. To deny water is to deny life. I woke with the consciousness of having denied someone the water of life. It was sad to have said no. In the most perfect of all worlds, I could have said yes. I count this among my abortions.

Every woman who says yes or no to her pregnancy, whether through sheer willpower, birth control, or abortion, steps into the role of priestess, shamaness, guardian of the threshold between the spirit realms and the embodied world. Her choice determines whether or not a soul will enter its next incarnation. With her ability to terminate a pregnancy, woman holds a tremendous power, the power to embody either the golden, life-giving goddess, or the devouring black Mother, who in Hindu images often appears garlanded with the skulls or corpses of children.

Anne Llewellyn Barstow says that in the sixteenth century, an accused witch was doomed if the charges leveled against her included the practice of any form of birth control. "The greatest sexual sin apparently was birth control, whether as contraception or abortion," she writes.[78] By criminalizing birth control and abortion, men tried to take control over women's awesome power over life and death. The evil, baby-killing witch of medieval man's imagination was none other than the dark goddess, seen through the distorting lens of unacknowledged fear. Reading the following description of the Hindu goddess Kali, we cannot help noticing how closely she resembles the European vision of a witch:

> Kali is always black or dark, is usually naked, and has long, disheveled hair. She is adorned with severed arms as a girdle, freshly cut heads as a necklace, children's corpses as earrings, and serpents as bracelets. She has long, sharp fangs, is often depicted as having clawlike hands with long nails, and is often said to have blood smeared on her lips. Her favorite haunts heighten her fearsome nature. She is usually shown on the battlefield, where she is a furious combatant who gets drunk on the hot blood of her victims, or in a cremation ground, where she sits on a corpse surrounded by jackals and goblins.[79]

While Hindus, even while projecting a fearsome image of the dark Mother, also acknowledged her divinity, European and American witch-hunters failed to realize that they were prosecuting their own shadows. To this day, Western civilization has not faced its deep fear of the dark feminine, a fact that is nowhere more evident than in the abortion debate. Patriarchy has tried to squelch the dark goddess within women, instead of acknowledging the primordial fear she evokes. The word "abortion" comes from Latin *aboriri*, to disappear. To abort a child is to make it disappear. Woman as the

ABORTION AS WORSHIP

I had two abortions. The first one was horrible. The second time, I went to a feminist women's health center, and it ended up being a wonderful experience. I had already grieved for the baby, and during the abortion, I felt so deeply connected with the Creator/Destroyer. It did not feel shameful but beautiful and joyous. The women who were with me held that sacred space together. It was a great gift. There was such a sense of being honored; it was like being part of a worship.

IRENE

dark abyss into which life vanishes without a trace—such an image is bound to evoke powerful responses. It is perhaps not surprising that today, as in medieval Europe, the abortion debate is deeply influenced by unconscious archetypal fears. The Catholic church, in particular, pays lip service to the sanctity of motherhood, yet refuses to honor the Mother in her whole, uncensored majesty, including both her light and her dark aspects, her life-giving and life-denying powers.

Donna, though she was single and poor, chose to keep her baby. For her, birth was an easy, joyful experience.

I had my baby at home. He came a month early. The night the labor started I had been drumming and dancing and having a good old time. I came home and started labor at midnight. I had read this article about how doctors hated to come and then find that the woman was in false labor. I was determined not to be one of those women in false labor. In retrospect, I am so thankful. My midwife was unavailable, and had I called, I would have been sent to the county hospital and would have had a horrible delivery. I just sat by the window and breathed. Then, around five, my midwife arrived. She took one look at me, without even examining me, and said I would be having my baby in half an hour. I just danced through my labor. I never even got into bed. I only pushed right before he was born. Fifteen minutes after the baby was born, I was up, coloring some birth announcements to send out and taking a shower. It was a wonderful, easy birth.

Her voice full of wonder, Donna continued describing the miraculous process of pregnancy. "To be pregnant," she explained, "is to share and incorporate consciousness, the consciousness of the other."

In order to accept a pregnancy, we have to nurture what is alien and would normally be rejected by the body. This is very primal and basic. The fetus is a foreign body that should trigger antibody reactions. Normally, everything would be geared to destroy it. But there is a psychic counterpart that accepts the other. We are able to take in, gestate, and nourish an alien consciousness.

Donna emphasized that a pregnant woman holds not only a second physical body within her own but also a second consciousness, with its unique energy and emotionality. She is an infinity that contains a second infinity. Her child is a spark of divine Light contained within another spark, a soul within a soul. This means that the opening required of her is not merely physical. Rather, pregnancy and birth involve a total opening through all dimensions of her being—physical, emotional, energetic, and spiritual.

No wonder, I thought as I listened to Donna, a woman's energetic circuitry is so incredibly complex, sensitive, and vulnerable. No wonder feminine energy is so porous and permeable. As a woman is geared to receive and nurture a second body within her own, so her energy body, too, has a quality of permeability and receptivity that differs from the denser male energy body. No wonder, also, that certain women describe their pregnancy as a time of spiritual awakening.

For Donna, the birth of her son was an initiation into her essential feminine nature. In theory, she had long known that the body of a birthing woman is a gateway through which Spirit streams into manifest form, and that she embodies the ancient, universal Mother who gave birth to the universe and all its creatures. However, in the

THE POWER OF PREGNANCY

The power of being pregnant was incredible. I remember walking down the street when I was seven or eight months pregnant and feeling every part of my body move when I walked. I remember how connected I felt, how I felt my hair and my skin and nails. It took me right to that place of my deepest core vibration. I didn't identify it as a spiritual connection at the time, but I do now. At that time, it was all instinctual. There was nothing intellectual about it. Now, I see it that I was tapped into the spirit within me that taps into the whole universe.   TARA

act of giving birth, Donna awakened to the immediate, overwhelmingly physical experience of this truth.

I once saw an ancient Indian statue that shows the goddess Kali giving birth to the universe. She is standing there and the universe is coming out with its palms joined in prayer. That is exactly how I felt when I gave birth to my son. I held a universe between my legs. I believe that every child is the reproduction of the cosmos, and for a moment, I understood and felt that. The universe was coming through me.

Anyone who has witnessed birth knows its ancient, primordial power. A birthing woman's bed is the original sacrificial altar, and she herself both the priestess and the sacrificial offering. We can see why, in cultures where it was believed that the goddess gave birth to the world, women were highly revered as her earthly representatives. Humanity's first priestesses appear to have been women, and women continued to function as the main mediators between the divine and the human realms for thousands of years. Though our society no longer honors mothers as vessels of the goddess, birth still remains a miraculous and breathtaking event.

Every woman, whether or not she has had children, possesses an innate knowledge of how to conceive, how to hold a pregnancy,

THE TRICKSTER BABY

When I conceived my daughter, I felt the fusion immediately, and I knew without a doubt that I was pregnant. But I hated the father; there was just no way I wanted his child. However, the doctors kept telling me I wasn't pregnant. I threw up every day, and they said it was just nerves and stress. Three pregnancy tests came out negative. My old family practitioner told me I had an ulcer. Another gynecologist gave me hormone tablets to induce my period, which is a very dangerous thing to do during pregnancy. Anyhow, I got my period. "Very good, congratulations," said the doctor. I felt safe again. But the next month, again no period. Another pregnancy test came out negative. By now, I was in my fourth month. I was still throwing up, and I had this hard little lump in my belly. I just couldn't figure out what was going on. I didn't find out I was pregnant until the fifth month. Then I knew that the spirit that was coming through had tricked me. She stayed in hiding for five months, because she knew full well that I would certainly have had an abortion had I known earlier. I have no doubt about this. But today, I love her more than my life.

MERCEDES

and how to give birth. Artist Meinrad Craighead, who has chosen a celibate life, says, "Whether we are weaving tissue in the womb or weaving imagery in the soul, our work is sexual: the work of conception, gestation, and birth."[80]

In my women's circles, the fact that women are involved in a ritual of birth is very obvious. When an important decision or a new consciousness wants to be born through us, it often emerges with the same tremendous urgency as a physical baby. Sitting in the center, a woman asks to be born once again. She is both the mother giving birth and the baby struggling to emerge. Something inside needs to let go, to open, to relax, but also to push, to stay with the process, to persist until that baby is out. Like any birthing woman, she is utterly focused. She doesn't care what she looks like or what others think of her. She is not concerned with what was yesterday or what will be tomorrow. Her mind has no choice now but to stay with her body, so consuming and intense are the sensations. As she struggles, the air vibrates with intensity. She is utterly absorbed in the process, surrendered to it. Nothing else matters. She talks, screams, sings, laughs. She sits silently, breathing, moaning. She waits. Her heart open, she asks for blessings. She prays. She struggles and curses. She bitches and complains that the pain is too much, that this is too difficult, that nobody told her it would be so hard or take so long. She despairs. And still, here she is, giving birth. What is she birthing? Is it freedom from an old relationship, freedom from an old addiction? Is she birthing a woman who has shed her old illusions, a woman grounded in truth? Or is she simply birthing the courage to continue living? Whatever it is, entwined with the birth is always a bit of death, a piece of letting go. Can we learn to approach our psychological labor with the same concern as we approach physical labor? We should not let the materialistic bias of our environment confuse us. Psychological birthing is important and valuable work. Without it, we will no more survive as a species than we would survive if women stopped birthing babies physically.

For some women, physical and psychological birth coincide. Valerie, a psychotherapist in her early fifties, shared how, in the act of birthing her son, she stepped into a new state of empowered womanhood. For her, giving birth triggered one of the most potent initiations of her entire life:

> At the time, the doctors did not approve of Lamaze. Women were mostly being drugged. But I was adamant. I wanted no drugs. My husband said, "You can't do it, you're afraid of pain." "Watch me," I said, "I can."
>
> My husband fainted early on in the labor. But I found my strength. Truly, in the experience of childbirth I found my strength as a woman. I did what I said I was going to do. This beautiful baby came out and he was totally alert, his eyes open, and we made instant contact. I will never forget that moment of looking into his eyes. He was right there, and then he looked at his father. It was astounding.
>
> After giving birth I was starving, and I demanded break-

fast. "Oh, no," said the nurse, "you just had a baby, now you go to sleep." "No!" I roared. "I'm awake and hungry, I feel great and I want some food." I felt charged, and I wanted to celebrate. I remember sitting in that bed alone, saying over and over again, "I did it. I did what I said I was going to do. The gynecologist said I wouldn't be able to do it, my husband said I couldn't do it, but I did it." It felt so empowering to have chosen something, maybe for the first time in my life, because it was what I wanted for myself. I stepped over a big boundary, and it was so physically marked, so linked to my female body. After that, I felt a great fullness as a person. It was an initiation and an empowerment through which I passed into womanhood.

Donna, too, experienced birth as a deeply sacred initiation. Later, however, she realized that for most women, birth was nothing of the sort. "When my son was two," she told me, "I went back to school to get my nursing degree. At that point, I saw birth in the hospital for the first time. I couldn't believe how fortunate I had been to have had my baby at home." Donna was appalled at the disrespectful way birthing women were commonly treated, and at the complete lack of awareness of birth as a sacred act. What she saw awakened her desire to support birthing women, especially those who were poor or underprivileged.

I felt great compassion, especially when I heard stories from black women about how hard their experience of childbirth was. Their complaints were never about the birth itself, but always about staff attitudes. They would say, "I told them the baby was coming, and they said it wasn't and they put me in a room all by myself, and there I had the baby all alone." Or: "They put me on a gurney in the hall, and I had my baby in the hall." Or: "They tried to shut my legs and wouldn't let me deliver."

I remember one woman in the delivery room, pushing. And the doctor snarled at the nurse, "Don't ever call me every time one of them thinks she wants to push," and he stormed off. It was horrendous. Later he was sewing her after the birth. It is very difficult to know whether the woman is completely anesthetized. Typically, if it takes long, the anesthesia wears off. This woman told him very timidly that she was hurting. And he said to her, in a tone of utter disdain, "That's what you Lamaze patients get for wanting to do it naturally." So often, I couldn't believe what I heard and saw.

I saw how the doctors would always try and tell a woman who wanted a home birth that she was doing something to endanger her baby. Things are still bad. They have improved, but not enough. The attitude toward women who have home births is still that they want something they don't deserve. Hospital and home birth are drawing further and further apart, primarily because of legal issues. Not because of safety issues, but because of the fear of getting sued.

Women of the most recent generations have conceived and given birth, as women of all times and ages have, but they have done so in a singularly bleak atmosphere. Probably for the first time in history, all sense of reverence for the mysterious power embodied in a birthing woman was stripped away. No longer are conception, pregnancy, and birth perceived as sacred mysteries, and no longer are birthing women honored for their sacrifice. In the recent past, mothers were declared incapable of mothering and advised to follow the well-meaning but often idiotic advice of male "experts" who injured an entire generation by discouraging mothers from breast-feeding their babies and from feeding them when they were hungry and cried for food. Yet women know, in a deep visceral way, that their babies should not be separated from them, should not be dragged away and put into boxes where they lie alone, their skin aching for touch and love. Joanne had two children, one in the hospital, the second at home:

I had my daughter in a yucky operating room, and they took her away and put her in the nursery. I don't think that's good. You have to have your baby right there with you. She had been in my body for all this time, and suddenly, she was gone. Even though it was only for one night, it wasn't good for me or for her. What a stupid thing to do!

The second time, I was prepared. I had my baby on my own, at home. I knew the intensity of birth, but I was able to stay very conscious the whole time, riding the waves, relating to them as intensity rather than as pain. At one point, I intuitively started making sounds. I kept sending the energy out through my voice, singing and shouting and chanting in a loud voice. That opened me up tremendously. It was a wonderful birth. It made a big difference that my husband was right there and caught the baby, and he never left me.

Deep in their bodies, many women hold an ancient rage at the way their gift has been denigrated and distorted to the point where birth is treated not as a sacred mystery but a medical condition requiring hospitalization. Shortly after giving birth, a friend told me that for her, the greatest gift of birthing, next to her son, was the intensity of anger it put her in touch with and the immense power that radiated from that anger.

The contractions felt like they were breaking me open, and I truly felt I was dying. And suddenly, all this fury arose. At first, I was furious with god, because I had no control. I had done everything I knew to do, and the pain was unbearable.

"I've had it," was the feeling. "I've been a good girl. I've done my breathing and my moving and my surrendering. I can't take any more. I'm fed up. I'm quitting, I'm stopping, I don't care, it's over, this is it." Which, of course, made no difference at all.

Then I started to throw up. It was like a volcano erupting. Everything was being spewed up, kicked out of the way. After that, the rage came back, but with far greater intensity. This time I was just livid. There are almost no words for it. I could feel with every fiber of my body that the only reason every being on this planet was here was because some female had gone through this and had been broken open in this way. I was just enraged that people didn't honor women for that. I felt that every mother should be treated like a goddess for having given birth. Not only are women not honored, respected, and revered, but they are denigrated. And though I had known this intellectually before, I felt that I was just as guilty as anyone else. I hadn't especially honored my mother for birthing me. The sanctity of motherhood had always been an abstract concept to me.

Earlier in my labor, a Tibetan monk who is a friend of my husband's had called. "Mothers should be honored," he had told my husband. "There is a whole Buddhist Sutra about honoring the mother." When my husband first told me this, I thought, "Oh, how sweet of him. Isn't that nice?" But when my rage arose, I just bellowed, "You better believe it! That's baseline, and you guys don't get any special brownie points for having figured that out!" It was as if I was breathing fire. In the midst of all this physical drama that was unfolding around me this rage was erupting not out of my mind, but straight out of my body. Now I see what a gift that rage was. But of course it's not what we write on our list to Santa.

It makes a big difference whether a birthing woman believes that she is merely doing one of the many things female animals are conditioned to do or whether she sees herself as an embodiment of the sacred feminine, enacting the most sacred goddess ritual of all—the ritual of birth. It also makes a big difference whether she is treated as a person involved in a difficult and dangerous initiation or as a patient undergoing an unfortunate and cumbersome medical crisis. When Donna talks about her work as a midwife, she speaks with the awareness of participating in a sacred process. A priestess disguised as a white-robed nurse, she approaches women's bodies with a deep reverence akin to worship. She sees sacredness shining forth through their bone and marrow, through the curve of their breasts and the flow of their blood. It feels good to know that such priestesses are among us, walking quietly down the hospital corridors.

27

THE FINAL INITIATION

For I am the first and the last.
I am the honored one and the scorned one.
I am the whore and the holy one.
I am the wife and the virgin. . . .
I am the barren one,
and many are her sons. . . .
I am the silence that is incomprehensible. . . .
I am the utterance of my name.

The Gnostic Gospels

A elderly woman examines her face in the mirror, gingerly touching the wrinkles around her eyes and the gray that threads its way through her hair. "I'm getting old," she thinks with a sudden pang of anguish. And she wonders whether her husband ever dreams of wandering off with a younger woman, a woman whose breasts are firmer, whose belly is flatter, whose skin is soft and fresh. Many of her women friends have turned to plastic surgery for help. Should she have a facelift? Smoothing moisturizer into the skin around her eyes, she sighs as she tries to make peace with her aging body.

Diane, now in her mid-forties, contemplates her own aging as she observes her mother's struggle:

I think the self-hatred is passed on from mother to daughter. In my mother's eyes, there's just the smallest window of what a sexual, physical woman is allowed to look like. The aging process has really pushed her up against the wall. It's hard for her to look at herself now. She was an absolutely gorgeous woman in her younger years, very beautiful. But like most of us, she felt her beauty was just skin deep; it was just on the surface, and now she's losing that. If you don't love yourself and your body deeply as a younger woman, then how are you going to love your body as you age? I think aging will be a struggle for me, too. I have always struggled to love my body. There is a deep self-hatred and a lack of self-acceptance. I can accept the imperfections of other women's bodies, but not my own.

These are feelings many women share, and it is good to name them. But Diane also acknowledges that aging has brought her other, more welcome, quite unexpected gifts:

My sexuality has deepened tremendously over the years. I have learned what pleases and satisfies me most, and I have learned to appreciate the infinite realms of pleasure. My sexuality has become less genital and seems to fill my whole body. Where in the past orgasm was always the main focus, now my lovemaking as a whole feels orgasmic. Orgasm is no longer an event, a moment. To my great surprise, sex has become far more satisfying.

Postmenopausal women are challenged to deal not only with their own physical changes, but also with the cultural prejudices and judgments that surround menopause. Many people still believe that it is somehow shameful or inappropriate for older women to be sexually passionate. In recent years, older women have been courageously battling this repressive belief. "We *are* passionate," they insist. "Don't deny our femininity just because our bodies are no longer young. Don't diminish us by ignoring our sexual nature."

Of course older women are sexual. But what exactly do we mean by "sexual?" If we define "sexual" as "desirous of genital intercourse," then we must concede that many older women are indeed less sexual than their younger sisters. Laughing, Donna remembered how just before she hit menopause, she told her husband that she wanted more sex.

Ten days later, I went into menopause, and suddenly, everything changed. I went back to him and said, "You know what?

I may not want to make love for a month or two." We still make love regularly, and it feels important to me that I do so, for reasons I can't exactly define. But for the first time ever, I no longer feel compelled to have sex. There used to be a dependency. I know the strength of desire. I know what it feels like to want to ask the first man you see on the street to bed with you. Now, I feel so much more freedom. I can chose to make love instead of needing to. I enjoy it, but I no longer depend on it. For me, menopause has been a very powerful initiation, the final initiation that my sexual body will guide me through.

As you may have noticed, quite a few of the women whose stories we have heard so far are well over fifty. Throughout this book, their voices have been inviting us to reexamine the meaning of that elusive word, "sex." Thoughtfully, Donna said, "Part of my life has been about plumbing what we call sex. Somebody once told me that there are a hundred words for 'love' in Sanskrit. In this culture, when we talk of sex, we mean the sexual body and the desire for genital union. But there are so many different ways to be sexual."

As Donna points out, our culture is wedded to a narrow definition of sex as genital activity. As a result, women who are not interested in genital intercourse are automatically identified as nonsexual. Every single one of the menopausal or postmenopausal women I interviewed objected to this narrow definition. When older women become less interested in sexual intercourse, they often feel as if their sexuality had become invisible and somehow unreal. We need a new understanding of sex that is less fixated on genital arousal.

As long as we equate sexuality and genital activity, we will naturally conclude that our most sexual years fall between puberty and menopause. But if we define sex as our body's way of opening to the life-force, a very different story about our sexual journey emerges.

Look at the energy system of a baby, and you will see that her circuitry is wide open; energy flows freely and encounters no resistance. Therefore, the child is a highly erotic being, open to every sensual pleasure. Within her small body, a complex web of energetic rivers, rivulets, and streams carries the life-force to every last cell. Then, slowly but surely, the child develops an ego, which grows stronger and more dominant as she approaches puberty. In the clear mirror of the body, all the ego's coping mechanisms and survival tactics are reflected as a complex system of energetic resistances, blockages, knots, and obstructions that cloud the child's original clarity. Gradually, she loses the energetic transparency of childhood—and the effortless ability to commune with spirit, which many children enjoy.

Then, in puberty, as the ego reaches its zenith, genital sex kicks in with a vengeance. From the perspective of harried parents, it may seem unfair that nature has added the problem of teenage hormones to the already difficult challenge of dealing with a teenage ego. But as far as nature is concerned, genital sex is the perfect medicine for ego-dominated creatures such as we. Children have less need for such medicine; their bodies are still luminous and translucent, and their energy is naturally light and porous. For adults, however, the situation is different. As a rocket needs a powerful push to help it lift off, so most of us require the voltage of sexual pleasure to raise our somewhat opaque, dense consciousness into the light-filled realms of ecstatic communion. Genital sex blasts open our blocked channels and purifies the inner streams of energy while lifting us out of the heavy tangle of adult roles and responsibilities into a lighter, more playful dimension. Nature, it seems, knew how much we would need this medicine, and made sure that unlike other mammals, who have sex only at certain points in their hormonal cycle, humans would be able to have sex anytime.

After menopause, women often begin to recapture some of the lightness and the magical ability to fly that they lost at puberty. With age, a woman's bones tend to thin, almost as if her body were preparing to take to the air. In fact, I have noticed that after they reach the age of forty many women become very interested in birds, or find birds flying through their dreams. As a woman's body changes, her psyche transforms as well. The ropes that bind her to the earth become thinner and more elastic. Her psyche may acquire a new lightness, an affinity to the spirit worlds. As a result, she may find that she no longer depends on genital stimulation the way she used to. Sara, now in her eighties, says:

I am finding that the older I get, the more I can experience sexual energy without having sex, without even touching myself. With age, the life-force has become more accessible. As I allow myself to breathe deeply and exhale deeply, I am more and more able to generate delightful feelings through my genitals all the way down my legs and through into my arms and hands. Sometimes, I can come to orgasm merely by charging my internal energy through deep breathing. On the one hand, I am living almost monastically, and yet I feel I am living a fully sexual life. That is possible. It's very different from the monasticism that rejects sex. It is possible to be simultaneously celibate yet fully sexual. For me, this has been a gift of age.

Conventional wisdom would say that Sara has become less sexual with age. But if we look upon sex as a means of opening to the life-force and channeling it through our bodies, then the opposite is true—she has become *more* sexual, rather than less so. Her sexuality is simply less genitally focused and less compartmentalized, as when a blinding spotlight broadens into a wide floodlight.

We can see, however, how some men might find the sexuality of older women intimidating and prefer to deny it entirely. Sara is typical of many women whose dependency on male lovers has decreased dramatically with age, as has her willingness to adapt to, compromise with, and coddle the male ego. The feisty, carefree independence that older women often manifest can easily evoke feelings of insecurity and even hostility in those who expect women to wait on them and cater to their needs.

We often think of puberty as a period of rebellious acting out. But menopause can trigger in us a far deeper, more mature form of rebellion, a rebellion of the soul rather than of the ego. With age, women often find that outer approval no longer interests them as much as it used to; nor does the specter of disapproval terrify them as it once did. Being a good wife, a pretty woman, a loving mother, or a responsible worker is no longer their first priority. As one menopausal woman said, "I may not be perfect, but I'm sick of trying to improve myself. People will just have to take me as I am."

Theresa told me that with menopause, her willingness to mother and nurture others, especially men, decreased dramatically.

In menopause, I started moving into the crone—the wise-woman, the knower. For three years, I found I wanted to be absolutely alone. It was the first time in my entire life I had ever been alone, and I loved it. My celibacy was never a problem. I was very possessive of my energy, and I was not about to give any of it away. Suddenly, I was saying no to people all the time. Before, I never knew when to stop giving. Even when I didn't have anything left to give, I would keep giving, just as my mother had done. It felt really healing and wonderful to close my boundaries. I felt very sexual but not genital, and I wasn't about to share my sexuality. This was new for me. Since I was twelve, I had never been without a main squeeze.

Like Sara, and like Theresa, every one of the older women I interviewed refused to equate sexuality with genital sex. "What is sex? What does the word mean to you?" I asked Hannah, in her late fifties. She considered for a minute and then replied, "Sex is the light that streams from the body." She went on to explain that since menopause, her sexual interest has shifted toward a more diffuse appreciation of the life-force as it streams through her being.

I went into menopause when I was forty-four, eight years ago. Some time in there, I became less interested in genital sex. What interests me very much, however, is the aliveness of the cells. At that level there are no compartments—the ecstasy is everywhere in your body and consciousness. I often think of Jesus' words in the Gospel According to Thomas: "Where is the kingdom? It's spread out inside you and outside you, but you do not see it." It's in the cells of my body and everywhere. The experience can no longer be identified as sexual. And yet it's the same energy, just not compartmentalized.

When I asked Anya, a woman in her fifties, the same question— "What is sex?"—she replied without hesitation.

I see the whole world as sexual, as an interaction of energies. As we sit here, our energies are making love, and out of that comes this conversation, and out of that will come this book. And I am aware that the tree is participating and the rug is participating. All these energies are multiplying each other, making love. This is Eros. What happens when you hug a tree? Not only does your energy blend with the energy of the tree, but they both expand. And if you are willing to open, you receive the blessing of that expansion. To me, sex is magic, a field of magic.

Sex is magic, says one woman. Sex is the light that streams from the body, says another. Sex is a spark signaling that body and spirit have caught sight of each other and are straining to unite. Sex is an angel that has been posted to remind us that the gateway to heaven will always be open. Sex is a fire that melts us down until we become streams of molten gold. Sex is a power that accumulates in the body, as when a rocket gathers speed for takeoff, until it shoots into outer space, headed for worlds of amazing luminosity and radiance.

Often, menopause brings a growing hunger for spiritual communion, a longing to explore inner worlds and to listen deeply to the quiet voice of the soul. "Since menopause," Anya told me, "I feel that I just want to be. Just to walk out in nature, to be in conversation with the sky and the trees. In the past, I was very goal-oriented. I had a long To Do list that I could never satisfy. Now, I want silence. I long for it more than ever before."

Mercedes, a beautiful Mexican-American woman in her sixties, tells me that since menopause she, too, has shifted toward a quieter, more introverted way of life. Today she expresses deep gratitude for the very physical symptoms that women often hate about menopause, symptoms that forced her to pay attention to her body in a whole new way.

Menopause was hard for me. I had always had so much energy, and I was competent and efficient. Suddenly, I became clumsy, and I was exhausted all the time. But that exhaustion was really valuable for me, because it forced me to reconnect with my body. All my life, I never really paid attention to my body. It was healthy and strong, and I took it for granted. I just was on the go all the time. My head decided what to do, and my body obeyed. Then suddenly, it wouldn't do what I wanted anymore. I had no choice but to slow way, way down. And gradually, I realized what an incredible gift my body had given me. I am finding such joy in doing small things in a conscious way, and honoring the natural speed of my own organism. I have become a much more relaxed, happy person.

More and more women, especially those who are creative and spiritually sensitive, are suffering from chronic fatigue syndrome, a disabling illness. Our entire culture is tired, exhausted, overwhelmed with fatigue. Our immune systems are breaking down, and the number of people with environmental allergies is skyrocketing. Addicted to activity and speed, we brutally batter the gentle goddess within, whose movements soothe and heal and evoke sweet, erotic feelings. Even though our bodies and souls might cry out for rest, we refuse to stop and pay attention to the slow, organic rhythms of our bodies. "I have to make a contribution," I hear my clients cry. "I have no time. I have responsibilities." But one can only force the body for so long. Then it will rise up in rebellion—and often, this occurs in our forties or fifties. Suddenly, our bodies collapse and refuse to do our bidding.

The erotic life is a slow life, a life lived in harmony with nature's rhythms. I can think of nothing less erotic or more deadening to a woman's sensuality than a schedule that leaves her no time to take long baths, no time to sit in her rocking chair and look out the window at the evening sky, no time to gossip and laugh with her friends. One of the most important choices we can make to support ourselves as sexual women and priestesses is the choice to honor the rhythms of our body. Can we give ourselves the rest and nurturance we need? Can we allow ourselves to move slowly and deliberately, with graceful, unhurried ease? Can we learn to say no to unnecessary and draining activities? And how will the young ones dare to resist the frenetic pace of our society, unless their elders model the possibility of a life lived gracefully, slowly, and harmoniously?

Like Mercedes, Joanne experienced menopause both as a difficult threshold and as a period of rebirth. She, too, has learned to pay attention to herself in a new way, to honor her own authority and to live life according to her own values.

Menopause brought me the discomfort of hot flashes and a lot of emotionality. I struggled with a low-grade depression. But at the same time, it was also the beginning of a new phase. I was leaving motherhood, and that opened up some space for me to reevaluate my life. I felt I was coming into my own, and that I was picking up where I left off in adolescence. Suddenly I saw that I could use my brain freely, and that I could live to please myself. I had known how to do that as a child, and then I had lost that knowledge during adolescence. I started obeying the rules that applied to women at those times. After menopause, I felt fuller. I was finding myself again, separate from being in relationship to anyone else—husband, children, or bosses.

It is amazing how little reverence we have for this important and intriguing threshold in our lives. Barbara Walker says that in ancient Europe, "it was believed that women became very wise when they no longer shed the lunar 'wise blood' but kept it within."[81] Why do we hear only about the hot flashes, the vaginal dryness, and the exhaustion, and not about the rich gifts that menopause can bring? How different we might feel about menopause if, instead of viewing it as a loss of sexual potency, we acknowledged it as a time of increasing wisdom, a time of opening to subtle dimensions of consciousness and to the formless, ever-present life-force! How wonderful if we could see menopause as a threshold into an exquisitely expansive, erotically vibrant state of being! How liberating it would be if, instead of approaching menopause as an unfortunate and embarrassing ordeal, we could honor it as a period of initiation into a circle of empowered elders, grandmothers, wise-women, and priestesses.

2 8

THE STORY OF A WISEWOMAN

Someday there will be girls and women whose name will no longer mean the mere opposite of the male, but something in itself, something that makes one think not of any complement, but only of life and reality: the female human being.

Rainer Maria Rilke

Upon meeting Sara, I was instantly charmed by her warmth and her delightfully irreverent sense of humor. Now in her late eighties, Sara exudes an extraordinary lust for life and a lighthearted wisdom that refuses to take life too seriously. "I don't believe in god," Sara said to me with a twinkle in her eye. "I believe in Life, with a capital L." Though she is no caster of spells, no mutterer of magic words, no rider of broomsticks, she would undoubtedly have been prosecuted as a witch had she lived in the so-called burning times. From a young age, she has insisted on speaking her sexual thoughts, feelings, and beliefs, even when they embarrassed or shocked others. Confident and feisty, she has never been one to bow to outer authorities.

The stories of older women are often rich and flavorful, like stews that have simmered for a long time. They have come a long way, and their journeys have transformed them. When they tell a story, other stories, other memories, other times and places resonate through their words. Sara was born in 1910; her childhood memories transport us to another era. The first weeks of her life, she remembers, were touch-and-go.

I was born on a farm. I was not nursed, and I nearly died because I was allergic to the formulas they gave me. Finally, a neighboring farmer came over and took my dad by the hand. "Look," he said, "here is the cow you ought to milk for that child." I don't know where that farmer got his knowledge, but he knew. So my father milked that cow and brought me warm milk straight from the udder, and I began to thrive.

We were brought up in a very free way and taught to be independent. There were bears up in the woods, and I clearly remember gathering huckleberries and meeting a mother bear with her cubs. We had a happy childhood, with lots of laughter and giggling. We learned to swim in the ocean at an early age, too. After swimming, we would take off our suits and lie naked in the warm sand, feeling very sensual. Nakedness was quite acceptable then, and everyone in my family was comfortable around nudity. My mother would bathe my brother and myself in the bathtub together, and I often saw my brother and my father nude. There was no prudery there.

Of course, they didn't equate nudity with sex at all. Life was not so sexualized. Sunshine on the body was considered healthy. People assumed that children were innocent and had no interest in sex, so we could do anything we wanted. The little boys and girls in my neighborhood would go out behind my grandfather's barn. We would take down our pants—supposedly to show our bottoms, but of course our bottoms weren't what we were really interested in. I laughed later when I read about penis envy, because I clearly remembered feeling sorry for little boys to have that thing hanging between their legs, and thinking how I would cut it off if I were a little boy.

My mother never talked to us about sex. No, never. I found out about sex once I went to college. This was in the twenties, and the first sexual revolution had started. The men were back from the First World War, after having experienced life in Europe, and there was a lot of flamboyance. I remember going home and telling my mother, "I found out how you can prevent having babies. "How?" she asked. So I told her what

I had learned about condoms. "Humph," she said. "Both you and your brother were born when condoms broke."

Sara's first sexual experience occurred in the context of a loving yet decidedly unorthodox relationship. In college, she started dating an art professor who was married, with two small children. He and his wife had agreed to each have their own lovers. This man acted as a mentor and sexual initiator to Sara. "I think that sexually, Stan saved my life," Sara said fondly. "He taught me to associate everything about sex with beauty—everything about the body was beautiful to him."

And yet neither he nor Sara had a clue as to the all-important function of a woman's clitoris. Listen to Sara talking about her first orgasm—in the 1920s—and you get a sense of the distance women have come in this century:

> Once Stan caressed my clitoris, and I had an orgasm. I was scared to death; I had no idea what an orgasm was, or what caused it. I shook and trembled and didn't know what was happening. After that, I never had another orgasm until I was married. I talked to Stan about it, but knowledgeable as he was, he too didn't know that stroking a woman's clitoris could cause an orgasm. You have to understand how ignorant even the most educated people were about sex in those days. There were no sex books available at that time, either. This generation of men grew up having not a ghost of a notion about women's sexuality. Most men believed that women never had orgasms, and of course, eighty percent of them didn't. It was the purest luck if a woman had an orgasm. Stan and I made love many times, but even though I loved it, I never had an orgasm through intercourse. So when I did have an orgasm, he just didn't know what it was.

Sara's first choice in love set in motion a pattern for her whole life. "All my life," she told me, "my love affairs have been with people I had enormous admiration for, and who, in many cases, were my teachers."

Sex was for me not only a great personal joy, but also a form of worship, if you want to call it that. Not worship in the religious sense, but a means of expressing my physical and spiritual love for another person, my reverence. I always gravitated towards greatness, and have always sought out people in whom I felt a greatness of spirit. Sex was my way of acknowledging their spirit and learning from them. I owe each of my lovers a great debt, and to me, sex was an important part of the growth that occurred.

Though we rarely think of our lovers as teachers, many of us would concede that the most important lessons of our life were learned not in school, but through our intimate relationships. Because our culture values intellectual learning so highly, we tend to believe that knowledge can be communicated only through concepts, thoughts, ideas, and words. But in other traditions, it is understood that consciousness does not depend on language. A teacher may initiate and enlighten her students with a gesture or a song, or through the gaze of her eyes, for the soul has a myriad ways of transmitting its knowledge. Intuitively, Sara recognized that by making love with Stan, she was uniting not only with his body but also with his energy and consciousness. In a very natural, effortless way, she was absorbing his wisdom through osmosis, as he was absorbing hers.

What happened next, Sara said, "was very important, probably the most important thing that ever happened in my life." As graduation approached, she became more and more desperate. She knew she would have to part from her lover, but the very thought seemed unbearable; she could not imagine living without him.

"What did you do?" I asked.

"Well," she said, "I thought (and this was a big mistake), that if I could just get myself to love somebody else, I would feel better about leaving my lover." And so, just before her graduation, Sara had a brief sexual contact with a man she neither loved nor intended to ever see again.

From this, I became pregnant. A month later I didn't menstruate, and I began to get very nauseated. Very, very nauseated. Another month later, I still hadn't menstruated. I didn't know what to do. That month I did every crazy thing I could think of to induce a spontaneous abortion. I leaped off of haylofts in the fields. I went swimming in ice-cold water. I went horseback riding for hours. No matter what I did, nothing happened.

Finally one night, I was feeling absolutely desperate. I went to a nearby mountain and I climbed up to the top. Up on top of that mountain, I made a promise. I guess you might say it was a promise to Life, because I didn't believe in god. I think when saints go into ecstasy, they're having a love affair with Life. They call it god, and I call it Life. So on that mountain, I made a promise to Life that if I got out of this catastrophe, I would spend the rest of my life doing something to make sex better for women.

And on the way down from that mountain, I began to bleed. My prayers had been answered.

Who would have thought that a woman's lifelong commitment to sexual liberation could begin with an abortion? Yet so it was. Spirit (or Life, as Sara prefers to call it) will use anything it can to initiate us and to turn our lives in the right direction. Sara's unwanted pregnancy inspired her to make a commitment that was to influence and define her entire life's work. Because of this vow, she took every opportunity to educate others about sexuality. She became a sex therapist, founded schools, spoke on the radio, wrote articles, and helped mothers through their pregnancies—to name just a few of the many ways in which Sara has fulfilled her promise. In a period when sex was laden with shame and guilt, Sara dedicated herself to supporting open communication in sexual matters. Though she might not define herself as a devotional person, her entire life has been an act of service to the life-force she holds sacred, and the direction her service took was determined that night when she climbed the mountain and cried out for help, and her plea was answered.

A few years after making her vow to Life, Sara met her husband. Once again, she felt attracted to an older man whom she admired tremendously. In the eyes of conventional wisdom, Sara's liaison seemed disastrous. "I would have pleaded with any of my women friends to reconsider, had they been in my shoes," Sara says of the match between herself and Thomas. Nonetheless, like many other women in the presence of their soul mates, Sara felt a joyful assurance so strong and unwavering that it silenced her doubtful mind. After having spent only two whole days with Thomas, she went ahead and tied the knot.

My friends were full of dire warnings. "He's twenty-two years older than you, has a different background, and it will never work." Well, I went to visit him anyway, and the very night I arrived, we decided to get married. Since Thomas was so much older than me, I said to myself, "This may be the only day we will ever have together, so I had best live it fully." I was aware that he would probably die a long time before I did, and that we had better make the best of what we had. And we had a wonderful thirty-seven years. We both felt sure. I can't tell you why, but I just knew it was right, even though I would have advised any of my friends against it. Our vow to each other was that we would live together as long as it made us happy. That was all. We made that vow, and then we announced we were married.

Our first night together, we had sex, but I did not have an orgasm. But the second night, Thomas decided he was going to change that, and he did. He just took all the time it took, probably about an hour, gently stroking my clitoris. It was a revolutionary experience for me. After that first orgasm that had scared me so, I never had another one. Now I wasn't scared. All my married life, we never made love without my having an orgasm. Thomas never left me without making sure I was satisfied. That was very, very rare in those times. Sex was wonderful between us, and we both loved it. Thomas was gentle and imaginative, an extraordinary man.

By now, the Depression was really on. Neither of us had a job, so we decided to stay on in the woods and build a little log cabin next to a lake. We had no running water and no electricity. I had maybe twenty dollars, and my husband didn't have much more. Soon I got pregnant. Winter had come, and it was getting very cold. The farmers couldn't sell much, so they let us help ourselves to what they had. By god, I learned how to cook apples and onions and potatoes! We piled wood around the cabin and wore long underwear.

When the local doctor told me I was pregnant, he said, "I would advise you to get legally married, if you aren't yet." So we found a justice who would marry us. He asked us whether we would promise this and that, all the usual marriage vows. We said no to all of them. No, no, no, no. Finally, he lost patience. "Well, what will you promise, then?" We told him the only promise we would make was to live together as long as we were happy. Many people believe in suffering as a way of personal growth, but Thomas believed in growing through pleasure and joy. "Well," our justice said, "I had a Jewish couple in here recently, and all I had to ask them was whether they cared to be man and wife." So we said, "Pretend we're Jews." That's how we got married.

In many ways, Sara's marriage conformed perfectly to traditional images. In her home, four children were raised lovingly and carefully, cats and dogs ran in and out, guests were warmly welcomed, and the kitchen was well stocked. Yet sexually, Sara and her husband were pioneers, revolutionaries, and rebels. From the onset, they agreed to have an open marriage, setting each other free to engage in outside sexual affairs. "I have had about twelve male lovers," Sara told me, "and three women lovers."

At eighty-four, Sara is not only the oldest woman I interviewed, but also one of the most unconventional, the only one who lived in an open marriage that satisfied both partners' needs and endured for almost four decades. What made this marriage work, when so many other attempts at open marriage failed, was a rare combination of deep, passionate, committed love between the partners, an innate lack of jealousy, and a high degree of maturity and sensitivity to the needs of the family as a whole.

Thomas made me promise I would always follow love's path, wherever it might lead me, and he assured me I would never have to worry about his jealousy. He said he really saw no difference between making genital contact and any other kind of contact. "You can love a person with your eyes," he said. Friends of ours were amazed and couldn't understand a man not being jealous. But Thomas truly didn't have a jealous bone in his body. When Thomas first talked to me about having an open marriage, I thought he was nuts. I couldn't believe that I would ever want to sleep with anyone else. The first time another man wanted to make love to me, I said no, and we just cuddled. I still felt ambivalent; I just didn't see how I could have sex with two people. In a way I had accepted the idea, but the reality of it was a different matter.

Though, over the years, we both had affairs, we were extremely careful in our choices. One man I had slept with was quite promiscuous. I thought this was unwise and told him that I really didn't want to pick up a disease. Of course, this was long before AIDS. But I said to him, "No way do I want to be involved with you. I love you dearly, but no matter how much fun it might be, it would not make it worthwhile."

Only once did I see anything like jealousy in my husband. I had always wanted a very beautiful opal ring. My husband would have loved to give me such a ring, but it was not something he could afford. One time, one of my lovers gave me an opal ring. A couple of days later, I found this cartoon on my desk. My husband had drawn a picture of an opal ring and he had labeled it "Jealousy." I gave that ring back to my lover right away. That was the only time I saw Thomas express anything close to jealousy, and it wasn't jealousy about my love affair, but about his inability to fulfill my material desires.

There were some rules to the game, which we discovered as we went along. We never allowed ourselves to make love to anyone who might try to drive a wedge between us. Also, we never did anything that would injure the family situation. Our kids were never aware of our affairs, and we were never gone overnight. We also discovered how important it was that our lovers should love both of us. When Thomas started having other lovers, it might have been hard for me had they not been so warm and friendly to me. Instead of feeling betrayed, I felt included. Thomas and I were always primary to one another, and our lovers remained on the fringe of our life. Over the years, I met men I was very excited by, but never anyone I preferred over my husband for the long haul.

Sara and her husband had four children, and her first acts of engaged social service evolved in direct response to her own experience of pregnancy. "At that time," she says, "natural childbirth was still unheard-of."

You were taken to a hospital, put on a table, and left alone. It was nasty. After the birth, the babies were taken away from their mothers, and women were discouraged from nursing. You really had to fight if you wanted to nurse your baby. I had all my four babies in the hospital except for the last one, which I had at home. What a different experience! Even though it was the longest labor of them all, it was just wonderful.

Just like Roseanne (Chapter 1), Sara found nursing a highly erotic experience. However, unlike Roseanne's Korean doctor, Sara's doctor flat-out denied that nursing could trigger an orgasm.

When I told my doctor that I could come to orgasm with a baby at my breast, he said that was impossible. Knowledgeable as he was, he didn't believe me. I think this is one of the most withheld secrets from women. After childbirth, they massage the woman's belly, trying to bring about the contractions that are necessary to realign the uterus. But when the baby starts nursing, it can trigger those contractions naturally. I didn't come to orgasm often that way, but nursing was always pleasurable. I loved nursing my babies. I nursed all of them as long as they wanted, until they turned me down, between one year and two and a half years.

As Sara became aware of the plight of birthing mothers, she realized that here was something she could do for other women.

I started looking at scenes of childbirth in literature, and realized it was almost always talked about as something horrible and painful. There was hardly anything that talked about birth as a marvelous, joyful event. The first time I saw a baby being born, I felt so awestruck. I saw what it took to make a human being. I felt that if every man could observe the birth of a baby, men would appreciate the preciousness of human life in a much deeper way. I started connecting with pregnant mothers and seeing them all through their pregnancy, recording everything that went on and everything they said. I would talk to them about their dreams and fears, and when they went to the hospital, I would go with them and stay with them. I wished that kind of support had been available for me when I had my babies.

As Sara and Thomas raised their children, they began to focus on the issue of childhood education. Together, they founded and directed several schools. The first one was a nursery school for about 150 children. Later, the couple decided to move to the country and start a school for older children, between eight and sixteen years. One of their main goals was to help the children develop enough self-love and self-esteem in order to make wise sexual choices. Sara remembers:

> We took bright kids who were having some kind of difficulties. We were like parents to them, and they all lived with us in a twenty-two-room farmhouse. We talked very openly about sex. We said if any kid could get their parents' permission, they were welcome to have sex. Of course, that meant it was no go. But they really didn't want sex; they weren't ready for it yet. We never had a pregnancy, and we never had a kid trying intercourse. What the kids wanted was body contact and cuddling. I think one of the great crimes against children today is that teachers no longer touch or hug them for fear of being accused of child molestation. In our school, we had lots of warm, cuddly times, lots of touching and stroking.

Sara is right. What messages do we give children when we teach them to fear human touch? Close physical contact of any kind, whether between men, women, or children, has become polluted with caution and prohibitions. When a friendly cat walks up to us, we pet her and stroke her fur. Instinctively, we know this is how she will absorb our love. Yet it has become difficult, if not impossible, to give our fellow human beings the same kind of affection. To deprive children of touch all day long can only stunt their development and well-being.

The average American child watches one hundred murders a month on television.[82] Compared to this thorough education in all the nuances of violence, most children know very little about sex, and few adults are willing to discuss its complexities with them. Sara, on the other hand, was determined that her own four children (who today are themselves mothers and fathers) would get all the information they wanted. As you might suspect, she was never your typical mother.

Because of my openness, lots of kids came to ask me for advice, and quite a few mothers asked me to talk to their kids about sex, because they felt uncomfortable doing it. With my own children, I was very open about sex. Once, when my son was two, he had an erect penis when I lifted him out of the bath. He looked down at himself and then he said, "Mummy, I have touched myself all over, so why does that part feel the best of all?" I told him this was a wonderful discovery, and that one day he would have a lot of fun with his penis.

Another time, I was talking with one of my daughters about how babies are born. She said, "I want to see the hole I came out of." So I showed her. Then she said, "Well, I want to climb back in." "It's really too small now," I told her. She didn't believe me. "How do you know it's too small? I bet I can get back in." "No, honey," I told her, "you really can't." Oh, she was so disappointed!

We would all have baths together. Bath time was fun time. Once, when my daughter was about six, my husband was sitting in the bathtub and his penis was flopping in the water. All of a sudden, she said, "Daddy, what a wonderful ship for the mermaids to ride on!" And she leaned down, kissed his penis, and popped up again. So far, so good. But one day soon after, her teacher started talking about the differences between girls and boys and asked whether any of the girls had ever seen a boy naked. Everyone said no, except our daughter. "Sure," she piped up, "I have even kissed my daddy's penis." Oh my god! Can you imagine? If that happened today, all hell would break loose.

It would indeed. It is of course essential that the general public be aware of the threat of child abuse and take steps to protect children who have no way of protecting themselves. However, it is a sad state of affairs when innocent, loving parents and teachers feel terrified of facing false accusations, as is the case today. Surely it must be possible to find a third option besides denial on the one hand and paranoia on the other.

Several years later, Sara's husband had a heart attack, and the couple closed their school. Not one to rest for long, Sara soon began to channel her energies into organizing an adoption program for unwanted babies. Unfortunately, the Catholic church felt extremely threatened by her work and involved her in a fierce battle which could easily have landed her in jail. Because of her outspokenness, and her refusal to comply with the forces of hypocrisy, she found herself viciously attacked by those whose complacency she threatened. Echoes of the witch-hunts still reverberate through our lives, and sometimes spoil our attempts to create a better world.

I began working with about ten unwed mothers at a time. If they wanted to keep their babies, we would help them find jobs after the birth, often as nannies, so they could stay with their babies during work. If they wanted to give up their babies, we would put them in touch with potential adoptive parents, so they could participate in the choice. Anyone who got a baby through us had to contribute enough money to take care of some other girl who needed help.

This system worked extremely well. But what I was doing enraged the Catholic church. Adoptions were a lucrative business for them. Mothers would simply give the church their babies, and the church would get enormous contributions from the adoptive parents, big endowments. It was legal, and it wasn't considered a baby trade, but the church was making a hell of a lot of money this way. So the Catholics were very upset about my work.

Unfortunately, most of the high bureaucrats in the state were Catholics. The cops, the judges, the head of the children's bureau were all Catholics. I discovered the state had put a detective on me who opened all my letters. Naturally, I was furious. Finally, they subpoenaed me. I thought they might put me in jail; I didn't know what might happen. They had ten counts against me, stupid things, such as the doors in the home being too narrow. They said we had lewd paintings on the wall, but much to their embarrassment, it turned out those paintings were from the Bruges chapel. In the end, they decided they would let me go free if I left the state. So I did. There was nothing else I could do.

Sara was close to sixty when her husband died. Grief-stricken as she was, she took comfort in the fact that for many years, she continued to feel his loving presence around her.

Like many older women, Sara was unable to find another compatible male partner.

I might enjoy having a male lover, but I have not met any man I would want to be with. Most of the older men who interest me are married, and I stay clear of them. Many of the available men at that age are unable to commit to a partner for one reason or another. They are very self-centered, still babies in some funny way. A woman who has lost her husband would much rather be alone than go out with an adult baby. She is done raising babies and tired of nursing a sick man.

However, Sara is neither lonely nor sexually frustrated. Today, twenty-five years after her husband's death, she is happily partnered with a woman, an old childhood friend with whom she has lived for the last twelve years. Having received much pleasure, comfort, and joy from female friends and lovers, she has become a strong and vocal proponent for women who turn to other women for emotional and sexual intimacy. Like Iris (Chapter 13), who found making love with a woman to be a revelatory experience, Sara emphasizes that although physical intimacy between women *can* be sexual, it does not need to be.

I am concerned about older women, who, on average, live eight years longer than men. There is practically no chance for them to find a true partner. Seven out of eight women are left with no partner in the last years of their life, and therefore without any physical contact. I think much of our need can be filled with touch, massage, and cuddling. Caressing becomes more important the older you get. I talk about self-caressing, too. I hate the word "masturbate." It means "to pollute with the hand." Isn't that awful? Some nasty-minded adult invented a nasty word for a lovely act.

After my talks, I am always surrounded by women who want to know how to make a contact with an older woman. As women, they have not been taught to initiate contacts, and everybody is scared of rejection. It's a problem I don't have an answer for. To approach a man is sort of acceptable today, but to approach another woman or to even bring up the subject is scary. Many women repress the physical expressions of their love for other women for fear of being called lesbians. I, too, would be uncomfortable being labeled homosexual in today's world. You don't go out and expose yourself to the rock-throwing that goes on. My partner is scared to death to have anybody know we have a sexual relationship. I ask her, "Do you think people are dumb? They know." But unlike men, women can get by without openly acknowledging their relationship. Still, she would be horrified if somebody in town knew. She is very protective about it. She has never acknowledged that she is lesbian to her friends in any overt way. Old maids have always slept together, and since they have been considered asexual, they haven't been stigmatized as much as men.

If I had to identify myself, I would call myself bisexual. I am drawn to women, but I don't think it's primarily sexual. Even though I live with a woman, my sexual fantasies are about men. But then, I think everybody is bisexual. I don't like those categories. I believe we love whom we love. If we start with love, rather than sex, it can go anywhere. It's love energy, and sometimes love translates into sex. I don't believe there is any kind of love that doesn't contain some element of sexual energy.

"Women can have wonderful relationships with other women," Sara said. Then she grinned and added,

Not everyone wants to hear this, though. At one of my talks, a more conservative woman leaped from the audience and cried, "I would rather sleep with my dog before I slept with a woman." I laughed and couldn't help but say, "Well, yes, some women do like dogs."

Sara has dedicated much of her time to broadcasting the message that people of all ages cannot thrive without intimacy. Without close, emotionally expressive relationships, the soul becomes parched and dry. Even the hardiest seed cannot grow without good, nourishing soil, water, and light. The soil the elderly need is community, the water they need is affection and love, and the light they need is a communal awareness of their value. Sara devotes a great deal of energy to communicating the message that being old does not mean being useless, unattractive, and burdensome, and that the elders need to be encouraged to come forward with their unique and precious gifts. As long as they are not appreciated, our whole community will suffer.

Sara has helped thousands of men and women find sexual fulfillment, and has acted as an ardent, sometimes outrageously outspoken advocate for the sexual and emotional needs of the elderly. With humor and stories, she energetically seeks to educate the public about the fact that sexuality does not disappear with age, and encourages people to let go of the idea that it *should* disappear. "I have devoted much of my life to teaching people about sexuality," she says. She is one of the pioneers of women's liberation who remembered the sanctity of sexual energy at a time when most had forgotten. Independent in her thinking, outspoken in her words, and effective in her actions, she has served many women as a model of strength and integrity.

"Looking back," Sara says, "I believe I have been true to that promise I made to Life as a young woman on the mountain. I took that promise very seriously. And in my lifetime, I think I have done quite a few things to make sex better for women." She pauses and then says, thoughtfully:

> In my lifetime, there has been a real emergence of women sticking together, supporting each other. When I was a child, even though women maintained strong friendships with other women, they tended to become competitors for men and status. I think that now, women are just beginning to learn how to be *real* friends with each other. Finally, we are learning how to really support each other.

Then, grinning mischievously, Sara leaned in and confided, "I have a fantasy of how I want to die. I want to die while all my closest friends massage and touch me. The only problem is, I think it might be so pleasurable I would want to stick around. It's such a magical world. If there is a heaven, I sure hope there is sex in it!"

EPILOGUE

It is God who yawns and sneezes
and coughs, and now laughs.

Look, it's God doing ablutions!
God deciding to fast, God going naked
from one New Year's Eve to the next.

Will you ever understand
how near God is
to you?

                    Lalla, fourteenth century C.E.

Six hundred years ago, a woman called Lalla saw who she really was, and from that moment onward, she walked naked through the streets of India, singing and dancing with joy. Will we ever understand how near the holy presence is to us, she asks? One glimpse is enough to transform our lives forever.

Look down at your hands, and see—there is the Holy One, manifest in these marvelously intricate sculptures of bone and flesh, skin and nails, fingers and knuckles, thumbs and palms. Science will tell you that despite their appearance of solidity, these hands of yours are in fact pulsating fields of energy. Every particle in your body has witnessed billions of years of history, and every particle consists of vibrating, intelligent energy. And what is energy? Here, science falls silent and the mystic responds: energy is the footprint of the Mother. Take a deep breath, and let her fill your chest. Feel her power as she lies coiled near your genitals, seat of her creative power. Bow down to that eternal presence and know that you are

That. You are spirit on a long journey of coming home to yourself.

The ancients pictured life as a great tree that had its roots in spirit and sent its branches through every particle of matter. Your spinal column is a branch of that universal tree, and in your sexual pleasure you feel its sap rising through you. You are a channel of this sacred sap, this divine love juice. Your sexuality is god's love letter to you, a miracle of biological engineering that could have been devised only by a mind of vast and humorous generosity, a mind that knew the pain and the sense of confinement earthly beings would feel and wanted to make sure you might always have glimpses of heaven. No matter what your sexuality has meant to you, no matter whether it has been a source of pleasure or of pain, of joy or of confusion, it connects you to the power that created the universe, and it is worthy of honor.

It is up to you to nurture your particular branch of the Tree of Life and keep it healthy. If you would save the planet, begin by honoring and loving yourself. Please stop feeding your ancient shame. Please stop telling yourself you are ugly. Please stop analyzing your physical imperfections. Your body is exactly as nature intended it to be. Your genitals are perfect and beautiful. You are worthy of all the love in the world, and your story matters.

When I first went to India, I received an invitation to live with a family. Though they barely knew me, they assured me with typical Indian hospitality that I was welcome to stay with them as long as I wanted. I accepted, and their house became my home for the next six months. I arrived with two suitcases stuffed full of supplies for the next year—clothing, gifts, bribes, and journals, as well as articles hard to come by in India, such as tampons and hair conditioner. I had barely walked in the front door when the whole clan descended on my suitcases like a flock of vultures on a carcass. Thrilled, they began unpacking, exploring, investigating, touching, and smelling. They discussed and argued and joked. They organized and asked questions. I was stunned. Had they never heard of privacy, of private property? At the same time, the instant sense of belonging I felt intrigued me. They had accepted me as a member of the family, and therefore my things had become theirs. This, I realized, was what it meant to become a member of a tribe.

Now, as I think about the way we hold our sexual stories, I remember this unpacking ceremony. I think that every woman should have the opportunity, at some point in her life, to set down her sexual baggage among people who respect and support her, and to unpack it with them. Our isolation has reinforced the assumption that nobody shares our feelings, or cares about our story, or wants to know. But our individual baggage is never just ours alone. Rather, it belongs to the collective. Other women have their own piece to carry. Maybe theirs is a little carry-on, a box, a parcel. Even so, we need each other. The time has come to speak of what we know.

In the temple, we now sit in silence, a circle of priestesses. One by one, each one of us has stepped forward to make her offering. Each one has given her gift, revealing through her story a beauty that made us catch our breath, a courage that renewed our own, or a compassion that warmed our hearts. Around us, we sense the spirits of many others: mothers and grandmothers, lovers and husbands, teachers and guides, the spirits of the ancestors and of future generations.

Who are we? Most of us carry no outer marks of spiritual authority; nobody has ordained us or given us any official credentials. After all, spiritual authority is not a gift that one person can bestow upon another or that can be earned with a graduate degree. It comes from within, from having walked our path, explored our truth, made our mistakes, and learned our lessons. We are the woman standing next to you in the supermarket, the woman who checks your pulse at the doctor's office, the woman looking out the window at the coffee shop, your son's third-grade teacher. Look at any one of us with jaded eyes, and you will say, "She's nothing special—a woman like any other. Just one among billions." You know us well; we are your sisters, daughters, mothers, lovers, and wives. But look more deeply, through the eye of your soul, and you will see that we are none other than the Holy One who walks among you, disguised as a businesswoman or a college student or a grandmother. Just like yourself, we are that sacred Presence, walking, talking, dancing, and making love, learning, forgetting, and remembering, again and again, until every particle within us knows the truth and we no longer forget.

NOTES

1. Robert I. Friedman, "India's Shame," *The Nation,* April 8, 1996, pp. 11–20.

2. Gradually the situation is reversing, and some girls are now being sent to dance classes because it is believed this will improve their marriage prospects. Unfortunately, this is not a sign that Indians are beginning to embrace the prosexual attitudes of their ancestors. On the contrary, the sexual history of temple dance has been repressed so thoroughly as to render it harmless in the eyes of the moralists.

3. In recent years, some important research on the devadasis has been published, most notably Frederique Apffel-Marglin's book *Wives of the God-King: The Rituals of the Devadasis of Puri* (Oxford: Oxford University Press, 1985), which examines the lives and rituals of nine living devadasis and provides valuable glimpses into a vanishing world.

4. Jay Livernois, "Aphrodite Goes to Haiti," *Spring: A Journal of Archetype and Culture,* vol. 57 (spring, 1995), p. 98.

5. Sobonfu and Malidoma Some, *Indigenous Views of Intimacy and Sex,* audiocassette distributed by Oral Tradition Archives, Box 51155, Pacific Grove, CA 93950.

6. *Reflections on the Art of Living: A Joseph Campbell Companion,* selected and edited by Diane K. Osbon (New York: HarperCollins, 1991), p. 163.

7. *San Francisco Chronicle,* "Childbirth death rate alarms UNICEF," June 12, 1996.

8. Anaïs Nin, "Eroticism in Women," in *The Erotic Impulse,* edited by David Steinberg (New York: Tarcher, 1992), p. 119.

9. Matthew Fox, *The Coming of the Cosmic Christ* (San Francisco: Harper & Row, 1988), p. 163.

10. Thomas Moore, *Soul Mates: Honoring the Mysteries of Love and Relationship* (New York: HarperCollins, 1994), p. 180.

11. *Sappho,* A Translation by Mary Barnard (Boston: Shambhala, 1994), p. 63.

12. Jean Shinoda Bolen, *Goddesses in Every Woman: A New Psychology of Women* (New York: Harper Colophon, 1984), p. 251.

13. James Hillman, *Loose Ends* (Dallas: Spring Publications, 1994), p. 54.

14. E. M. Forster, *A Passage to India* (London: The Abinger Edition, 1973), p. 72.

15. The goatish attributes of the Christian devil—his horns, beard, cloven feet, and tail—were taken over from the goat-god Pan, the horned god of pre-Christian religion who presided over the fertility of earth and all her creatures, and cavorted in joyful abandon with the forest nymphs. By identifying the horned god with Satan, Christianity attempted to convince the common people to view their ancient gods as evil and demonic. However, the original Pan was by no means an agent of evil, but a god who safeguarded the creative and procreative energies of life, evoking lustful joy and exuberance, laughter, play, and ecstatic sex. Pan, in turn, is often associated with Dionysus, who turned water into wine, as did Jesus, thus unveiling the intoxicating presence of spirit within physical matter.

16. *Women in Praise of the Sacred,* edited by Jane Hirshfield (New York: HarperCollins) 1994, p. 132.

17. Many Jungians also define Eros as feminine, and Logos, the creative intelligence, as masculine, as if Logos were the fertilizing semen of a male creator-god.

18. Author's translation from: *Das Stundenbuch* (The Book of Hours), 1899–1903.

19. *The Peacock's Egg: Love Poems from Ancient India,* translated by W. S. Merwin and J. Moussaieff Masson (San Francisco: North Point Press, 1981), p. 123.

20. Esther M. Harding, *Women's Mysteries: Ancient and Modern* (New York: Harper Colophon, 1971), p. 159.

21. Frederique Apffel-Marglin, *Wives of the God-King,* p. 315.

22. Marion Woodman, *The Pregnant Virgin: A Process of Psychological Transformation* (Toronto: Inner City Books, 1985), pp. 180f.

23. Joseph Campbell, foreword to Maya Deren, *Divine Horsemen: The Living Gods of Haiti* (Kingston, N.Y.: McPherson & Co, 1988), p. xvii.

24. Janet Adler, *Arching Backward: The Mystical Initiation of a Contemporary Woman* (Rochester, Vt.: Inner Traditions, 1995), p. 124.

25. Julie Henderson, *The Lover Within: Opening to Energy in Sexual Practice* (Barrytown, N.Y.: Station Hill Press, 1987), p. 8.

26. Harry Maurer, *Sex: An Oral History* (New York: Viking Press, 1994), p. 289.

27. Robert Bly, "The Humming of Eros," in Steinberg, ed., *The Erotic Impulse,* p. 289.

28. Mary Condren, *The Serpent and the Goddess: Women, Religion, and Power in Celtic Ireland* (San Francisco: Harper & Row, 1989), p. 7.

29. Unlike actual sex, the metaphor of sacred union always centers around the image of heterosexual union. Much of India's erotic art juxtaposes voluptuous, big-breasted, curvaceous women with strong-shouldered, handsome men. This is not a symptom of homophobia or prejudice; in fact, ancient Indian culture appears to have been quite accepting of homosexuality. Images of union between men and women are not to be taken as a literal prescription, but as a metaphor for the union of all possible opposites—life and death, light and darkness, good and evil. Ultimately, the union of male and female stands for the union between ourselves and all that we perceive as "other." In medieval alchemical imagery, the contrast between the two partners was sometimes emphasized even further by depicting one partner as white, the other as black. Polarity acts as a powerful sexual stimulant in any relationship, be it hetero- or homosexual. However, in real life, the polarities may be psychological and energetic rather than physical.

30. The location and function of each chakra and basic practices for opening the flow of life-force through the appropriate channels can be found in any book on Tantra, Kundalini, and the chakras, for example Ajit Mookerjee, *Kundalini: The Arousal of the Inner Energy* (New York: Destiny Books, 1983).

31. Richard Katz, *Boiling Energy: Community Healing Among the Kalahari Kung* (Cambridge, Mass.: Harvard University Press, 1982), p. 41.

32. Hirschfield, ed., *Women in Praise of the Sacred,* p. 89.

33. *News of the Universe: Poems of Twofold Consciousness,* chosen and introduced by Robert Bly (San Francisco: Sierra Club Books, 1980), p. 277.

34. Jane Hirschfield, ed., *Women in Praise of the Sacred,* p. 18.

35. Osbon, ed., *Reflections on the Art of Living,* pp. 51f.

36. Nin, "Eroticism in Women," in Steinberg, ed., *The Erotic Impulse,* p. 122.

37. Rainer Maria Rilke, *Letters to a Young Poet,* translated by Stephen Mitchell (Boston: Shambhala, 1993), pp. 80, 86f.

38. Martha Heyneman, "The Whirr of His Wings," *Parabola,* vol. 20, no. 4 (winter 1995), p. 76.

39. Riane Eisler, *The Chalice and the Blade: Our History. Our Future* (San Francisco: Harper & Row, 1987), p. 189.

40. This is true, if we equate feminism with a unisex approach that denies the differences between men and women and expects women to be-

come high achievers in the outer world. However, in its more enlightened manifestations, feminism encourages men and women to own the full spectrum of who they are, their introversion as well as their extroversion, their quiet, gentle side as well as their assertiveness. Nonetheless, it is true that initially, the marriage was not based on "a feminist model" because Iris did not take her own perceptions and desires as seriously as her husband's.

41. Arianna Stassinopoulos and Roloff Beny, *The Gods of Greece* (New York: Harry N. Abrams, 1983), p. 162.

42. Moore, *Soul Mates,* p. 30.

43. *The Collected Dialogues of Plato,* edited by Edith Hamilton and Huntington Cairns (Princeton, N.J.: Princeton University Press, 1961), p. 542.

44. Ibid., p. 544.

45. Barbara Ann Brennan, *Light Emerging: The Journey of Personal Healing* (New York: Bantam, 1993), p. 186.

46. Jack Kornfield, *A Path with Heart* (New York: Bantam, 1993), p. 7.

47. *The Kabir Book,* Forty-Four of the Ecstatic Poems of Kabir, Versions by Robert Bly (Boston: Beacon Press, 1977), p. 31.

48. It seems to be one of the strange ironies of history that the very areas where strong goddess-worshipping civilizations once thrived are today centers of religious fundamentalism and male dominance.

49. Diane Wolkstein and Samuel Noah Kramer, *Inanna, Queen of Heaven and Earth: Her Stories and Hymns from Sumer* (New York: Harper & Row, 1983), p. 37.

50. Ibid., p. 38.

51. Ibid., p. 43.

52. Ibid., p. 55.

53. Ibid., pp. xvif.

54. Ibid., p. 60.

55. Ibid., p. 58.

56. *The Book of Job,* translated and introduced by Stephen Mitchell (San Francisco: North Point Press, 1987), p. xxvii.

57. Judith Wallerstein and Sandra Blakeslee, *The Good Marriage* (New York: Houghton Mifflin, 1995).

58. Ibid., p. 91.

59. From an interview with John Gray in the *San Francisco Examiner Magazine,* May 28, 1995, p. 27.

60. Deren, *Divine Horsemen,* p. 36.

61. Stratford Caldecott, "I Thirst to Be Thirsted For," *Parabola,* vol. 20, no. 4 (winter 1995), p. 81.

62. Deren, *Divine Horsemen,* p. 145.

63. Ken Wilber, "The Way Up Is the Way Down," *Parabola,* vol. 20, no 4 (winter 1995), p. 86.

64. Marion Woodman and Elinor Dickson, *Dancing in the Flames: The Dark Goddess in the Transformation of Consciousness* (Boston: Shambhala, 1996), p. 7.

65. The unconscious seems to understand that in order to survive an onslaught of pain, the individual needs some form of outer container—a family, a relationship, a job, a marriage. The psyche will generally hold onto its dark, festering knowledge until it senses the presence of some outer support, and only then does it relax its hold. First, just a few toxic bubbles rise to the surface—episodes of depression, irritability, and discontent. Later, the dams may break. Problematic as Naomi's marriage was, it provided just enough of a safe container to keep her alive when her unconscious began broadcasting its terrible knowledge.

66. Miranda Shaw, *Passionate Enlightenment: Women in Tantric Buddhism* (Princeton, N.J.: Princeton University Press, 1994), p. 41.

67. Chögyam Trungpa, *Shambhala: The Sacred Path of the Warrior* (Boston: Bantam Books, 1986), p. 20.

68. Thich Nhat Hanh, *Being Peace* (Berkeley, Calif.: Parallax Press, 1987), p. 64.

69. Joan Halifax, *Shamanic Voices* (New York: Dutton, 1979), p. 11.

70. "Helping Teens Say No to Sex," *San Francisco Examiner,* January 29, 1995.

71. Ellen Bass and Laura Davis, *The Courage to Heal* (New York: HarperPerennial, 1994), p. 143.

72. Wolkstein and Kramer, *Inanna,* p. 12.

73. Barbara G. Walker, *The Woman's Encyclopedia of Myths and Secrets* (San Francisco: Harper & Row, 1983), p. 197.

74. Ibid., p. 409.

75. Betty Dodson, *Sex for One: The Joy of Selfloving* (New York: Crown, 1987), p. 55.

76. Ibid., p. 65.

77. St. Hildegard of Bingen, *Symphonia: A Critical Edition of the Symphonia armonie celestium revelationum,* edited and translated by Barbara Newman (Ithaca, N.Y.: Cornell University Press, 1989), p. 125.

78. Anne Llewellyn Barstow, *Witchcraze* (San Francisco: Pandora Books, 1994), p. 134.

79. David Kinsley, *Hindu Goddesses* (Berkeley, Calif.: University of California Press, 1988), p. 116.

80. Quoted in Sherry Ruth Anderson and Patricia Hopkins, *The Feminine Face of God: The Unfolding of the Sacred in Women* (New York: Bantam, 1991), p. 192.

81. Walker, *The Women's Encyclopedia of Myths and Secrets,* p. 187.

82. Marty Klein, "Erotophobia: The Cruelest Abuse of All," in Steinberg, ed., *The Erotic Impulse,* p. 176.

THE DESCENT OF INANNA: A JOURNEY THROUGH THE ANCIENT SUMERIAN GODDESS MYTH

To learn more about the myth of Inanna's descent to the underworld, discussed in Chapter 16 of this book, you can order an audiocassette on which Jalaja Bonheim retells the myth for contemporary listeners.

The Descent of Inanna: A Journey Through the Ancient Sumerian Goddess Myth costs $10 per tape, plus $2 shipping and handling for the first copy and $1 for each additional copy. To order, write to:

Musimedia
20 Sunnyside Ave. A 235
Mill Valley, CA 94941

Please indicate the number of tapes you are ordering and include your clearly printed name and mailing address along with a check or money order.

ABOUT THE AUTHOR

Jalaja Bonheim, Ph.D., is a counselor in private practice and a workshop leader. Raised in Germany and Austria, she spent several years in India studying Indian temple dance, and has lived in the San Francisco Bay Area since 1982. She is the author of *The Serpent and the Wave: A Guide to Movement Meditation* (Celestial Arts, 1992).

If you would like to receive information on author events and workshops, please write to:

Meetings in Sacred Space
P.O. Box 9446
Berkeley, CA 94709–0446

The author welcomes letters and responses from readers, but regrets that she is not able to respond to every letter.